History, Sex and Syphilis

Famous Syphilitics and their private lives

Tomasz F. Mroczkowski

Hardcover ISBN: 978-1-63490-828-3
Paperback ISBN: 978-1-63490-829-0

Published by BookLocker.com, Inc., Bradenton, Florida, U.S.A.

Printed on acid-free paper.

BookLocker.com, Inc.
2015

First Edition

DISCLAIMER

This book details the author's personal experiences with and opinions about the history of syphilis and private lives of famous syphilitics. The author no longer is a healthcare provider.

The author and publisher inform that all details concerning private lives of famous syphilitics are based on books, biographies and other publications on certain individuals (see references) and all medical information are in accordance with contemporary knowledge on Sexually Transmitted Diseases.

The author and publisher are providing this book and its contents on an "as is" basis and make no representations or warranties of any kind with respect to this book or its contents. The author and publisher disclaim all such representations and warranties, including for example warranties of merchantability and healthcare for a particular purpose. In addition, the author and publisher do not represent or warrant that the information accessible via this book is accurate, complete or current.

The statements made about products and services have not been evaluated by the U.S. Food and Drug Administration. They are not intended to diagnose, treat, cure, or prevent any condition or disease. Please consult with your own physician or healthcare specialist regarding the suggestions and recommendations made in this book.

Except as specifically stated in this book, neither the author or publisher, nor any authors, contributors, or other representatives will be liable for damages arising out of or in connection with the use of this book. This is a comprehensive limitation of liability that applies to all damages of any kind, including (without limitation) compensatory; direct, indirect or consequential damages; loss of data, income or profit; loss of or damage to property and claims of third parties.

You understand that this book is not intended as a substitute for consultation with a licensed healthcare practitioner, such as your physician. Before you begin any healthcare program, or change your lifestyle in any way, you will consult your physician or other licensed healthcare practitioner to ensure that you are in good health and that the examples contained in this book will not harm you.

This book provides content related to topics physical and/or mental health issues. As such, use of this book implies your acceptance of this disclaimer.

Acknowledgments

I would like to express my sincere gratitude to Wojciech A. Krotoski M.D., Ph.D., M.P.H., formerly Director, National Ambulatory Hansen's Disease Program, U.S. Public Health Service, for his indispensable work in the preparation of the English edition of this book. His expertise, knowledge of the Polish language, and overall linguistic advice in this project cannot be underestimated.

I also want to thank my wife Emilia ("Emi") Mroczkowska, M.H.Sc. for her continued support and critical comments during the work on the manuscript, as well as for her unyielding encouragement and involvement during the publication phase, freely admitting that without such personal engagement it would never had been completed.

Table of Contents

Illustrations

Figure 7.4 Portrait of Heinrich Heine, by Moritz Daniel Oppenheim

PREFACE

Five hundred years ago, Christopher Columbus reached the New World, and from there he brought back to Europe a previously unknown venereal disease, which was subsequently to be called syphilis. From the very beginning, this disease caused fear and consternation, due to its violent course, repulsive skin manifestations and high mortality.

Over the course of years, syphilis, also called lues, became a disease of increasingly protracted, yet less dramatic course, although, as a result of an absence of effective treatment – penicillin did not appear until the twentieth century – it remained incurable, causing death in more than half of those contracting it. Many people died not only from syphilis itself, but also as a result of the side effects of the remedies applied; this led to the conviction that, in the first phase of the epidemic, the cure was worse than the disease in many instances.

People from all social classes became ill, beginning with peasants and concluding with their monarchs. Information on the subject comes mainly from biographies or stories about the latter, but such sources are not always credible. Often, they were written many years after the events, by authors governed by their personal inclinations either to glorify or to embarrass the persons described. The signs and symptoms provided by these sources are frequently imprecise, and are similar to those occurring in non-venereal diseases; this could lead to pinning the label, "syphilitic," onto persons suffering from other maladies. For the same reason many true syphilitics might not have been recognized, and could have been treated for other diseases, e.g. general paresis or *tabes dorsalis,* not knowing that they were the signs of late syphilis.

The more credible accounts of syphilis and syphilitics do not appear until the middle of nineteenth century, when lues began to be distinguished from other diseases. It is worth mentioning that, until then, even gonorrhea was considered simply a milder form of syphilis. The biographies of well-known syphilitics of the later period, particularly those of artists, are more credible, and allow readers to learn about the lives of those suffering from lues. It must be added, however, that, due to the character of the disease (from the very beginning of the epidemic, syphilis was regarded as embarrassing and disgraceful for the patient), accounts are sparse and often avoided, with the aim of protecting the good name of the person described

In chapters devoted to well-known artists who suffered from syphilis, the reader will find accounts of their ailments and the signs and symptoms that appeared in them, as well as suggestions regarding when they became infected. I permitted myself to expand these chapters with information on the private lives of the subjects, underlining the risky behavior that most probably led to their infection. Writing about known artists suffering from syphilis, I could not avoid providing information about the works that made them famous, the more so, as, in the nineteenth century, a view prevailed that it was the lues that was the source of their talent.

In addition to a history of syphilis and accounts of the lives of renowned syphilitics, in the last chapter of this book I included some of my own recollections acquired while working with those ill with the disease, bringing attention to current problems such as change in sexual behaviors, and emphasizing the threat that a carefree attitude toward sex carries. One of the new elements changing sexual behaviors of our patient are recent anatomic discoveries and tremendous popularity of Internet, especially porno websites, which became the primary source of sexual education. These changes have resulted in noticeable diversification in sexual practices, some causing previously rarely seen lesions of primary syphilis.

One of the aims of this book, in addition to a review of the history of the syphilis epidemic that has plagued humanity for the last 500 years, is to remind the reader that, despite the availability of prophylactic methods and inexpensive, effective medicines, the number of cases of syphilis in the world is still very high and, what is really troubling, has started to increase in recent years.

Tomasz F. Mroczkowski, M.D.

CHAPTER 1

SOUVENIR FROM A TRIP

The end of the fifteenth century to the beginning of the sixteenth was a period of long sea voyages and many geographical discoveries. In these, mainly the Portuguese and the Spanish specialized. In 1488, the Portuguese sailor Bartolomeo Diaz rounded the southern promontory of Africa, later named the Cape of Good Hope, thus opening the possibility of reaching India by sea. Four years later, Christopher Columbus set out with the same goal, hoping to find a shorter route to Asia, but in the opposite direction. In 1497, the Portuguese monarch, Manuel I, commissioned the well-known sailor, Vasco da Gama, to sail to India by a route around Africa. On May 30th, 1498, da Gama reached Calcutta on the western shore of India, becoming the first European to reach Asia by a sea route. Several years later, Ferdinand Magellan set off on the first voyage around the world, which would take close to three years, and which he would never complete. Magellan was to lose his life in April, 1521 in the Philippines, where he meddled in a conflict between local tribes, for which he paid with his life. His expedition returned to Portugal in September 1522, but now under a different leader, one of his captains, Juan Sebastian de Como.

All of these expeditions had the goal of discovering the very shortest route to Asia in order to institute trade with India, China, and Japan, and to replenish the reduced stores of gold in the treasuries of the rulers of Portugal and Spain. Trade by the land route had been practically stopped by the growing Ottoman Empire, which was in an adversarial mode toward Christians.

Without a doubt, the most important event of that period was Columbus' expedition and his discovery of America, even though it was somewhat unfairly attributed to him: the Vikings had arrived there long before he did, although farther to the North, and about 560 years earlier.

Christopher Columbus was born in Genoa, one of many city republics on the territory of what later became Italy. His family name was actually Colombo, which is the Latin form. As a child, being the oldest of five children, he assisted his father in a textile factory, despite being attracted to the sea even from his early years. The fact that Genoa was at that time an important seaport, where sailing ships called from many parts of the world, was not without meaning; it doubtless fed the young boy's imagination. Columbus' interest in later sea voyages began to crystallize when he moved to Lisbon, one of the more developed and wealthy cities of Europe at the time. There, young Christopher was to meet his future wife. As a good Catholic (although some claim that he was Jewish)(1) he attended Mass regularly, and there met the comely Felipa Moniz de Perestrello, who was from an excellent family with Italian roots, which had settled in Portugal for two generations, while Felipa's grandfather came from Piacenza. The young couple married in 1476 or 1477 – the exact date is not known – and soon thereafter, their first son came into the world. Thanks to his marriage to the daughter of an influential family, Columbus improved his social position by several levels, and simultaneously entered the company of people who took part in maritime expeditions for business purposes. As in Lisbon, so in Madeira, the relatives of Felipa's mother and father had significant standing, and thanks to Bartholomew II, Felipa's brother, Columbus gained access to a variety of documents, in which the history of Portuguese navigation on the Atlantic was consolidated. (2) (Fig.1.1.). It was not without meaning that his younger brother, Bartolomeo, a later companion on sea expeditions, had a shop with maps and instruments needed for marine navigation. We should remember that this was also the time when Portuguese sailors reached the Azores and Madeira, while Bartolomeo Diaz, mentioned earlier, had already sailed around the southern tip of Africa.

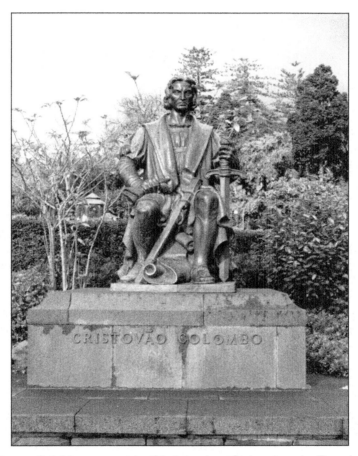

Figure 6.1 Monument to Christopher Columbus in Funchal, Madeira. Photo: E. Mroczkowska

This was also a time of intense searching for a sea route to the countries of Asia, also known as the Indies-a time

3

when more enlightened people already knew that the earth was round, and wondered what existed to the West of the Iberian Peninsula, across the "Great water." Columbus also belonged to these, and resolved to find out. After much geographical computation, he arrived at the conclusion that voyaging in a westerly direction would reach the Indies – and would be a lot closer than travelling around Africa (3).

To accomplish such a voyage, several ships plus their provisioning would be needed, hence a large sum of money. By 1482, Columbus had tried to interest the Portuguese King, John II, with his idea; however, when the latter heard how much it was going to cost, he removed his support. In the meantime, he improved his sailing abilities by voyaging to Madeira and the Bay of Guinea. In 1485 Columbus journeyed to Spain in order to interest that country's rulers with his plans. Simultaneously, his brother, Bartolomeo, sailed to England in order to persuade Henry VII, then to France, where he presented a similar proposal to Charles VIII. While Bartolomeo was unable to persuade either English or French monarchs to provide funds for an enterprise that was uncertain, in their opinion, Christopher managed to win over Queen Isabella to his ideas (4). Nonetheless, he had to wait a while, as, at the time, the Catholic Kings of Spain were busy with dispatching the Moors. However, after the fall of Granada in January 1492, they had more time, and were ready to undertake the expedition. At the start, there were such problems obtaining suitable means for the endeavor that Queen Isabella was ready to pawn her jewelry for it; in the end, that turned out not to be necessary, as the Royal Treasurer recognized a good investment and gathered the needed funds. (Fig.1.2.)

Columbus was so certain of his success that, as a reward for discovering a shorter route to the Indies, he requested the bestowal of a nobleman's title, the rank of admiral, the status of governor of the newly discovered territories, and, in addition, a percentage from trade with them. (5)

The expedition sailed on August 3, 1492; it consisted of three ships: the *Santa Maria*, the *Niña* and the *Pinta*, (Fig.1.3.) as well as a crew of 90, constituted mainly of people from *Palos de La Frontera*, the place from where the expedition left. Today, not far from Palos is a small village, *La Rabida*, where there is a Franciscan monastery housing a museum dedicated to Columbus' expedition.

Although the majority of the expedition's members believed the earth to be round, they did feel some insecurity: what if it were otherwise? The duration of the voyage was also troubling, and gave birth to the question of what would happen if, after sailing several weeks, the expedition didn't reach the Indies, and would have to turn back. Would there then be enough water and provisions? Nevertheless, after a somewhat lengthy stay on La Gomera, one of the islands of the Canaries archipelago, the expedition left San Sebastian on September 6; three days later, its members saw the shores of Hierro, the westward most extension of the archipelago of the Canaries.

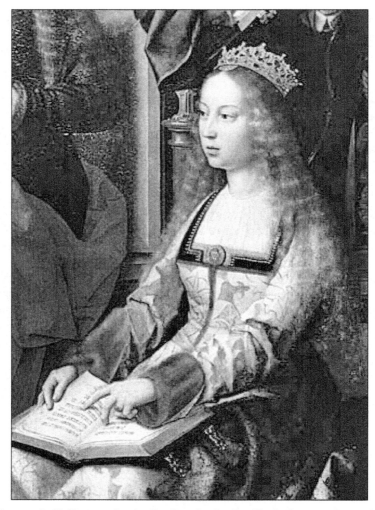

Figure 1. 7 Queen Isabella the Catholic (Painting attributed to Gerard David)

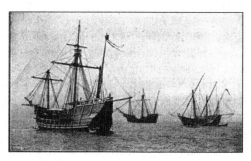

Figure 1.3 Replicas of Pinta, Niña and Santa Maria

After twenty-one days of sailing with good weather and advantageous winds, some of the expedition participants begin to express their fears aloud. They unanimously let it be understood that their patience was at an end and would allow Columbus no more than three days to reach land. Two days later, during the night of October 11th to 12th, they sighted a coastal outline. Before noon on October 12th, boats were arriving on the shores of the island, which was given the name San Salvador by Columbus. In this way, he wished to give thanks to his Creator for the success of the expedition – as well as for saving his skin, for no one knows what would have happened to him if the voyage had taken even a few more days!

The newly discovered island turned out to be one of the smaller islands of the archipelago now known as the Bahamas, and to this day we do not know which of them it actually was. After several days' stay on San Salvador, the ships sailed southwest, and landed on the shore of Cuba. On the basis of its size and geography, including its mountains, Columbus was convinced that he had arrived in China. He even sent a group of his crew into the interior of the island to find the road to Peking, as he wanted to deliver a letter from King Ferdinand and Queen Isabella as quickly as possible to the Chinese Emperor.

After some time Columbus and his Spanish crew began to realize that perhaps they were not in China! The local population, though disposed in a very friendly manner, was, after all, ethnically different from the Chinese. They had a different skin color, different facial features, and a different diet. Reconciling himself to the fact that he was not in China, Columbus then sailed in a south-easterly direction, and reached an island whose shoreline reminded him of Spain-- thus, its name of "La Isla Espagnola" (Hispaniola), now known as San Domingo. Sailing past current Cap Haitien, Columbus' biggest ship, the Santa Maria, struck some submerged rocks and sank. After saving what was possible, with the help of the local "Indians," it was decided to establish a fort in the area, based on the inhabitants' friendly disposition. Significant at this point was the fact that there had arisen a need to leave behind a portion of his crew, 40 persons in all, as it was not possible, based on the size of the remaining ships, to take them back to Spain. On January 16, 1493, just two ships began on the return journey.

Unfortunately, this time weather conditions were very bad. They encountered opposing winds and a storm on the Atlantic that almost sank the tiny Niña, while the small flotilla, now consisting of but two ships, became separated at the latitude of the Azores. When the Niña, with Columbus on board, reached the Portuguese island of Santa Maria, her governor almost threw the Spaniard into jail. The suspicious Portuguese did not give credence to Columbus' account that he was returning from an expedition across the Atlantic, and wanted to imprison them all, suspecting the Spaniards of piracy along the west coast of Africa, which was then under Portuguese control. After an acerbic exchange of words, and with a threat to shoot up the port, Columbus and his crew were allowed to sail away in the direction of the Iberian Peninsula, where, again, violent storms on the ocean forced the ship to change course and land in Lisbon. Following several days of rest and an audience with King John II, to whom Columbus introduced the "Indians" he was transporting, they sailed in the direction of Spain. The Niña arrived at Palos on the 15th of March 1493. The following day, the Pinta also arrived. As quickly as possible, this time on horseback, and accompanied by several officers as well as a group of the Indians, Columbus arrived in Barcelona, at that time the residence of King Ferdinand and Queen Isabella.

As one might expect, Columbus' reception at court took place with great pomp. The promised title, Admiral of the Open Sea, was ceremoniously conferred on him, thus giving him wide powers pertaining to sailing laws and matters related to the sea. He also received the title of Viceroy of the Indies, and was assured of preparations for his next, larger voyage (7). Finally, a great parade was organized in the city, during which Columbus had the opportunity to present to a wider audience a group of the Indians, as well as unknown birds (parrots), samples of gold, and unknown fruits and spices from the New World.

This joyous atmosphere was not disturbed by the minor fact that some of the members of the crew, including the captain of one of the ships, were showing signs of a strange malady, unknown to Spanish doctors.

The first reaction was that this was a new form of plague, or even of leprosy (Hansen's disease). The apparent likeness to the latter was based on their remembering that that disease appeared in Europe after the return of the crusaders from the Holy Land. However, other signs, plus the violence of the new disease's course, quickly eliminated leprosy from consideration, particularly as the first signs of the former appeared on the genitalia in the form of ulcers and pustules surrounded by induration. Soon after the appearance of these first signs and symptoms, there appeared scaling pimples, sometimes reminiscent of warts, on the skin of the whole body. During this phase of the illness, patients experienced violent pains in their bones or joints. After a year or more, pustular swellings appeared on the skin, as well as indurations (hardenings) of a solid consistency that were extraordinarily painful, especially at night when the pain was so intense, that they provoked yells from the sick. Following this, in almost every case, effects on bones were seen, which, when involving the extremities, left them permanently bent and shortened. The disease frequently progressed to destruction of the uvula, the nasal cartilage and trachea. Later, the victims lost their minds, behaved as though deranged, began to have trouble with moving around, and finally became unable to walk. In this manner, more or less, did witnesses of the time describe their patients (Gasparis Torellae 1497, Petrus Pindor 1499, Jacobi Catanei de Lacumarino 1504, Antonii Benivenii 1507, Juan de Vigo 1514). (8)

After the first cases appeared in Spain in 1493, the number of those ill from *las bubas*, as the new disease came to be called, began to increase dramatically in succeeding years. The cause of this is attributed to Columbus' second voyage, during which at least two convoys were sent to Spain under the leadership of Antonio Torres; in 1494, he brought back, in addition to gold and other goods, first 26 Indians of both sexes, and then, in the spring of 1495, about 300. It was said that Columbus himself recommended the capture of Indians together with their wives, as the men – he wrote in his diary – will withstand captivity in Spain better when they have women from their own country with them. Many of the women who survived the voyage and reached Europe later found themselves in brothels where they worked as prostitutes and become the source of infection for their clients (9).

At this point, it must be clarified that Columbus' second voyage to the New World differed in many respects from the first discovery voyage. The sweetly idyllic relations that existed between the ships' crews and the native inhabitants ended very quickly during the second voyage, when the

10

Spaniards saw that the settlement established by the crew of the Santa Maria had been leveled to the ground and the sailors murdered. From that moment, the Europeans began treating the Indians as enemies: they were forced to work the land, and to search for gold. The men were now treated as slaves and the women as slave women, despite instructions received by Columbus from Queen Isabella, who spoke clearly of the obligation to evangelize them and treat them well as free subjects of the crown.

Although it was suspected that the new illness may have come from the New World, even from the first months after its appearance in Spain a bit more time had to pass before this view was established. In this regard, following several personal testimonies from those times:

Gonzales Fernadez Oviedo, who from 1513 on was the royal superintendent of gold and silver mines in the New World, and where he remained for over ten years, recorded that "the serious illness, *las bubas*, which appeared in Spain after Columbus' return comes from the Indies, where it is widely distributed among the local inhabitants, yet is not as violent and dangerous as in Europe . . . ." Another account was provided by a contemporary of Oviedo, the physician, Diaz de Isla, who called the new disease *morbus serpentis,* or the snake disease, and wrote that "it appeared in Barcelona in the year of Our Lord 1493, yet which has its origin from the island of Hispaniola." Diaz de Isla recorded his own observations as he took care of and treated sailors from Columbus' first voyage, and also treated instances of *las bubas* in Barcelona. Similarly, Bartolomeo de las Casas (1498), a priest caring for Indians in the New World, described numerous cases of 'las bubas' among the local population (10, 11).

The question arises of why a disease, which coursed through the native population in a mild manner, and was a chronic illness that did not threaten life, once transferred to Europe produced a major pandemic of serious, painful and

11

life-threatening disease, first after introduction to Spain, then farther, to the remainder of Europe and the rest of the world. The answer would seem to be simple. This disease, which from the middle of the seventeenth century will be known as syphilis, appeared in virginal (European) territory, in which the population, not having had any earlier contact with it, had not developed any mechanisms of immunity. In an analogous manner, diseases known for many years in Europe, such as chickenpox, measles, diphtheria or whooping cough, and later, tuberculosis, reduced the Indians, who had never had earlier contact with them, to a tenth of their original numbers in the newly discovered lands.

With the appearance of innumerable new cases of this new, serious disease, other questions arose: what is its cause and what produces it?

As I already mentioned, it was first considered possibly to be a new variant of plague or leprosy. But, there also arose many fantastic theories, of which I will name only a few. One was a theory stating that the fundamental cause of the disease was the cohabitation of a leper with a courtesan; another, sodomy in the form of humans copulating with monkeys; or the addition of the blood of lepers to wine. Yet another theory belonging to a sexual, hence *sinful* method of becoming infected, spoke of "the anger of God, who permitted that this disease should befall the human species as a way of restraining its lustfulness and unchecked covetousness" (Ambroise Pare, 1575) (12).

The greatest number of adherents, however, subscribed to an astrologic theory professed by many authorities of the time. Experts on the stars considered that the epidemic, among other occurrences was caused by an unfortunate arrangement of the planets, to wit the November 1484 conjunction of Saturn and Jupiter in the constellation Scorpio and home of the god Mars (Grunpeck, Hutten, Villalobos) (13). With the passage of time, however, theories closer to the truth appeared, some of which were not encountered before the start of the twentieth century. Earlier, the French doctor and mathematician, Jean Fernel (1497-1558), court physician to King Henry II, formulated a theory that attested to his shrewd observations. He asserted, "the cause of venereal illness is a pernicious venom acquired by contagion or touch, that lives in some 'body' that serves as its support and transmitter." He compared it to the venom of a scorpion or rabid dog, which, beginning first from an infected part, spreads over the whole body. Fernel added that "the disease receives its start there where there was contact, provided that a breach has been caused in order to allow passage of the venom, which is rather weak [by itself], in order for it to beat a path on its own [strength]" (14). This theory was already very close to what we know today, as, for infection with syphilis to occur, at least a small disruption of the integrity of the skin surface is necessary, whereby bacteria (the pale spirochete) get into the skin and then extend to the circulation, to produce a generalized infection. Ambroise Pare, theorized similarly as early as the sixteenth century, writing that the "venereal virus" carried by the blood distributes itself over the whole body, beginning with primary changes, and developing at a later period of the disease to include such sequelae as ocular and nasal destruction, a perforated palate and a loss of hearing and sight."

While generally holding Columbus accountable for the transfer of syphilis to Europe, we cannot neglect other opinions suggesting that the pandemic of the disease that started in the sixteenth century, had nothing to do with him, and that there is abundant evidence that it was known in Europe and Asia almost "forever." The dispute over the origins of syphilis really began in the seventeenth century. In order to support their thesis, the opponents of an American origin cited the biblical description of the disease of Job (boils on the body, accompanied by pain in the bones at night) as fitting the picture of lues. They also cited the works of Hippocrates, Celsus and Galen. Likewise suspected were descriptions of lues in the Babylonian poem of *Gilgamesh* in the papyrus of Ebers, and the writings of Paul of Egina and the writings of Pliny the Younger. They quoted ancient Arabic physicians writing about skin changes in the genital and anal areas. The well-known French physician from the time of the rule of Ludwig XIV, Guy Patin, who was Dean of the Medical Faculty in Paris, maintained that, in addition to Job, David and Solomon were also infected with venereal disease, and that its descriptions may be found in the works of Hippocrates and Herodotus (15).

Citing the Bible and ancient thinkers, the opponents of an American origin for syphilis forget that the use of the equivalent terms "lues" or "venereal disease" addresses at least several or more than a dozen diseases in which changes occur in the areas of the genitalia or anus. These could have been any of a number of other diseases transmitted by the sexual route, including, in addition to lues, gonorrhea, chancroid, genital herpes, infections caused by the human papilloma virus (HPV) and tuberculosis or leprosy, or even other afflictions producing changes on the genitalia and other areas (16). Many of these diseases have been known since ancient times, and their signs and symptoms could suggest syphilis, but that does not mean that they were, in fact, definitively the former. The dispute over the origins of syphilis that began in the seventeenth century lasts to this day.

Contemporary adversaries of an American origin of lues cite, as evidence, that it existed in the Western Hemisphere even before Columbus, the results of tests on bones and skulls, which, in their judgment, indicate syphilis, yet which come from archaeological sites dated from before the fifteenth century. These findings come from such disparate regions as Central Russia, Upper Egypt or China, and from such separated periods as before 2000 B.C. or the Neolithic. Bones with changes characteristic of syphilis coming from 500-2,000 years ago, have also been found, among others, in the state of Colorado in the U.S.A., or the territory of the Dominican Republic, the last in places visited by Columbus during his first voyage to the West.

Very recently, there appeared an English report, presenting the results of studies of human skeletons from the thirteenth and fourteenth centuries found in the cemetery of St. Mary's Hospital in London, England, which showed features suggestive of syphilitic changes. Despite the fact that the age of the bones was well-documented, the changes attributed to lues could also have been caused by other diseases. The dispute, as though still alive, continues with another, recently published study from Emory University in Atlanta, Georgia. By the use of genetic analysis, it was established that bacteria responsible for syphilis, as known currently, were most closely related to those seen in South America suggestive of the endemic treponematoses called yaws (17).

I believe that the dispute of the origin of syphilis will continue yet a while longer, but am also of the opinion that there are far more arguments in favor of an American origin of lues than of any another. First, there is the time relationship. The epidemic of syphilis in Europe exploded shortly after the return of Columbus from the New World and the arrival of first Indian women in Spain. The speed of spread of the disease and its unusually serious and dramatic course, testify to a lack of immunity inherited from forebears. And, finally, there is the evidence obtained by the use of genetic analysis, namely a description of genetic structures that appear to confirm a close relationship of modern bacteria of syphilis with an endemic form originating in South America from places where Columbus landed for the first time.

Without prejudging who is right, we will examine how the epidemic that exploded in Europe from Columbus' time developed, and what the fate of this disease was in succeeding years.

CHAPTER 2

THE NEAPOLITAN DISEASE, THE FRENCH DISEASE, THE SPANISH DISEASE ...or... The Syphilis Epidemic in Europe.

The discovery of new lands in the Western hemisphere by Columbus produced a new political situation on the Iberian Peninsula. Until then it was primarily Portuguese sailors who traced new paths and discovered new lands along the way to Asia on the route around Africa. But now, the Spaniards joined them, and despite the fact of uncertainty as to what precisely would be found on the other side of the Atlantic, it was prudent for them to protect their freedom of action.

The previous Pope, Callistus III, granted the Portuguese monarchy the right to all non-Christian lands abutting the new discoveries, which, according to Portugal's understanding, meant a right to the whole New World. The Spaniards questioned this division, maintaining that the Pope had in mind only the lands on the eastern shore of that ocean, and not the newly discovered territories to the West, about which the papacy of Callistus had never heard.

Both Queen Isabella and the Portuguese king were equally interested in a peaceful resolution to the dispute. Not insignificant in this regard were the numerous family relationships, since Isabella, as a daughter of Portuguese mother, was brought up in that country, while her first-born daughter, also named Isabella, had married Alphonse of Portugal in 1490, and, after Alphonse's death, became the wife of his successor, Manuel I, known as Manuel the Fortunate.

For a resolution of the dispute, they turned to then extant Pope Alexander VI, Rodrigo Borgia [of the notorious Borgia family] who was a good friend of the Spanish rulers. Borgia was from Spain, where he had been a cardinal, and at the time, had granted a dispensation for the marriage of Isabella and Ferdinand, despite their close familial relationship. The marriage permitted the unification of the Kingdoms of Aragon and the Kingdom of Castille, which widened the power of the House of Aragon considerably. Personal contacts and earlier endeavors at the papal court were also fruitful, and before long the Spaniards were in possession of five papal bulls protecting the Spanish fleet directed westward (1). The final understanding, named the Treaty of Tordesillas, which was signed by both sides and underwritten by the Pope, divided the regions of influence between the rival nations.

According to the Treaty, the line dividing the sailing areas of both nations ran 10 leagues to the west of the Azores and 370 leagues from the Green Cape. The ocean and lands lying to the west of this line belonged to Spain, and to its east, to Portugal. It also divided the territories within which both nations were to conduct evangelical efforts among the inhabitants of the newly discovered lands (2).

As it later turned out, the Spaniards did well – and the Borgia Pope did also. His s on, Juan (Giovanni) Borgia married his closely related Spanish queen, Maria Enriguez de Luna. Additionally, the Pope depended on the support of Ferdinand, and possibly on obtaining the military help of Spain, should the French King Charles VIII decide to attack Italy. Concerns about the latter were not without foundation, as much led to the conclusion that this would happen. After the death of Ferdinand I (Ferrante I), the king of Naples, a new situation arose in the region. The succession of Ferdinand's son, Alphonse, required coronation by the Pope. Naples was a papal feudal state, and only the Pope, as sovereign of its kings, had the right to crown him. In the meantime, Charles VIII announced himself to be an heir to the throne of Naples, and sent a warning to Rome, giving the Holy Father to understand that he would deprive him of his position, and would name a new Pope were the latter to crown Alphonse (3,4). (Fig.2.1.) The Pope knew well that French rule in Naples would be a mortal threat to the independence of the Church's territories (papal states). The French king also announced that he was considering conducting a new crusade to regain Jerusalem from pagan hands, and, besides, would have to occupy Naples as a first step, since it was on the road to the lands occupied by the infidels.

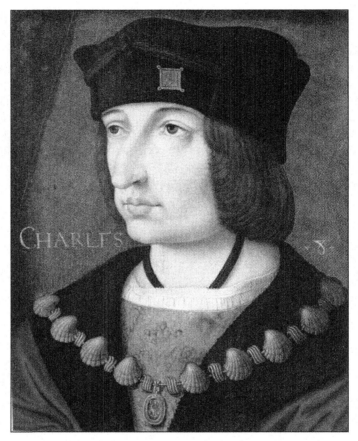

Figure 2.1 Charles VIII of France (1470-1498) (Musée de Conde Chantilly)

On the first of September 1494, Charles VIII entered Italy at the head of a forty thousand-strong army, composed mainly of mercenaries. On the side of the French were the Flemish, the Gascons, the Swiss, the Spanish, and even the Italians. As early as December, the army threatened Rome, which found itself in this unenviable situation as a result of the treachery of the leader of the Neapolitan forces that were supposed to defend Rome, but which, at the last moment joined the French. Pope Alexander considered how to prepare for a defense. The fortress of Castel Sant'Angelo had a secret passage to the Vatican, as well as stores of enough food and water for several months. Unfortunately, the city itself would find itself under the lash of the invaders, and without a doubt would be plundered, while his rule as Pope would come into question. Influencing Alexander's decision, however, was an event that took place on the road from Capodimonte to Rome. On this road, the French apprehended two well-born, young women; one was Giulia Farnese, Alexander's latest love. Giulia had left Rome several weeks earlier at his urging because of concerns about her health in Rome, as cases of plague had appeared there, and had sent her, together with his daughter Lucrezia, to Pesaro in southern Italy, in order to wait out the epidemic. By bad luck, Giulia decided to take advantage of the situation just then to visit her husband in Capodimonte, which is where she fell into the hands of the French (5).

Alexander could have reconciled himself to the destruction of Rome's treasures, the plundering of the town, and maybe even to the loss of his papal position, but not to the loss of his very young paramour. A decision about changing strategy was needed. On Christmas Day, the Pope ordered the remaining Neapolitan detachments to abandon Rome without delay, and sent a delegation with a letter to Charles VIII stating "His Holiness, Pope Alexander VI wishes to greet him, while travelling through Rome on the road to Naples" (6).

At the end of December, the French entered Rome. Charles forbade his armies to plunder, and announced that all acts of violence there would be punishable by death. Of course, the prohibition did not apply to taking advantage of various delights such as the city had to offer, not excluding the brothels, of which there were plenty. It must be noted that, according to some historians, the proportion of prostitutes to honest women was the greatest there.

The agreement that Alexander VI made with Charles VIII allowed the French to pass freely through the territory of the Church lands, and stated that, if Charles managed to conquer Naples, Pope Alexander would grant him the Church's approval in all his undertakings. On top of this, Charles was promised that he would be named the principal leader of the planned Crusade, in return for which, the French king promised Alexander his obedience and acknowledgment as the true vicar of Jesus Christ. As a sign of his loyalty, the Pope was to place his beloved son, Cezar, into Charles' hands as a guarantee; this was the very same Cezar Borgia who, holding the position of Cardinal was entitled to crown Charles VIII as King of Naples, when that city was taken (7,8). And so, thanks to the beautiful Giulia, who received the title, "the Betrothed of Christ," Rome and its treasures avoided destruction, the inhabitants of the city avoided plundering and Aleksander remained Pope.

At the end of January 1495, the French moved on Naples. The prohibition regarding rape and plundering did not, after all, apply to games and revelry, which took place in innumerable public houses and bordellos in Rome. In the army, one could note a reduction in discipline and also the loosening of morals, which were already very liberal. Behind the army, as always in those times, followed a flock of women camp followers and prostitutes, as well as crowds of beggars.

On the 22nd of February, the French armies entered Naples without firing a single shot. King Alphonse II abdicated his throne and fled the town. The population had no intention of opposing the new rulers; rather, the citizens fraternized with the victors. The French soldiers gave themselves without restraint to the delights of Naples, after having tasted the delights of Rome but a few weeks earlier.

The ceremonious entry of Charles into Naples and formal assumption of his rule over the City took place, much delayed, on May 12th. The French king, clothed in the style of a Byzantine emperor, rode through the streets on a chariot drawn by four white horses, only to leave eight days later, without any proclamation, and in great haste. His army, with greatly reduced discipline, behaved so scandalously that the earlier friendliness of some of the princes, as well as a large proportion of the inhabitants, changed to open enmity. All had already had enough of the presence of the French, and were wondering how to get rid of them. Not without influence on their decision was the summoning at this time, and under the patronage of the Pope, of the anti-French coalition known as the "Holy League," which, in its composition, included, among others, Republic of Venice, the Prince of Milan, the Catholic rulers Ferdinand and Isabella, and the Emperor Maximillian I. (9) In addition to all this, Ferdinand sent his army to Sicily under the orders of the famous leader, Gonzalo Fernandez de Cordoba, who, after finally driving the French out of Southern Italy, entered triumphantly into Rome, and was later decorated by the Pope with the Order of the Golden Rose, a decoration intended exclusively for princes and kings.

What caused the change in plans by Charles VIII, and the decision to retreat from Naples?

Aside from the military threat produced by the landing of the Spaniards on Sicily and the threats from Venice and Milan, which had entered the Holy League, the main cause of the sudden retreat from Naples was the appearance there of a new and unknown disease, which reduced the ranks of the French army to one tenth. The first written accounts of this malady come from Venetian military doctors from the time of the battle of Fornovo, not far from Parma. The battle in which the French suffered an ignominious defeat [some maintain that the result was actually a tie! (10)] took place on the 6th of July, 1495. The physicians wrote that they saw many French soldiers who had pustules on their faces and over their entire bodies. These changes, similar in size to millet grain, first appeared on the penile foreskin, on its inner surface, or on the glans. Often, a single pustule would arise first, and, if broken, would cause a deep ulceration to develop. After several days, pain in the arms, legs and feet would appear, accompanied by a dramatic eruption of pustules, which then remained for a year or longer.

"The sick looked repulsive, and suffered greatly, especially at night. The judgment of witnesses was that this illness struck terror with its ghastliness similarly as then-incurable leprosy or elephantiasis, and threatened life. There was agreement that it had its beginnings in the sexual act and it was assumed that it came to Italy from the west, namely from Spain" (Marcellus Cumanus, Alexandri Benedicti (1497), Natalis Montesauri (Veronensis) (1498), Nicolo Leoniceno (1497). (11).

The next mention of the disease, by then called *La Verole* or the" infirmity from Naples," appears at the beginning of 1496, coming from places lying along the marching route of the French armies. In Lyon, the authorities issued an order to remove from the town those "ill with *La verole*, as well as lepers, in order to protect them [the towns] from contagion, and to maintain the citizens in good health." In January 1496, the rulers of Geneva prohibited foreigners infected with this disease from entry into the town and from moving about [in it]. In Paris, the first reference of illnesses come from the hospital, Hotel Dieu, from which, for the good of those ill with other conditions, removal of those with the new disease to shelters near cloisters or even beyond the city was attempted.

In 1497 the illnesses had already appeared over practically the whole of the territory of France. The first cases of the *French disease* appeared in Nuremberg and Strasbourg at the end of 1495. Fault was attributed to the peasants serving in the army of Charles VIII. In subsequent years, in the majority of German towns, there appeared instances of *Bosen Blattern* or *Malicious pox*, which was said to have originated in France and Italy. One of its victims was

Emperor Maximilian himself, who supposedly was infected in Italy (12). The Emperor suffered greatly, as painful ulcerations appeared in his oral cavity; although, according to reports, he testified to a miraculous cure as the result of his intense prayers at one of the German shrines. With all due respect for his Imperial Majesty, it is more likely that in this instance the *cure* had more to do with remission of the disease to the symptomless phase, that is, concealed syphilis (*lues latens*).

In Italy, despite being spoken of as the French disease, everyone knew that it had come from Spain, where it was called *las bubas*. Both young and old, rich and poor were afflicted, but especially those who led a dissipated lifestyle, cavorted with courtesans or took advantage of the services of bordellos.

The loosening of morals after the period of the Middle Ages is clearly evident. It pertained equally to secular people as to people of the Church. Before the epoch of the Renaissance, sex and sexuality were considered as sinful, with sexual contact being solely to serve procreation. Religious principles controlled almost every aspect of daily life, the goal of which was to attain salvation. During the epoch of the Renaissance, however, love and sexuality were perceived as elements bringing salvation nearer. According to neo-Platonic philosophers (Lorenzo de Medici), „growing fonder of one's body is a step in the direction of growing fonder of wisdom, and consequently of God." The idea that one should be happy with life and take advantage of its charms was common. But, don't we, in this context, have to do something about turning the pendulum in the opposite direction? Unfettered sexual freedom can have sad consequences. We must also remember that in those times, much more was allowed men than women. In regard to extramarital relations of men, one looked aside at taking advantage of the services of women of loose morals, not seeing anything wrong. Male homosexuality was tolerated, but not a word was said about lesbian eroticism. Even in the Church, licentiousness was tolerated, and its dimension was astonishing insofar as modern morals of the institution are concerned. Almost all the popes from the Renaissance epoch had children, with the exception of Pope Leo X who was said to have been a homosexual. It is likewise considered that Popes Alexander VI, Julius II, and Leo X had syphilis. Not differing at all from the type of entertainment arranged at the royal courts or among the higher aristocracy, orgies with the participation of prostitutes also took place at the papal court, especially that of Alexander VI. The infamous Pope Borgia gave away his daughter, Lucrezia, in marriage several times with the aim of political advantage, and when they failed to be comfortable marriages, annulled them. It was said, likewise, that he was the father of her child, although that was also suspected of his son, Cezar, who was supposed to have infected her with syphilis. There is no clear proof, regarding the last assertion, although it is accepted that one of Lucrezia's husbands, Alfonso d'Este, as well as one of her lovers, Francesco Gonzaga (the hero of the Battle of Fornovo) were ill with this disease. (13a)

Not everyone approved of such behavior by the servants of the altar. The loudest critic of the Pope's morals was the Dominican friar from Florence, Savonarola. In his sermons, he stigmatized these transgressions by the Church hierarchy, particularly those of Alexander VI, calling him an adulterer, and denying him his right to be a true pope. For his words, Savonarola paid with his life. He was burned at the stake as a heretic (14). Alexander got rid of the monk after consulting his son, Cezar, who went to Florence in order to personally convince himself how dangerous for the papacy were the monk's public criticisms (15).

Pope Alexander VI lived many years in a relationship with the beautiful and intelligent Vanozza dei Cattanei, with whom he had four children acknowledged as legitimate: Juan, Cezar, Lucrezia and Jofre. (Fig.2.2 and Fig.2.3.).

Cezar Borgia, the second of Alexander's children, was nominated by his daddy to be cardinal at age 16, but did not feel right in the position. Released from his crimson robes after a number of years (the first resignation from this position in Church history), he became the commander of the papal army. A favorite with women, he often frequented the city, where he contracted the French disease. Cezar developed severe pains in the genital area and a facial rash. His court physician, Gaspare Torella, tested a new method of treatment developed by himself (16, 17). For many weeks he soaked the pustules, now covering Cezar's entire body, with a variety of herbs, then rubbed them off with hot pumice stones. The bigger pustules were lanced, squeezed out, and again soaked with herbs. The wounds healed, leaving small scars. The patient was delighted, and the physician received a handsome reward.

Not all had such good fortune, however. The sick without money had to suffer. Their appearance was ghastly, although in many, their pustules retreated. The richer Romans paid olive oil merchants huge sums for permission to soak in barrels of the oil. Multi-hour soaking in the fat did bring relief. The skin stopped shedding, and some pustules disappeared. However, not many people knew that the same oil was later sold in elegant shops as virgin olive oil. (18)

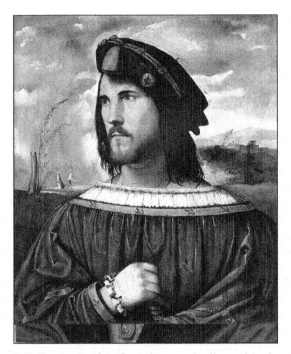

Figure 2.2 Portrait of a Gentleman believed to be Cezar Borgia (Painting by Altobello Melone 1490-1543)

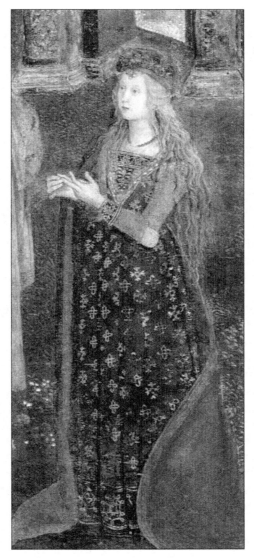

*Figure 2.3 Lukrezia Borgia as St. Catherine of Alexandria
(Fresco by Pinturicchio (Vatican)*

However, let us return to Cezar Borgia. Several months after his successful treatment, Cezar was infected with syphilis for a second time. (19) That, at least, is how authors engaged in writing about this disease, nicely put it. Today, we know that it isn't true. In syphilis there exists the phenomenon of *premunition*, which does not permit repeat infection in people who already suffer from the same disease. Periodic remission of symptoms is typical of syphilis, and temporary absence of skin changes does not signify cure. Periods of remission [latency] can last many months, and it is only a matter of time before new signs appear, which can signify advancing disease.

In Cezar's case, there doubtless appeared a recurrent rash typical of the second stage of syphilis, which is characterized by more abundant skin changes, and also the loss of hair from the head (20). Horrible pustules and erosion covered with puss appeared again on Cezar's face, this time with visible scars. Accustomed to complements about his handsomeness, the 25-year-old former cardinal was desperate. He couldn't show himself in the city, visit his lovers, or even have a drink in a public place. Everyone immediately knew that they were dealing with a person suffering from syphilis, and could scarcely hide their disgust. Cezar ordered his servants to cover his mirrors with a dark cloth. He slept during the day and worked at night. He rode horseback around the region, but only at night. In the end he decided to wear a mask, which he took off only when alone (19,20). At the age of twenty-five, he became practically an invalid, and that, not only as the result of ugly skin changes, but also as a result of psychological derangement. Always impulsive and inconsiderate, without scruples about his methods in regard to realizing his ambitions, he became unusually cruel later in life. Suspected earlier of the murder of his older brother, and, later, his brother-in-law, the husband of Lucrezia, Cezar raped/violated and tortured his enemies without pity. In 1500, at the head of his army, he conquered the fortress at Forli, which was defended by 37-year-old Catherina Sforza. Cezar raped her multiple times, not making any secret of it, and even joked that she defended her charms with far less passion than the fortress he conquered. (22) A year later, Cezar raped the wife of one of his officers, and imprisoned her for over two years, taking advantage of her sexually. When he became bored with her, he sent the poor woman to a convent (23). Some historians attribute his type of brutal behavior to the changes observed with late syphilis, described by name as *general paresis*.

In mid-September 1503, a splendid reception was held in Rome on the occasion of the 11th anniversary of the ascent to the papal throne by Alexander VI, as well as to honor the latest victories of Cezar, who conquered Romania, and the taking of the Senigallie port on the Adriatic, which belonged to the family of Cardinal della Rovere, later Pope Julius II, an obstinate enemy of the Borgia family. Taking part in the reception were virtually all the members of the papal family, their closest friends, and selected members of the Roman aristocracy. Even during the banquet, in the course of which everyone drank and ate in abundance, the Pope felt ill. He was pale, had chills, and perspired in copiously. Similar symptoms occurred in Cezar, which thus could have indicated poisoning. A trusted physician was summoned, and after an examination, stated that the symptoms pointed to a malarial infection, but that poison could not be excluded. He recommended the application of leeches, to which, at first, Cezar did not want to agree. Unfortunately, the treatment had little effect. The Pope, after a short time, died, although Cezar, being younger and stronger, coped with the illness for a long time, being at the brink of death for many weeks. Finally, he recovered, and joined a campaign to prevent the election of Cardinal della Rovere as Pope. (24)

It is a shame that we do not have a record of Cezar's state of health from this time, as we could then have determined whether or not he had malaria, which, characterized by recurring high fever, could have affected positively the syphilis from which he had suffered for a long time. (Several hundred years later, in fact, malaria was used to treat *general paresis* resulting from syphilis, and that with considerable success). Unfortunately, we will never find out, as our 'hero' was killed soon thereafter during the siege of Vienna on March 12, 1507, the result of treason by the armies he commanded (25).

The entire Borgia family, and particularly individual members became the heroes of many books, film plots, and television serials. Many painters immortalized their figures on canvas. Supposedly, Lucrezia posed for the famous Botticelli painting, *The Birth of Venus* and is the heroine of the opera *Lucrezia Borgia*, by Gaetano Donizetti, who, three hundred years later suffered from syphilis, and from which he, also, died. Currently, it is felt that Cezar Borgia was the original model of a hero of the political treatise of Niccolo Machiavelli, *The Prince*, in which are glorified violence, outrage, artifice, trickery, and hypocrisy in the sense that *the end justifies the means*.

Just as the ideas of the Renaissance, were born in Italy, from which they spread to other countries, so the epidemic of syphilis, which appeared on a massive scale there after the invasion by Charles VIII, spread, first in Europe, then to other regions of the world. In less than ten years after the battle of Fornovo, the epidemic covered all of Europe. In England, the first hints of illnesses due to syphilis appear in 1497. It was known as the *Sickness from Bordeaux*, which suggests that it was transported to the British Isles from France. In the same year, it appeared in Scotland under the name *grandgor*, which similarly indicates its French origin. Upon the recommendation of King James, the City Council of Edinburgh ordered the isolation of those ill with *grandgor* until their complete recovery. The City Council assured free transport of the sick to the Isle of Inchkeith in the Firth of Forth estuary, simultaneously warning that if any of the sick refused to go willingly to Inchkeith, an appropriate brand would be made on their cheeks with a red hot iron, which would make possible their identification and permit involuntary expulsion from the city.

In what today is Holland, and, specifically in the Netherlands and Flanders, syphilis appeared in 1496. This is linked with the expedition of the Spanish fleet, consisting of twenty sailing ships, which, in August of 1496 was carrying the daughter of Queen Isabella, 16-year-old Infanta Joanne, to her wedding to Phillip the Handsome. Remember that journey by land was not considered, as a result of the war with France. Such a large number of ships for the transport of the Infanta not only had the goal of showing Europe what a power Spain was at that time was, but also of ensuring the safety of its passengers, who were to sail many days along the coast of France. This same squadron, on its return journey, was taking the betrothed of the Spanish King Juan, Margaret of Flanders, to Spain. Sailors often do not lead a virtuous life. Shortly after the visit of the Spanish fleet, the first instances of the *Spanishe pokken* (Spanish pox) appeared in Ganda and in Leyden.

In Denmark, syphilis had already appeared in 1495 or 1496. The chronicle of John the Dane speaks of the appearance of a major disease called the *French mange*, not known until then among the Danes nor the Germans. It is said that many thousands died, and that never before had it been seen (Parvi Rosaefontani, 1560).

As we can see, every country in which syphilis appeared, gave it a name indicating suspicion of export from a neighbor. In France, one spoke of the Neapolitan disease. In Italy, they spoke of the French disease, because of the explosion of the epidemic that appeared after the invasion by the armies of Charles VIII. The people of Flanders and the Netherlands, similarly to the people of Northern Africa, called it the Spanish disease. The English and Germans spoke of the French disease, while Poles, first of the German disease, then later changed it to the French disease, also known as *Franca*. In Russia, syphilis was known as the *Polish disease*, in Portugal, the *Castillean disease*, while in Japan and India one would speak of the *Portuguese disease*. Only in Spain is it still spoken of as *las bubas*!

CHAPTER 3

A CURE WORSE THAN THE DISEASE

The appearance of previously unknown and life-threatening diseases at the juncture of the fifteenth and sixteenth centuries caused consternation and panic. The society of the time, having experienced epidemics of plague (the Black Death), leprosy and smallpox, found itself confronted with a new contagion with which it had never had to deal with before. It urgently began to seek avoidance measures, methods of prevention, and methods of treatment.

A certain wise Englishman once said, "The history of medicine is a monument to human stupidity." (1) In this assertion, there is a lot of truth, but also untruth. Physicians, if I may so call my sixteenth century colleagues, were neither more intelligent nor more stupid than the rest of society. One has to say with honesty that, in many instances, they demonstrated very sensible observations and an ability for logical conclusions. Were there among them fools, charlatans or cheats? Of course there were; but aren't there such now, even in the 21st century? Always, where scientific medicine is ineffective or helpless, there appears an opportunity for activity of those who take advantage of others.

Combatting diseases depends on their prevention and cure, but in order to be able to apply one and the other, there has to exist a minimum of knowledge of what one is dealing with. After the outbreak of the epidemic in Europe, it was recognized very early that the new disease was transmitted by the sexual route. Of course, other possibilities were entertained, one example   "through the air" – mostly because many infections occurred among professed celibates and among young women coming from honored families that could not allow such a loss of respectability. Disregarding *exceptions*, it is most likely that the majority of society recognized that the means of infection was sexual intercourse. This was corroborated by the absence of the new disease among children prior to puberty, and among the very old. Other evidence included the signs of the disease, which initially appeared on the genitals.

The first recommendations regarding prophylaxis, inasmuch as the disease is transmitted by the sexual route, were that in order to avoid it sexual contact with ill persons should be avoided. As early as 1497, Gilinus of Ferrara recommended that "in no instance should one unite with women infected with this dangerous disease, as I have seen many who became infected with this infirmity, as they experienced the greatest suffering." (2) What was also observed even more was what is currently called the *chain of infection*, and recommended avoiding sexual contact even with healthy women who had recently had contact with infected men. (3) Likewise enjoined were contacts with dissolute women and prostitutes, who, based on behavior or profession, were more likely to be exposed to venereal diseases than other women. Can one deny common sense in these recommendations? After all, they are exactly the same counsel we share with our patients now – 500 years later!

Another preventive method proposed was the isolation of those who were sick, based on their forced separation from the rest of society, as was attempted in, for example, Scotland or France. The models for this type of prophylaxis were doubtless the leprosaria and other places of isolation in which were kept those suffering from leprosy. I will only remind the reader that similar types of ideas arose in some minds even in the twentieth century, in the beginning phase of the AIDS epidemic.

In addition to these reasonably effective prophylactic recommendations, other methods were also proposed, which today appear to be senseless, if not amusing. One of these was a recommendation for application *post factum*, namely in situations in which contact with an infected person, or with one suspected of being infected, had already occurred. Its author proposed „careful washing of sexual organs with water or white wine, using clean linen for this purpose, and not using towels taken from prostitutes." Making even less sense, but appealing to the patient's imagination in case of the appearance of ulcerations on the male organ, recommendations were to "cover it from top to bottom with soft soap or the fat of a rooster or a pigeon plucked alive and skinned, or with a live frog cleaved in two."(4) The mechanism whereby this type of treatment was to be effective was based on the belief that the bleeding flesh of a sacrificed animal, thanks to its living heat, was said to disperse and absorb the toxin which had penetrated the organ. There was also no lack of more risky advice such as, for example „tying the organ at its base, in order to prevent, by this means, the penetration of the luetic toxin into the body." (5) One can easily imagine the consequences of an exaggerated application of this recommendation, which, in addition to causing problems with urination, gave the subject great confidence that he would never again be able to become infected with any disease transmitted by the sexual route – unless he uses a technique which doesn't require the use of his organ! Another recommendation now provoking laughter was one asserting that:

> [O]ne should not stay too long with a corrupt woman, and that one must quickly wash and dry [one's] organ immediately after intercourse, and that one should not keep the [one's] organ without [its] being drawn up into [its] sheath, as this organ, in this state, will absorb infection like a sponge. (6)

This recommendation clearly implies that the penis, in a state of complete withdrawal (flaccidity) is less susceptible to infection.

There was no shortage of preventive recommendations based on religion. Those, who considered the disease to be a punishment from God for licentiousness and lack of adherence to the Commandments, organized religious celebrations (as, for instance, the Canon of Notre Dame in Paris), who, in the last years of the fifteenth century led processions with the reliquaries of St. Marcel and St. Genevieve, to ward off "this dangerous and contagious disease, for which doctors and physics cannot offer a [curative] medication." (5) Others recommended fasts or other types of penances, and also suggested flogging before beginning treatments, asserting that medications used after this type of endeavors would be more efficacious.

And now, the medicines. In the introduction to this chapter, I wanted to remind the reader of the known fact that the level of medical science is a function of the development of basic sciences, such as biology, physics, or chemistry. At the juncture of the fifteenth and sixteenth centuries, the level of such sciences was very low, and the methods used for the treatment of diseases known earlier were very primitive. The appearance of a new, rapidly spreading disease was a surprise for all, not excluding physicians of the time, and it is no wonder that the first methods of treatment were not different from methods applied to diseases known earlier. These were sweating medicines, bloodletting, blistering agents, pills of *swallow's herbs* (*Chelidonium majus*), and aloes. Barber-surgeons used corrosive substances for ulcerations, with the goal of "burning out the ulcers," and also tried to cut them out. There now appeared ointments containing mercury, which from forgotten times was used in the treatment of skin diseases, including leprosy. Very quickly, then, mercury became medicine number one; its preeminence in its application to syphilis, already in 1496, is attributed to the Venetian physician, Georgio Sommariva. (7)

Accounts of the application of mercury in the treatment of syphilis during its early epidemic freezes the blood in one's veins, and it can be said without great exaggeration that, in most instances, the medicine was worse than the disease. Unfortunately, this was the only medication, which in the opinion of physicians of the time, produced a cure—perhaps one in a hundred. That *cure* is also problematical, however, because, as I first mentioned, the signs of lues, were frequently confused with other venereal diseases, such as gonorrhea, soft chancre (chancroid), genital herpes or skin diseases arising in the area of the genitalia and anus, hence not at all subject to a single cure. In addition, one should remember that, in syphilis, the primary chancre, as well as skin lesions in the secondary stages of the disease clear up by themselves – which does not mean a cure.

Regarding all this, the following is a description of one sixteenth century mercury treatment:

> The patients were rubbed with a mercury cream once or many times a day, and were enclosed in a steam bath during which a constant, very high temperature was maintained. The treatment lasted from 20 to 30 days. During such a regimen, the patient began to weaken. The ulcerations, which were accompanied by huge swellings, appeared in the throat and the oral cavity. The gums swelled, the teeth loosened, and fell out, while from the mouth flowed an unending, disgusting stream of saliva. (8)

The author of this account, Ulrich von Hutten, himself ill with syphilis, underwent this regimen eleven times (hard to believe!), and was a witness to the deaths of many patients. It is probably from this period that comes the famous saying, *A night in the arms of Venus leads to a lifetime on Mercury.*

I saw a certain healer while in the steam bath, for which he constantly ordered the raising of the temperature, which led to the deaths of three poor craftsman. These sufferers, who were convinced that the greater the heat they could withstand, the more certain and quicker would be their cures, were suffocated before they realized their unfortunate fate. I also saw others with swollen throats that did not allow passage of the already pussy mucus, which needed to be coughed up or vomited, as they struggled in the horrors of a cruel agony, and as they suffocated by the rotting humors. (8)

Von Hutten died in 1524 at 35 years of age, but it is unknown of what cause: whether as a result of lues, or maybe its treatment, or even of a completely unrelated cause.

Many other authors from this time drew attention to the side effects of mercury treatment. They write about the signs of shivering death agonies, paralyzed nerves and staggers, and loss of teeth. One writes of loss of hearing and disturbances of speech caused by the appearance of ulceration in the oral cavity. Evidence of how curious were the ideas of some of these physicians, is the fact that to reduce the unending flow of saliva caused by the mercury treatment, it was proposed to place a hot iron onto the skull of the patient "with the aim of irritating the brain, the organ directing the mucus, the lymph or the 'humor,' which produces the saliva." (9) Situations are described in which "as a result of the untempered application of mercurious balsam to the genitalia, there arose the need for their amputation." (10)

Torrela (11) accuses the followers of mercury treatment of the death of numerous prominent people of that time, who lost their lives not as a result of the disease, but rather of its treatment. Another physician of the time, Villalobos, called the adherents of using mercury "complete asses," and advised the use of analgesics (pain medications), frequent enemas, baths, and blood-letting. He was also a proponent of using arsenic in the treatment of syphilis.

Of long duration, not bringing any salutary effect, and destructive in regard to health, mercury treatments were the cause of financial ruin of many patients. Simultaneously, the treatment of syphilis became a very lucrative occupation and a source of the fortunes of not only physicians, but also of charlatans and quacks.

One cannot be surprised that, with such a low effectiveness of treatments with mercury and their horrific side effects, alternative methods began to be sought after, ones which might bring at least a minimum of relief to the ill, yet would not create the risk that patients would die as a result of the treatment. And that is how guaiac appeared.

Guaiac is a tree (*Guajacum officinale/lignum vitae*) growing on the Antilles Islands and in Central America. It was used in artistic carpentry due to its compactness and hardness. In the sixteenth century, guaiac was also employed in medicine as a purgative and diaphoretic (sweat-inducing) medium. Additionally, it had "special anti-luetic characteristics" because it came from the same geographical regions as the syphilis brought by Columbus from Hispaniola at the end of the fifteenth century. Guaiac used in the treatment of syphilis was prepared from the bark of this tree by grinding it to a powder, and after soaking it, preparing an extract by boiling over a small fire. Before beginning treatment, the diet of the sufferer was changed, and simultaneously mild laxative agents were administered. Before administering the guaiac, the patient was put into an unventilated, well-heated room, and, upon starting to perspire, was given a large dose of guaiac. Treatment lasted a month, sometimes longer, and the patient, who was often tottering on his legs as a result of the fasting, was then considered cured. Therapy with guaiac, while doubtless less drastic, had about the same effect as treatment with mercury, meaning almost none; yet despite this fact, it was used for a time with full vigor. The importation of guaiac in Europe was undertaken by the well-known Fugger banking family from Germany, who obtained a royal monopoly for bringing it to Europe. This privilege was obtained from Emperor Charles V who, thanks to loans received from the Fuggers, won election and became the ruler of the Holy Roman Empire, as well as the King of Spain and controlled trade between Europe and the New World. I will remind the reader that Charles V himself was accused of having syphilis, and was a competitor of the King of France, Francis I, who presumably died of syphilis. The Fuggers greatly enriched themselves from the import of guaiac, selling it to centers for the treatment of lues that were organized by themselves, and in which this preparation was used. (12,12a,12b.)

A great proponent of guaiac was the above-mentioned Ulrich von Hutten, after receiving several treatments with mercury, became enamored of the new medicine. He was one of the first to use it, while his work, *De guaiaci medicina et morbo galico*, from 1519 consists of a tribute to this expensive wood. (13)

In addition to guaiac, in the middle of the sixteenth century there appeared many other medications derived from the sarsaparilla plant (*Aralia species*), which was used for many years, first as the main, then as a secondary medium in the treatment of lues. This medication had already been known in ancient Greece and Rome as an antidote to various types of poison. In Central and South America, it was used by the Indians to treat skin and the urinary tract diseases, as well as a generally invigorating agent, and one increasing libido. Importation of sarsaparilla from Jamaica and Mexico was begun by the Conquistadors, and this agent was transported to Europe up to the end of the nineteenth century. The seventeenth century specialist in herbal treatments, herbalist Nicholas Culpepper from England, named sarsaparilla the treatment of choice for the *French disease*, and this agent appeared in the American Pharmacopoeia between 1820 and 1910 as a remedy for lues. Even in the middle of the nineteenth century, it was imported to England in a quantity greater than 150,000 pounds annually, of which a large portion was consigned for the treatment of syphilis, although it had already been said for a long time to have no influence on the course of this disease. (14)

Just as was mercury, guaiac was also used as a post-coital preventive for syphilis. A recommendation written by Fallopio stated: "If you did such a foolish thing, and had intercourse with a beautiful and infected siren, after washing yourself after the sexual act you should cover the member with a piece of cloth soaked in a mixture consisting of wine, shavings of guaiac wood, flakes of copper, mercury, root of gentian, red coral, ash from an elephant's bone [ivory?], burned deer antler," and several other strange things. This potion was to be applied for four or five hours, and was supposed to protect the patient, although I don't know from what—infection or development of the disease? Fallopio likewise recommended that persons who were unable to refrain from risky love should always carry several of such (prepared) cloths, and to use them at the appropriate time. (15)

Despite the wretched therapeutic effects and dangerous side effects of mercury (guaiac and sarsaparilla were more often used as add-on agents, it remained the basic treatment of lues for many centuries. Over the course of years, however, there appeared newer methods for its use. One of these was anti-venereal underwear, smeared on the inside with a mercurial cream, and used mainly in Italy. In Sicily, Tommaso Campailla (1668-1740)—the poet, philosopher and physician—treated his patients with mercury in self-designed wooden *botti (*barrels) in which patients sat while inhaling mercury infusions. The idea was pioneered in France, where the patient's head would project from the top of the barrel while Campanilla's design was squarer, and the patient's whole body sat in the *cabin*. Near the end of the eighteenth century, there appeared oral preparations containing mercury, considered until now, as dangerous poison. Nevertheless, these were used as helping agents next to the traditional, external treatments with mercury preparations. One new agent for oral use, sublimate (bichloride) of mercury, considered for many years as controversial, grew in popularity, because it was recommended by the famous Gerhard van Swieten, (Fig.3.1.) the physician of Maria-Teresa, Empress of Austria; it is said that he invented a drink consisting of grains of the sublimate dissolved in water and alcohol. This preparation, later called *liquer of van Swieten*, had a dizzy career, mainly for two reasons. Those ill with syphilis could treat themselves in their own homes, and, afterwards, were in far better moods than after mercury rubs; the second no doubt depended on the stimulating effect of the alcohol in the liquor. Among other forms of the oral use of mercury, one must remember the mercury syrup of Dr. Bellet, mercury cookies, a tonic water of the pharmacist Marbeck, and libido-enhancing chocolates containing a measure of sublimate, which was supposed to ensure its antisyphilitic activity. (16) The appearance of medicines that could be taken at home had an important psychological meaning, as it allowed patients to have hopes that the fact of their becoming ill with syphilis would remain their secret, or under the worst of circumstances, would be limited to the closest members of one's family.

Aside from various forms of mercury for oral use, mercurial preparations for intrarectal treatment in the form of enemas also appeared. These were adapted for combined use with mercury pomades for rubs, or alone, as the single form for dispensing the mercury. Claude Quetel cites the report of a Dr. Horne from 1775, who describes the case of 21-year-old Rosalie, a prostitute from Normandy, who, as a result of her syphilis, received at least 148 anti-venereal enemas containing mercury, as well as many rubs with mercury pomade, which, as he wrote, „achieved all possible results." (17) One has to congratulate the poor woman for her good health, and express surprise that she withstood such tortures! One can equally consider whether we were not dealing here with a case of the sexual deviation, *klismafilii*, in which the patient obtains sexual pleasure produced by the enema.

Treatment of syphilis was a very lucrative occupation. Involved with it were physicians and charlatans. Both groups made huge amounts of money for two reasons: the huge number of ill with syphilis, and the very long duration of treatment utilized, lasting practically a lifetime. Regarding how profitable treating those ill with syphilis was, let the following humorous anecdote be a witness: A dying doctor calls his son, also a physician to his deathbed, and apologizes to him, saying that he will not inherit any fortune from him, as he squandered everything by taking advantage of life's charms. At the same time, he consoles him, by relating that he is leaving him an inheritance of three patients ill with syphilis, which should ensure him a sufficient life-style for many years.

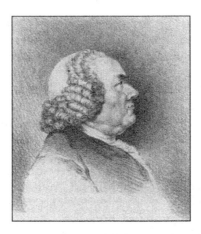

Figure 3.1 Gerhard van Swieten (from the Office of Medical History. US Medical Department and Medical History).

During the eighteenth century, aside from experimentation with new medications for lues (arsenic, antimony, lead), which turned out not to be effective, new prophylactic agents appeared. The most important of these, without a doubt, was the condom, whose national origin was most probably England. In texts from this period, (18) one finds reference to sacs made of very thin membranes, without stitches, in the form of a covering. These were most probably animal intestines, most likely from sheep. The name of the device, *the condom*, does not come, as some might wish, from any Dr. Condom, the supposed inventor, but rather from the Latin word, *condere,* which means "to hide or to protect." As a result of their place of origin, condoms were called *English jackets*, or *English cloaks*.

One of the first users of condoms was the famous eighteenth century eternal seducer Giovanni Giacomo Casanova, whose problems with health attest to the poor effectiveness of the condoms of the time, or of their unsystematic use by the owner. According to his own memoirs, the famous seducer, an object of sighs of unsatisfied wives, suffered venereally, and that not just once.

(19,19a) The first time he became infected with syphilis was most probably in London, and the course of his illness was so dramatic that he thought he would die. He later received treatment for it in Dresden for six whole weeks. It appears, however, that that infection with purported lues (he supposedly had more than twenty) was most likely gonorrhea or another disease, which either remitted after treatment with mercury, or remitted spontaneously. As can be seen from his reputation, frequent infections did not especially influence the state of his health, as he died at age 73, and not at all due to a venereal disease.

Having named the condom as a new prophylactic agent for men, one must add that, also in the eighteenth century, there appeared sponges for women, which, when introduced into the vagina, were supposed to guard against disease. Both of these means, condoms and sponges, which in the technologic state of the time could only protect partially against venereal disease, had one fault – they were also agents of contraception. They prevented pregnancy, and that, according to all Christian religions until the mid-1930s, was a serious sin. The view that condoms and sponges prevent the gametes from reaching the womb and thus waste life arose from the multi-century-old conviction that only the male, and, more precisely his sperm, is the carrier of new life, attributing to the woman an exclusively passive role. In many theological concepts, the woman did not contribute anything more to the formation of a new human being beyond that of acting as a formative medium to the shape of the dust of the earth, a flower pot, into which the male inserts the seed, from which seed alone, a child arises (20). This concept should have already had a basic revision in 1827, when the German physician from Konigsberg and professor at the University of Saint Petersburg, K.E. von Baer, discovered the female ovum, and determined that not until the ovum and male sperm join does a new human life begin. Unfortunately, even a hundred years later, one would hear the opinion that wasting the seed is virtually homicide. I remember how strongly I felt and how I sympathized with my friends, when we were in our maturing period, and learned during a certain lesson in school that we could be *murderers*! It is a regrettable that, even in the twenty-first century, and despite thousand-fold evidence that condoms may prevent infection with venereal diseases, including AIDS, their use could be forbidden for purely doctrinal reasons.

During the eighteenth century, there appeared the first hospitals for treating venereal diseases. I am not sure whether the word *hospital* in today's understanding of the word is adequate, as these were centers below any acceptable standards of today. Until this time, general hospitals did not accept those ill with venereal diseases, and only a few of them, depending on the country, agreed to provide care to these patients outside the hospital. One of the first of these specialty hospitals, as we would call them today, was founded by the Russian Tsarina, Catherine II, a fifty-bed hospital for those with venereal diseases, in St. Petersburg. It is said that the same Tsarina suffered from lues, and from this came her understanding for the sick poor (21). In mid-1756, the first hospital designated for venereal diseases on Polish soil was established in Warsaw, and several years later, a similar one in Krakow (22). At about the same time, there began to arise hospitals or hospital departments for those venereally ill in Denmark and in France. In England, they took advantage, for this purpose, of beds designated for those with leprosy, whose numbers had been rapidly falling from the fifteenth century. In London, St. Bartholomew's, St. Thomas' and St. George's hospitals accepted patients with venereal disease. They were called *Lock hospitals*, from the word, *loque*, meaning rag or binding, which patients with leprosy used to wipe their ulcerations before crossing the threshold of the hospital. (21) In Vienna, a hospital for syphilitics, by the name of St. Mark's, accepted those ill with advanced syphilis, who for various reasons could not be treated at home. Emperor Joseph II ordered their wards to be opened to visitors, most probably so that they could view the consequences of the disease. Apparently, there was no lack of those willing to look, as „equally men and women – in pursuit of a cheap thrill, came to this hospital to laugh at the sufferings of the patients." (22a)

Descriptions of conditions existing in centers treating patients with venereal diseases scared away, rather than welcomed, those wanting to take advantage of them. Visiting such a hospital, Bicetre, in Paris, a visitor wrote that the conditions existing there were more suitable for a prison than a healing institution:

> The ill are there like a load of Negroes on an African ship .... Betwen two rows of beds, the center of the floor is covered with the sick. This is mainly the result of a shortage of space, but sometimes, equally to the fact that the poor and emaciated prefer the hard floor to an infected and dirty bed (23).

In Bicetre, in the second half of the eighteenth century, about 100 patients at a time were being treated, each for about five weeks. The list of patients awaiting a free place was so long that some, and those primarily prostitutes, signed up even before they were attacked by the disease. The overfilled wards were saturated with the vapors of mercury to such a degree that specific signs associated with its use, such as sweating, sialorrhea (drooling), etc., appeared in the sick even before the start of therapy. It was noted that the most varied, risky treatments were allowed, and to the extent that fatal cases of syphilis had been rare earlier in the eighteenth century, so in Bicetre they occurred mainly as a result of treatment. To this type of hospital also came the sick referred by police order. This applied primarily to prostitutes serving the army, for which they constituted a danger for its readiness for battle. In the same army, venereal recidivism was punished with fines, and from 1778, every French soldier treated more than twice for venereal disease had to serve in the army for an additional two years. (24)

At the end of the eighteenth century, the first shelters for children with congenital syphilis appeared. This was not yet the time when the causes of births of children with signs of lues were known. It had been recognized for a long time that in women infected with syphilis, miscarriages and stillbirths occur *en masse; however,* only in small numbers, and those being in the later stages of the disease, do they give birth to children with the characteristic appearance of old age, and covered with blisters or pimples. As to causes, a plethora of opinions ruled, beginning with the theory that infection of the child occurs at the time of birth, since, on the sexual organs of the mother are found venereal ulcerations (25); through the theory that the venereal toxin may be transferred to the child by the parents at the time of impregnation; to an opinion saying that the infection occurs through the father's seed. It was asserted equally that the infection may occur during the time that the unborn child is in the womb, or that the infection may be transmitted from an ill wet-nurse, and even by a kiss from an infected person. It should be added that there were opposite situations when healthy mothers were infected by children with syphilis transmitted in the course of nursing. With this in mind, in Parisian shelters for children in Vaugirard were posted warnings that syphilitic children should be nursed only by their birth-mothers, and wet-nurses were given mercury, in reduced doses, under the belief that their milk, saturated with mercury would act therapeutically on the newborn (25).

The nineteenth century brought new ideas for the treatment of syphilis, or, maybe one can perhaps say, venereal diseases, because in that century, there appeared a distinct ability to distinguish among them. One has to admit that already earlier, beginning with the sixteenth century, many tried to prove that syphilis and gonorrhea are two different diseases (Fernel 1554, Sylvius 1614-1672, Cockburn 1715 and many others (26), yet this view did not attain universal acknowledgment, particularly after the unfortunate experiment of Hunter in 1776. John Hunter, a Scottish physician, deliberately infected himself (some say a volunteer), with the pussey secretion taken from a patient with a discharge from the urethra (a typical picture of gonorrhea in a male). Hunter did not know that this same patient was simultaneously infected with syphilis, but did not yet have any symptoms of the latter, as he was in the incubation period, averaging two to three weeks. Hunter experienced signs of gonorrhea, and then syphilis, which corroborated the thesis that gonorrhea is just one of the manifestations of syphilis (27). In 1812, a French physician, J. F. Hernandez, conducted a similar experiment inoculating a volunteer from prison in Toulons, producing gonorrhea with none of the added signs characteristic of syphilis. Another French researcher, a known venereologist and physician to the Emperor Napoleon II, Philippe Ricord (1800-1889), distinctly separated the signs of lues from venereal warts (*condylomata acuminata*) produced by the HPV virus, and acknowledged that gonorrhea and syphilis are two distinct diseases. Ricord, as one of the first to do so, divided syphilis into several, successive stages of the disease, but did not shield himself in this from certain errors. In 1852, Leon Bassereau confirmed that soft chancre (chancroid) and syphilis are two distinct diseases. (28)

As always in times when new theories arise, there was no dearth of persons who did not agree with them. There were still many educated people, who believed in a syphilitic gonorrhea and that soft chancre is a manifestation of lues of lesser virulence (29). The foremost proponent of this theory, Dr. Auzias-Turenne moved ahead, and proposed so-called *syphilization*, which indicates nothing less than vaccination, of those suffering from syphilis, with infectious material obtained from those ill with "syphilis of reduced virulence," that is, those suffering from soft chancre (chancroid). This measure was supposed to effect a cure of syphilis, or, in the worst case, ensure its having a mild course. Even worse, he intended that, should he vaccinate healthy persons with this same material, he would induce a resistance to infection with syphilis. He wanted first to vaccinate prostitutes to protect them from syphilis so that their clients would avoid infection and take advantage of the services of only these 'ladies,' who would legitimize themselves with a certificate of syphilization. Fortunately, the ideas of Dr. Auzias-Turanne were not accepted, as the Academie Imperiale de Medecine recognized syphilization as too dangerous. To the author of syphilization one must nevertheless acknowledge that he was an honest man. Despite his absurd ideas, as it turned out that he himself submitted to syphilization, keeping this fact a secret; it came to light only after the opening of his last will and testament (29).

Alongside such ideas as syphilization there appeared in the second half of the nineteenth century experiments in the treatment of venereal diseases with new preparations such as potassium iodide and compounds of arsenic, cauterization, and even surgical treatment. The last consisted of the excision of the primary chancre, which, as it shortly turned out, didn't prevent the development of the disease nor its transition to the next phase of disease, secondary or tertiary. Mercury was still in use, although together with the already classical rubs, mercury pills and high-percentage liquors of van Swieten, there appeared mercury injections as well as other compounds of mercury, such as the acetate, nitrate and phosphate of mercury, and mercuric sulphate.

More or less in the same time period, a new direction in medicine – homeopathy appears; the name was derived from two Greek words, (homois), meaning similar to, and (pathos), meaning suffering. Its beginnings went back to the first half of the nineteenth century, the leader of the new trend being the German physician-venereologist, Samuel Hahnemann (1788-1843) (Fig.3.2.). Homeopathy is one of the unconventional forms of medicine, whose adherents use diluted substances that are supposed to cure diseases with symptoms that are similar to those that arise from their use. The father of homeopathy, Dr. Hahnemann, came to these conclusions by experimenting with quinine – a treatment for malaria. He noticed that after taking quinine, he experienced symptoms seen in those ill with malaria. After many experiments with different substances, he formulated the principal of similarity, known as similia similibus curentur, or "treat similar with similar." He believed that producing certain signs/symptoms by the use of medicines strengthens vital forces for fighting the disease, and that artificially developed effects abate together with removal of the medication. Still another principle – there are more – was the principle of potentiation, which said that the efficacy of a medication increases together with the degree of dilution connected with an appropriate disturbance. (30).

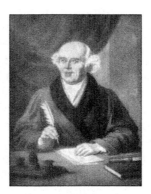

Figure 3.2 Samuel Hahnemann - the founder of homeopathy.

And so, because some signs of syphilis resembled signs of mercury poisoning, homeopaths prescribed greatly diluted mercurial agents named *Mercurius, Mercurius corrosivus,*

Cinnabaris, Mercurius dulcis, and so forth. Other popular agents recommended for the treatment of syphilis were compounds of arsenic used in great dilution. In one homeopathic work titled *Materia Medica,* published in 1854, there is a description of a very popular agent, *Feltz's Anti-syphilitic Decoction,* containing dilute arsenic, the use of which "assured the cure of syphilis." Potassium iodide or potassium bromide were recommended as obligatory therapeutic agents in late, third-stage syphilis, while potassium iodide was also given to children with the congenital disease. Along with already known agents used in the treatment of lues – except that here, they were used greatly diluted – homeopaths proposed news ones, such as *Hepar sulfur,* – especially for persons previously treated with mercury, Nitric acid, in first and second stage syphilis, *Aurum,* (gold) – in cases of second stage disease developing changes (ulcerations) in the oral cavity, and many more, whose identity is difficult to establish. (31)

It is an amazing thing that, despite the variety and, particularly, methods of preparation of homeopathic products (multiple dilution, special method of shaking, etc.) that are reminiscent of black magic, this medical offshoot found many adherents/ proponents, and was especially popular in the second half of the nineteenth century. One of the patients of a homeopathic physician was the German composer, Robert Schumann, who, ill with syphilis, was treated with homeopathic doses of arsenic. Regardless of much evidence that the action of homeopathic agents is equivalent to the action of placebos, even today the method originated by Dr. Hahnemann has its followers who believe in the efficacy of this type of therapy. Insofar as treatment of lues is concerned, it is certain that homeopathic doses of mercury or arsenic used in the nineteenth century were less harmful to patients than the formerly traditional ways of using these agents. As can be seen, the nineteenth century, despite many attempts to introduce new medicines, and also of ways in which they were used, homeopathy did not manifest itself as a turning point in the treatment of syphilis. The great breakthrough, not yet in treatment, but in approach to the etiology of venereal diseases, resulted from the work of Louis Pasteur, which heralded a dramatic development of bacteriology in the seventies of the nineteenth century. In 1879, Albert Neisser, a German physician from Wroclaw (Breslau), discovered the presence of small bacteria in smears from the urethras of those ill with gonorrhea, which, to honor the discoverer, later received the name, *Neisseria gonorrhoeae*. Ten years later, August Ducrey discovered the Gram-negative bacterial rod now known by his name, *Haemophilus ducreyi*, which is responsible for soft chancre (chancroid). The cause of syphilis, however, remained a mystery.

In February 1905, the director of the Institute of Zoology at Berlin University announced that Dr. Siegel, an assistant at the Institute, discovered, in blood, as well as in material obtained from syphilitic lesions, the presence of protozoa, to which he gave the name, *Cytorryces luis*. The Berlin Sanitary Bureau ordered two zoologists, Drs. Schaudinn and Neufeld, as well as a young dermatologist, Erich Hoffman, to confirm this discovery (Fig.3. 3,4). After less than a month's work, Schaudinn confirmed the presence of a small, mobile creature of spiral shape, in one of his specimens, which was unusually difficult to test. Several days later, Schaudinn and Hoffman found the same spiral creature in the lymph node accompanying the primary lesion, in skin lumps and in the blood of a patient with syphilis. (31a). On April 6, 1905, Fritz Schaudinn and Erich Hoffmann published their work under the title, *Vorlaufiger Bericht uber das Vorkommen von Spirochaeten in syphilitischen Krankheitprodukten und bei Papillomen* (Preliminary report on the presence of spirochetes in syphilitic disease products and in papillomas) as an undertaking of the Imperial Health Office (*Arbeiten aus dem Kaiserlichen Gesundheitsamtes (Berlin)* vol. 22, pp.

527-534, 1905). Six weeks later, at a meeting of the Berlin Medical Society, Schaudinn and Hoffmann demonstrated to its members, gathered in a crowd for this meeting, a new bacterium, which for over 400 years had been the cause of suffering and death of many millions. From this moment, physicians and patients knew their adversary. It was a pale spiral, T*reponema pallidum* (Fig.3.5). *Treponema*, because it has the appearance of a twisted thread, and *pallidum*, because it is of pale color. The adversary was now known, but how to conquer it?

For an effective medication against the adversary, we still had to wait several decades. In the meanwhile, the first tests appeared, which, after examination some blood, allowed confirmation or exclusion of the disease. So-called serodiagnosis was born, initiated by Bordet and Wassermann, and called the BW test. First attempts at cultivation of the pale treponeme were undertaken, as well as exploration of ideas for developing a vaccine. Studies on new medications continued in parallel, as those available were not only of little efficacy, but also very toxic. In the same year in which Schaudinn and Hoffmann discovered the cause of syphilis, Drs. H. Wolferson Thomas and Anton Breinl of Liverpool, in the course of studies on African sleeping sickness, confirmed that atoxyl, (the sodium salt of arsenic acid) had an effect on trypanosomes, unicellular organisms that had morphological similarities to the pale treponeme. As we remember, tests of arsenic preparations in the treatment of syphilis had already been undertaken earlier, and similarly to then, new studies demonstrated that the medications were too toxic. (32)

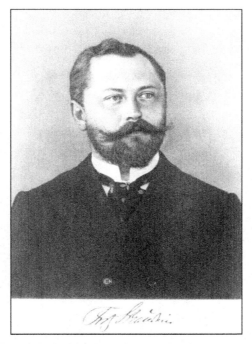

Figure 8.3 Fritz Schaudin, co-discoverer of Treponema pallidum

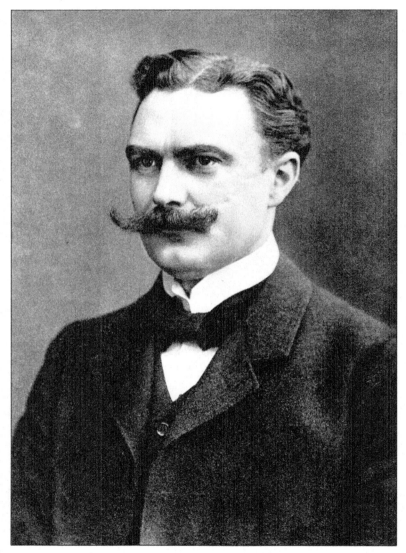

Figure 9.4 Paul Erich Hoffmann, co-discoverer of Treponema pallidum

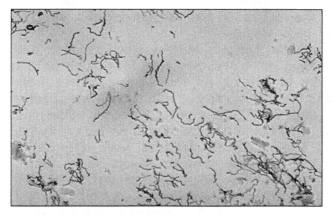

Figure 3.5 Treponema pallidum (microscopic view)

In 1909, Paul Ehrlich of Frankfurt, Germany, together with the Japanese, Hata, worked on a new preparation based on the alternate (trivalent) state of arsenic, and so began the era of the so-called *arsenobenzenes*. First to appear was Salvarsan (arsenobenzol), or *Preparation 606*, and later, Neosalvarsan (novarsenobenzol), *Preparation 914* (from the 914th trial). At almost the same time, Sazerac and Levatidi confirmed the treponemocidal effect of bismuth. Even at the end of the nineteenth century, trials using bismuth in those ill with syphilis had been undertaken (Balzer 1889), but these were discontinued, because of serious poisonings occurring in persons to whom the medication was given. At the start of the twentieth century, however, bismuth was resurrected, and, used with arsenic preparations speeded up the healing of the primary chancre) the disappearance of the rash of secondary syphilis, and the earlier resolution of gummas. Most important, however, was the fact that the new treatments were less toxic than mercury. For the first time in the century, patients and doctors equally perceived light at the end of the tunnel, and began to believe that syphilis could be cured, and, what follows, the extent of the epidemic could effectively be limited.

And epidemiologically, there was something to fear! According to statistics from 1874, one in nineteen inhabitants of the city of New York suffered from lues. According to other studies, one in twenty-two citizens of the United States was ill with syphilis at the end of the nineteenth century, and in other places, it was no better. In the same period, 17% of the French had lues, while in England, one in five soldiers, and one in seven sailors of the British Navy were ill with syphilis or gonorrhea. In the British army stationed in India, it was even worse, as more than half of the army was being treated for venereal diseases. (33) At the time of World War I, half of the adult population of some European cities was ill with syphilis, and in just one year 2,300 British soldiers were hospitalized for an average of seven months due to venereal diseases. In France alone, from the start of the war, that is from August 14, until the summer of 1917, over a million persons suffered from syphilis. Other venereal diseases were not registered. Reportedly, in some instances, soldiers deliberately infected themselves, using matchsticks passed from one to another, in order to avoid serving on the front lines. (34) These data should not be surprising, since, beginning with the end of the fifteenth century, every war was a happening that worsened the epidemiologic situation – remember how syphilis is indebted to the Italian campaign of Emperor Charles VIII! This applies not only to syphilis and gonorrhea, but also to other infectious diseases associated with a poor level of hygiene (typhoid, typhus, tuberculosis, dysentery, etc.). It also applies to other diseases transmitted by the sexual route, such as scabies and pubic lice, the numbers of which are subject to great multiplication during periods of war.

In the years between the first and second World Wars, treatment of syphilis depended generally on arsenicals. However, trivalent arsenicals of the first generation, such as novoarsenobenzol, were gradually replaced with pentavalent arsenicals (Treparasol, Acetylarsan, Stovarsol), which were considered less injurious. These were used together with preparations of bismuth, mercury and iodine, which permitted all types of combinations. They were given in the form of subcutaneous, intramuscular and intravenous injections, in the form of tablets and pills, and some in the form of skin rubs. Treatment appeared to be more efficacious, and was less toxic, but it lasted a very long time – years. Pessimists asserted that the syphilitic had to be treated practically for his or her lifetime.

In 1927, the Viennese psychiatrist, Julius Wagner von Jaurreg became a Nobel laureate in the field of physiology and medicine for introducing so-called malariotherapy to the treatment of syphilis. (Fig.3.6). This was based on injecting malaria parasites into those sick with syphilis, with the aim of producing bouts of fever. (As late as the 1950s, both human and simian parasites were being used, the latter for their sometimes greater fever production while lacking any proclivity to produce relapses in humans: W.A. Krotoski M.D.-personal communication). The method proved itself effective beyond all expectations, although its actual mechanism of action has not yet been completely defined. The simplest explanation would be an acknowledgment that maintaining a high body temperature for a period would be deadly for the treponemes. But whether this is for certain, or whether other phenomena that occur in the body of a person during high fever play a role, is difficult to say.

Dr. Wagner-Jaurreg, was an assistant with the Hospital for Nervous Diseases in Vienna, occupied with studying the influence of fever on some psychiatric diseases. He had noticed earlier that during an epidemic of typhoid, malaria, or smallpox, the psychologic state of patients ill with depression, mania and general paresis underwent an improvement that was not understood. Wagner-Jauregg came to the conclusion that *therapeutic* infections of this type, including with malaria (already widely known to be curable with the help of quinine), could produce a cure, or, at least an improvement in the psychologic state of those ill with signs of general paresis (GP) also known as progressive paralysis. Near the end of World War I, he had on his ward a psychiatrically ill soldier, who had contracted malaria at the front. He took some blood from him, and injected it into nine patients with GP. After 7-11 attacks of high fever, these patients received quinine, which caused a remission of the fever. Among six patients who agreed to this experiment, there was a dramatic remission of the symptoms of general paresis, with three returning to a normal life. Wagner-Jaurreg's experiment was repeated in several other psychiatric centers with similar results, meaning that a complete cure was seen in 30-40% of patients with GP. It is worth noting that, to the extent that treatment of syphilis with arsenobismuth preparations produced a degree of improvement in patients with primary and secondary syphilis, late syphilis, of which GP was one of the clinical forms, was practically incurable. Practically all patients with GP at the time – and they comprised 15% of all the sick treated in psychiatric hospitals – died, usually within 3-4 years of establishment of the diagnosis. Malariotherapy, which began to be used commonly in the '20s and '30s of the last century, was a deliverance for these patients. (35,36)

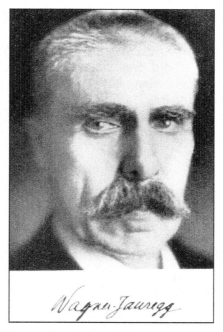

Figure 3.6 Julius Wagner-Jauregg

Like all new methods, this one also had its skeptics. Some considered that infection of a human with a disease in order to free him from another is not ethical, particularly as the method was effective in barely one-third of patients. Others considered that infecting an already ill person with malaria could perhaps produce an epidemic of the latter in large residential areas, which would be very difficult to control. Regardless of the skeptics' opinions, malariotherapy was the method of choice – practically the one – for the treatment of late syphilis, and, used together with injections of Salvarsan or Neosalvarsan, provided a chance of almost complete cure of syphilis. Tests using high temperatures in the treatment of lues by means of other methods (use of preparations containing sulfur, or of so-called *fever cabinets*) did not fulfill expectations, and malariotherapy was considered the best method in cases of advanced syphilis up to 1941.

After an interval of 500 years from the beginning of the pandemic, studies on syphilis, despite a distinct advance in knowledge about this disease, had not attained a fully effective treatment for this horrible malady, and patients with lues were still awaiting a treatment that would ensure them a rapid and 100% certain cure.

CHAPTER 4

DISEASE OF THE COURT - " THE ROYAL POX"

From the onset of the syphilis epidemic in Europe, it was felt that the disease occurred more frequently in rulers and in those of noble birth. Among the many names used to describe it (the word syphilis didn't appear until the middle of the sixteenth century), there also appeared the terms "Royal pox" or "disease of the court," which, itself implied that those suffering from the new affliction were primarily kings and their courtiers. Nothing could be farther from the truth! Everyone, from the peasant to the king was ill with the disease, the difference being that the peasant and his closest ones would know that they had it, whereas concerning their rulers, only whispers abounded at court, gossip was spread in public houses and eating places, while accredited ambassadors included such facts in their reports. Gutenberg's invention of the printing press was already known, and permitted the more rapid and widespread dissemination, not only of important news, but also of gossip and suppositions concerning the lives of persons highly placed in the social hierarchy.

The terms *Royal pox* or, later, *syphilis*, and even later, *lues*, were used very imprecisely. Not only were they used for cases of *true* syphilis, but also for other venereal diseases, and many diseases of the skin whose symptoms appeared in the genitourinary area. These latter had nothing to do with venereal diseases, but the low level of medical knowledge at the time did not allow them to be differentiated.

One of the first monarchs to be associated with syphilis was Emperor Charles VIII, whose Neapolitan expeditions gave rise to the epidemic of the disease in Europe. (1) To whatever extent it is true that Charles VIII's soldiers could have spread syphilis over all of Europe, to that same extent any confirmation that Charles had it, and that he died from an overabundance of sexual activity is more likely pure fantasy. The majority of chroniclers maintain that Charles died as the result of an unfortunate accident. He hit his head on a doorframe in his own palace in Amboise on the Loire River, and as death occurred within several hours after the accident, one may assume that the real cause could have been a subarachnoid hemorrhage.

Much has been written concerning lues in Cezar Borgia, whereas far fewer authors have written about his father, the head of the infamous Borgia family (and, later, Pope Alexander VI), or his sister, Lucrezia, as also suffering from the disease. Unfortunately, there is no evidence worthy of belief to support this. I wrote earlier that one of Lucrezia's husbands, as well as one of her lovers, suffered from syphilis, although whether or not Lucrezia herself had it, we do not know for sure. Supposedly, the successors to Alexander VI—Popes Julius II and Leon X—also suffered from syphilis, (2) but in these cases also there is a lack of convincing evidence. It may surprise the contemporary reader that there are so many churchmen among the syphilitics of the Renaissance period. Morals existing at that time at the papal court did not differ, or differed very little, from those adhered to in the courts of secular rulers. They were condemned equally by representatives of the Church, and doubtless became one of the reasons for the later popularity of Martin Luther's teachings.

Reading about the social interplays occurring at the beginning of the sixteenth century, one is left with the impression that almost all the rulers of the time supposedly suffered from lues. I write *supposedly*, as the majority of authors dealing with this subject and writing about diseases (not only the venereal ones) of many crowned heads use the words *probably* or *supposedly*, underlining the fact that based upon the level of medical knowledge of those times, as well as the lack of exactitude of the descriptions, one can do no more than surmise that a given person suffered from one of the distinct diseases that we recognize today. Among the best known reported syphilitics of that time are included the French king,

Francis I (1494-1547), the king of Spain and simultaneously the Holy Roman Emperor, Charles Vth (1500-1558), as well as the English king, Henry VIII (1491-1547) (2). All three were entangled in numerous intrigues and wars with each other, and also in inter-family marriages. Supposedly Henry III (1551-1589), the king of France and Poland, had lues, of which he was cured by the Spanish physician, Dr. Pena, who gave him a "decoction of Barden root," a medication used in Turkey. (2) Just the fact that Henry III was cured of syphilis by drinking some "decoction" requires one to doubt the veracity of this account.

Francis I

Francis I (Fig.4.1) became the king of France at the age of twenty-six, upon the death of his father, Louis XII. He was an ambitious man, somewhat perverse, but open to new ideas, a lover of the arts and protector of artists. He was interested in new trends in literature and the arts. He was considered a handsome man, adored by women. He valued numerous amusements, liked to hunt, to play tennis, and took part in balls and masquerades. He loved beautiful surroundings, particularly beautiful women. He supposedly used to say "a palace without beautiful women is the same as a garden without flowers." He took pains to make sure that in his garden there was no shortage of "beautiful flowers," and reportedly surrounded himself with a retinue of women acknowledged as the most beautiful in his kingdom. He took part in many wars, both successfully and unsuccessfully, but perhaps is best remembered for his defeat at Pavia in Italy, where, overcome by the armies of Emperor Charles Vth, he was imprisoned by the Spanish. He is said to have sent the famous message, "All is lost except my honor," to his mother, Louise of Savoy. It is not known whether the year-long stay at the Spanish court was able to curb the monarch sexually, or whether other factors were the cause, but after his return to France, Francis became even more dissolute than before. He acquired the conviction that he had the right to take advantage of the services of not only those ladies of his court, who had not yet married, but also the wives of his courtiers. He is said to have remarked that the husbands of the court ladies who became royal mistresses should be proud of the fact that their wives were warming the royal bed. As Branthome wrote, (3) he nightly had to threaten a jealous husband with a sword if the latter stood in his way to the bedroom of his wife. One of the king's mistresses supposedly was Mary Boleyn, the sister of Ann, who became the wife of Henry VIII, and who was also suspected of sleeping with Francis while she was staying at the French court. Francis is said to have infected Mary with lues, and she, in turn, to have transmitted it to Henry, with whom she later had a romance, and even became the mother of his son. Tales, or if one prefers, legends, of this type are not rarities; it is only a shame that they are not based on any evidence worthy of belief. (4)

The well-liked favorite of Francis I was Anne d'Etampes, whom the king gave in marriage to a very ugly man, in order to maintain the appearance of propriety. This husband became jealous, not of the king, but of other courtiers, whom the beautiful Anne also did not refuse at night. The king's favorite, irritated by this fact, is said to have confided to a certain lady, whose husband had recently died, that "not every woman has the good fortune to become a widow." For a long time, Francis escaped the consequences of his romances until he happened on a lover whose jealous husband determined to seek revenge. Not, however, to kill the king, as that would have been difficult to accomplish and, even if successful, its perpetrator, sentenced with a valid judgment, would have perished accompanied by terrible tortures. This jealous husband, Monsieur Ferron, was a lawyer, and thus knew what could await him for regicide; instead, he chose another method. He decided to infect the king with a venereal disease; but, how to accomplish this? The jealous and vengeful husband knew not the boundaries of self-sacrifice. He went to a bordello and asked for a prostitute with syphilis in its most infectious form! The astonished madam fulfilled his wish without asking about his reasons, and so the husband of Lady Ferron infected himself with syphilis. Next, he infected his wife, who, not suspecting a plot, then slept with the king. After a time, there appeared a small, painless ulcer on the king's genitals, which, after several weeks, underwent a rapid healing – to the king's joy. Unfortunately, after another while following this occurrence, a rash appeared on Francis' body. The doctors summoned had no doubts: the king had been infected with syphilis. This account comes from the seventeenth century, namely 100 years after all this supposedly took place, and there is no certainty that it was not manufactured. (3,4)

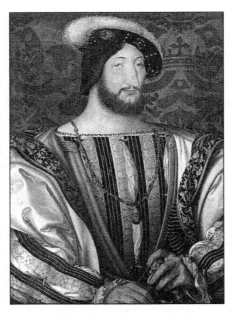

Figure 4.1 Francis I of France (Painting by Jean Clouet)

We do not know exactly of what the treatment of Francis I consisted. One medicine used in the treatment of syphilis at the time was mercury, whose effectiveness was doubted and its side effects frightened patients away from treatment. Supposedly, Francis sent an expedition to South America with the goal of bringing back the bark of a tree that the local population used in treating the disease. This was doubtless guaiac – whose effectiveness was even less than that of mercury. The medicinal was brought back, but the treatment did not bring about any effect. Francis I died four years later, probably as the result of his lues, although some suggest that the true cause was the result of an infection of the urinary tract. His sister, Margaret, the Queen of Navarre, contributed to publicizing Francis I's illness in a collection of short stories titled *Heptameron*, by trying to deny her brother's disease, as had been related by others – by which attempt she brought attention to that fact.

Charles V

Charles V Habsburg, King of Spain and Holy Roman Emperor of the German nation, was the grandson of the Catholic Monarchs, Ferdinand and Isabella, who sponsored Columbus' expedition to the New World (Fig.4.2). While it is suggested in several publications that Charles V suffered from syphilis, in my opinion, there is a lack of convincing evidence in support of this hypothesis. (2) Betrothed first to Princess Mary, the daughter of Henry VIII and Catherine of Aragon, Charles ultimately married Isabella, the daughter of the king of Portugal. This marriage was very happy, despite frequent and long marital separations caused by the need for the king to take part in innumerable war expeditions. Many chroniclers compete in praising the virtues of Charles' wife. They speak of Isabella as a person of wise, warm, and gentle character, yet one of self-denial in difficult moments, always a prudent counselor, and honorably representing her husband. (5) During the early years of their marriage, their first two children, Phillip and Mary arrived, then a daughter, Joan. Their second son, John, died in early childhood, while Isabella's last pregnancy ended in a miscarriage, the results of which left the queen very much weakened, and which produced a sudden fever, most likely due to influenza, or of puerperal origin, to end her life. However, it does not appear that the early death of Prince John, or the final miscarriage, could have had any connection to syphilitic infection. Charles V also had children with other women, yet this progeny had no signs of congenital syphilis. With regard to the Emperor himself, during the beginning of his reign he was blessed with good health, except for an episode in 1532, while living in Germany, when he became ill with, most likely, erysipelas.

On a certain night he felt an itch on his leg, which had been bruised, and scratched it vigorously. There then appeared blisters, a reddening of the skin, and a fever, which lasted a long time. His legs hurt so badly

71

that he started to think of wooden ones, although he related to his sister, with a measure of humor that he preferred his own, made of blood and bone! (6)

Descriptions of the state of his health during the last years of life of Charles V also do not indicate that he suffered from lues. He constantly complained of gout, the attacks of which began many years earlier, and which bothered him for a long time. One efficacious treatment was a diet ("Gout does not like food!"), but the king did not want to adhere to it. After his abdication in 1555-6, when he was living in Uste, symptoms and signs that could indicate diabetes appeared, which to a certain extent, would explain his lack of moderation at table. He drank much beer, despite the orders of his physicians, and complained of hemorrhoids. In 1557, at age fifty-seven, he was already an infirm old man, who was barely able to walk or use his hands as a result of advancing gout. Unfortunately, Uste, the town in which he lived in his old age, was regarded as malarious, and Charles contracted malaria. As could easily be foretold, the letting of blood was employed in its treatment, and did not bring any relief. Charles V died on the 21st of August 1558. (7)

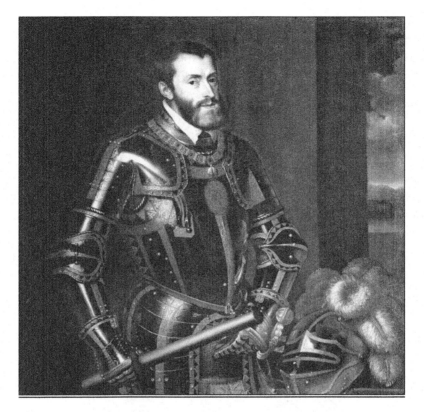

Figure 4.2 Charles V Holy Roman Emperor (Carlos I, King of Spain)

Henry VIII

The third European monarch of this period who has been described by the term, syphilitic, is Henry VIII Tudor, King of England (Fig.4.3). This is discussed in many biographies, and even serious handbooks of venereology place him at the top of lists of famous syphilitics (8). Henry VIII was an unusually colorful historical figure, and prompted innumerable biographies; he was the subject of many

73

historical tales, and the hero (main character) of films, both fictional and historical. The story of Henry's second wife, Ann Boleyn, became the theme for the libretto of one of the better-known operas of Gaetano Donizetti, *Anna Bolena.*

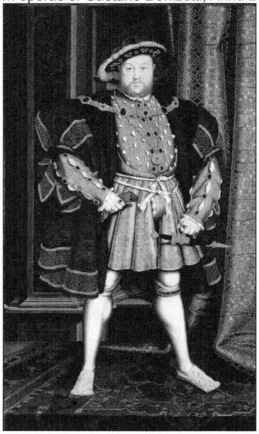

Figure 4.3 Portrait of Henry VIII by Hans Holbein the Younger

Henry VIII ruled almost 30 years, and opinions of the period of his rule were extremely varied. Many authors underline his merits, such as intelligence and personal charm, spontaneity, joviality and sense of humor – which led to the people calling him "Bluff King Hal." (9). He was undeniably a born leader and possessed organizational talents. He was intelligent, a reformer of his country, and organizer of England's army and navy. He was passionate and ruthless. He did not waver in regard to personal causes and breaks in conventions with Rome, nor in naming himself the head of the Church in England – which gave him a free hand in matters of divorce and the confiscation of Church estates. All this allowed him to decide about his own marriages and divorces, while the fortunes he acquired from the sale of Church goods permitted the bribery of opponents, the purchase of followers and the manipulation of court factions. Henry ruled by means of terror and artifice. He exterminated nearly 150,000 people in a country with a population of 2.7 million. He did not hesitate at beheading his inconvenient wives, the mothers of his children. He tortured his former friends and pronounced sentences of death on the basis of false testimony or of testimony obtained under the coercion of torture, which, as an otherwise intelligent man, he must have recognized. He knew no limits to the appeasement of his sexual wants, taking advantage of the services of his own and others' wives, of more or less willing ladies from the court, and even, as some whispered, those of prostitutes. He had six wives, of whom two died a natural death, two he had beheaded, and two survived him. One can say that Henry VIII didn't have luck with women, and conversely, that they lacked success with him. His first wife was the Spanish princess, Catherine of Aragon, the widow of his older brother, Arthur. Henry married her nine months after his coronation as King of England, and it would appear that the marriage was arranged, to a large extent, for political reasons. The new ruler depended on the strengthening of his position in regard to France, and even with England, through marriage with an influential family among the European dynasties. On the other hand this allowed his wife's father,

Ferdinand II, to have influence over England through his daughter. Queen Catherine's first pregnancy ended in a miscarriage. A year later, a son was born, but he lived less than two months. In sum, Henry and Catherine had six children, of whom only one lived through infancy. This was the Princess Mary, later, herself to be Queen of England, who, as "Bloody Mary," became famous for her revengeful cruelty in regard to the apostate opponents of the Catholic faith in that country. The question arises as to why the young marriage (the King was six years younger than his wife) did not result in more numerous living progeny, despite the fact that Catherine became pregnant at least seven times. There are many medical causes of miscarriage, abortive pregnancies, stillbirths, or deaths during infancy. One of these could have been syphilis, which, in those times had a distinctly more virulent course, as we are speaking of the early years of the sixteenth century – the beginnings of the epidemic of this disease in Europe. But syphilis in the English Queen? It is of little likelihood that the Spanish princess, an unusually religious person and the daughter of devout Catholic monarchs, brought it to England with her from Spain. Could her first husband, Arthur (Henry's brother), have infected her? This cannot be excluded, but is of low probability, as Arthur, at the time of his marriage, was only 15, and if one is to believe the accounts, he died as the result of tuberculosis. There is no certainty that Catherine suffered from syphilis, just as beyond the six unsuccessful pregnancies, there is no evidence to suggest lues. None of her biographers mention any skin changes, which, in the early stage of the disease would have had to be noticeable to those surrounding her. There are also no medical reports on the subject, nor any prescriptions in the royal pharmacy that would indicate that the Queen was treated for syphilis. Could Henry have been the source of an infection?

Many authors maintain Henry VIII had syphilis, supposedly affirmed by some signs of the disease that appeared in him in later years. Unfortunately, they provide neither the time frame nor any circumstances of the infections, which, in this instance are germane. We know that Henry was fortunate in his good health up to 1513, when, at the age of 22 he became ill with chickenpox or German measles. Inasmuch as the signs of these infections could suggest syphilis, proponents of the syphilis theory of Henry's problems assert that he could have been infected at this time, either in the course of a military campaign in France, or during innumerable carousings in England. Nonetheless, there is a lack of either direct or indirect evidence that would corroborate this thesis. There is no evidence on the subject of possible treatment, nor of the administration of mercury – unless we accept that the disease went unrecognized. It is worth noting that, at the same time, he suffered a first episode of malarial fever, which recurred even seven years later (10). As we know, malaria, and more precisely, the bouts of high fever that accompany that disease, were used with considerable success at the beginning of the twentieth century in the therapy of late syphilis, particularly in the treatment of its advanced stage (general paresis). One cannot exclude that a coexistence of these diseases could have erased the clinical picture of one of them. In 1527-1528, an ulcer appeared on Henry's leg, which the proponents of the syphilis theory describe as the rupture of a syphilitic gumma – a sign of third-stage syphilis. Opponents, however, remind us that in the same year the king hurt his ankle during a game of tennis, and as a result, had problems with walking. Another report about the King's sojourn in Canterbury says that "Henry had to stay in bed as the result of a painful leg, which was translated as the appearance of an ulcer, based on a varicosity that was said to have been caused by wearing rather tight breeches, or the result of a knightly joust." (11) Despite disagreements about the cause of the illness, the fact remains that non-healing ulcers on his legs became a serious health problem for the King, and accompanied him to his death, despite a variety of attempts at treatment.

While still in the course of his marriage to Catherine of Aragon, Henry flirted with numerous court ladies, the fruits of which were the births of two sons out of wedlock: Henry Fitz Roy, born in 1519, whose mother was Elizabeth Blount, and Henry, born in 1520, whose mother was Mary Boleyn, the sister of his future wife, Ann. It was Ann, in fact, who became the next object of the King's sighs. She was, however, more worldly and ingenious than her sister, as she "promised" to bear him a son, but only after marriage and her crowning as Queen of England. It is obvious that, in the way of Anne's attaining this goal would stand the existing queen, Catherine, who despite numerous problems with her pregnancies, lived and was well. The idea of *"matrimonium non consummatum"* (an unconsummated marriage) did not enter the picture because Princess Mary lived, and was a living contradiction to the concept. It was decided, instead, to annul the marriage with Catherine, based on the idea that its consummation was invalid from the very beginning. Catherine had earlier been the wife of Henry's brother, and this would render impossible the consummation of a legal marriage. There remained a certain problem: the Pope would have to be persuaded of that. It was supposed that persuading His Holiness of such a solution would be no problem; unfortunately, this was the time when the Spanish army had occupied Rome, and Pope Clement VII was practically a prisoner of the Spanish king, Charles V. We must remember that Catherine of Aragon was Charles' aunt, and he had not the least intention of supporting the "de-throning" of his own cousin. The Pope took advantage of this delay, and sent his emissary to England for an "examination of the matter." After numerous, months-long legal skirmishes, Henry lost patience, and Thomas Cranmer, the Archbishop of Canterbury appointed by Henry, announced that the marriage of Henry and Catherine was invalid, and confirmed the validity of the "secret marriage" undertaken earlier with Ann Boleyn. Catherine's daughter, Princess Mary, was acknowledged as his child of an illegitimate bed, his then-wife, Catherine, as Duchess-dowager of Wales. Ann Boleyn became the official Queen of England, while her daughter, Elizabeth (Ann did not keep her promise to bear Henry a son!) was nominated heiress to the throne. In response, the Pope excommunicated Henry, the early consequence of which was the overthrow of the Church in England, and immediately thereafter, Parliament voted-in several bills, which officially sealed the breach with Rome. From this time, more or less, dates the beginning of the Anglican Church, at the head of which stood Henry VIII.

On January 7, 1536, Catherine of Aragon died of cancer, and three hours later, Ann Boleyn prematurely gave birth to a long-foretold, yet still-born son.

This was too much for Henry, who had already had enough of his current wife, and had been flirting quite seriously with another woman. It appears that the loss of his long-awaited heir to the throne and continuer of the Tudor dynasty, who arrived stillborn, sealed the fate of Ann Boleyn. As we know, Henry had no scruples when it came to satisfying his own caprices, often clad in the robes of dynastic needs of the monarchy. He decided that the king must have a different wife, who would ensure a male heir. The candidate was already there. He only had to get rid of his existing wife. Ann Boleyn was accused of using spells with the aim of seducing the King and inducing him to marriage, as well as of adultery with five men, including her own brother. In contrast to Catherine of Aragon, whom, thanks to her relationship to Charles V, he let die in her own bed, Ann could not count on that. In May, 1536, the court under the leadership of her own uncle, Thomas Howard, the Duke of Norfolk, condemned Ann and her brother to death by burning at the stake – or by beheading, depending on the King's will. There remained four men, so-called lovers of Ann, who were to be hanged and quartered. One has to admit that Henry demonstrated "uncommon mercy" and permitted his wife to be beheaded, sparing her breathing-in the smell of her own flesh burning. It is interesting to speculate whether, if Ann had borne a healthy male heir, she would have saved her own head. There is yet another question: why, from the three pregnancies she had with Henry, only one was born alive, the later Queen of England, Elizabeth I.

Adherents to the syphilitic theory regarding Henry VIII explain that the King could have infected Ann with syphilis, and the miscarriage and premature birth of the dead boy could have been the consequence of an intrauterine luetic infection. Moreover, they suspect signs of congenital syphilis in Elizabeth I, interpreting that the leg ulcerations as well as her own hair loss (she wore a wig) could be signs of the disease. We know also that Elizabeth I never married, which is interpreted as a sign that she had a fear of infecting a future husband, or eventually bearing syphilitic children. Shortly after the execution of his second wife, Henry undertook a "quiet marriage" with Jane Seymour, who was already pregnant. This was his third attempt at ensuring the succession to the throne of the Tudor dynasty. A new Act of Succession from 1536 announced that the children of this union would be heirs to the throne and acknowledged Henry's living daughters, Mary and Elizabeth, as illegitimate progeny.

On October 12th, 1537, Jane Seymour gave birth to the longed-for son, but died 12 hours later, most probably from sepsis after a long, debilitating childbirth. The child, named Edward, was tiny and weak, but alive. The King and all of England celebrated the birth of the heir to the throne. Rigorous rules guarded the health of the royal child. Henry feared poisoning. Caring for Edward were specially chosen noblewomen, while the door to his room was guarded 24 hours a day by specially chosen guards. Edward was a sickly child, and often had declining health. Henry was already thinking of his next male heir with the aim of doubling his chances in the event of some kind of tragedy. Loneliness began to torment him; he was getting bored. He had neither a wife nor a mistress, and was getting fat; his legs hurt, and he felt unwell. His trusted counselor, Thomas Cromwell, advised yet another marriage, and suggested as a candidate, Anne of Cleves, the sister of the ruler of the Duchy of Cleves, which was located on the Rhine.

The Duke of Cleves was a Protestant, who could be an ally of England in the event of her conflict with Catholic countries. After seeing the portrait of his future wife, painted by Holbein the Younger, Henry confirmed that the chosen one was pleasing to him, while the flattering opinions of people who knew her, supported his persuasion that he had made a good decision. After the arrival of Anne in England and her presentation to Henry as his future wife, it turned out that the reality was far removed from the image that had so delighted him. Henry acknowledged that the chosen one was unusually unattractive, stating "I like her not," yet the wedding had to take place in accord with the agreement. His future ally, the Duke of Cleves, had, in the meantime, embarked on a conflict with the Emperor, which was also not to Henry's liking. Henry planned to divorce Anne, while the new Queen had nothing to say about it. She received the title of "Royal Sister," two splendid official palaces with beautiful parks, and a pension of 4,000 pounds annually.

Anne appeared satisfied with this, as her position and comfort were doubtless better than she could have expected in her fatherland. It was worse for Cromwell. He took the blame for the entire mix-up connected with the unfortunate marriage. He was fabulously wealthy, and had numerous enemies. He had made a fortune, including a huge estate, mainly at the time of the dissolution of monasteries and confiscation of Church lands. He was accused of treason, heresy, bribery, forcing of bribes, and abuse of finances. Additionally he was reproached for objecting to the King's rule, as well as illegal acquisition of the King's prerogatives. Half of these accusations were enough to receive a death sentence. Cromwell was beheaded, similarly to Ann Boleyn, whom he hated, plotted against, and to whose downfall he had contributed significantly.

On the very day on which Cromwell lost his head, Henry married the young Catherine Howard. This was already his fifth marriage. The bridegroom was almost fifty years in age, weighed 300 lbs. (about 140 kg) stank of the pus coming from the ulcers on his legs, had difficulty walking, and was carried about in a litter. The bride was less than twenty (the exact date of her birth is not known), was an attractive woman, supposedly pregnant by the King, something that proved untrue. Thomas Cranmer, Henry's right hand man at the time, was opposed to the wealthy and Catholic Howard family, which did not bode well for the new Queen. He informed the King that he had evidence of the young Queen's infidelity, to which Catherine admitted at trial. She was beheaded similarly to Ann Boleyn, who was her cousin. A year later came Henry's next wedding to wife number six, Katherine Parr. She was a wealthy widow, younger than her new husband by only twenty years. The new Queen took care of her husband more like a mother than a wife, nursing him in his illness, and assisting him in ruling the country. She mothered not only Henry, but also his two living daughters, and his son, the successor to the throne. At a certain point, as a result of interfering with matters of religion, she saw the executioner's axe over her head, but, fortunately for her, the incident was forgotten. She died in her own bed, having outlived the King by a little over a year.

Presented greatly abridged, this account of the "family" life of Henry VIII doesn't permit one unequivocally to confirm that his marital life and dynastic plans were affected by syphilis – which Henry has been suspected of having since the second half of the nineteenth century. There is much evidence to speak against this theory. First of all, it should be stressed that no prescriptions have been found in the royal pharmacy to indicate that Henry was ever treated with mercury, the remedy commonly used in the treatment of lues in those times. Also, treatment with the metal lasted many weeks, and caused the appearance of side effects that would have been readily noticeable by everyone around him, especially by all the meddling ambassadors tracking the King's every step. Another medication given to those ill with syphilis in Henry's time was guaiac, but here, again, we have no trace of its having been used for the King. In one of the proceedings against the former assistant to Henry VIII, Cardinal Lord Wolsey, he is accused, among other things, of wishing to infect the King with syphilis, "blowing a dangerous and infectious breath at him." It is of little likelihood that such a dangerous subject would have been broached if Henry had indeed had lues and had tried to hide the fact. There is also a lack of description of signs that would have spoken convincingly of congenital syphilis among his children or signs of syphilis among his many wives or mistresses. Multiple miscarriages or repeated stillbirths may, but do not have to suggest syphilis in their mothers. It must be remembered that in those times situations of this type were nothing extraordinary and were caused by a tragic state of hygiene, a low level of medical knowledge and recurring epidemics of infectious diseases that did not spare pregnant women.

The favorite argument of adherents to the theory of lues in Henry are accounts of features of King's character or his behavior in his later years; these are supposed to be evidence of late syphilis, and more specifically, general paresis, such as frequent changes in mood, cruelty, and indifference toward those close to him and to friends. I must remind the reader that cruelty, particularly among rulers of that period, was quite common. Other rulers besides "Henry" punished excessively, tortured, and murdered. The harsh rule was done to frighten potential criminals, while explaining this as the "right of the State" or "caring for the good of the monarchy."

The final years of Henry VIII, descriptions of his appearance, of diseases tormenting him and of his behavior attest to the fact that he suffered from various illnesses, but probably not syphilis. Excess weight, corpulence, a fat neck (so-called *buffalo hump*), swollen face (moon face) and bags of fat beneath the eyes could indicate Cushing's syndrome or disease, which is associated with an overproduction of steroid hormones. These diseases are most commonly caused by an adrenal tumor, or, as is the case with Cushing's disease, a tumor of the pituitary gland causing excess production of hormones of the adrenal cortex. In both instances, in addition to noticeable physical changes, there are psychological changes such as irritability, depression, panic attacks, excessive suspiciousness, emotional indifference, even in regard to close ones, as well as uncontrolled aggressiveness. As the result of a heightened production of 17-hydroxycorticoids, one notes disturbances of electrolyte balance, an increase in blood sugar, osteoporosis, hypertension, and petechiae (a flat rush on the skin). (12) Yet another theory is that Henry VIII could have had McLeod's syndrome, in which red blood cells bearing the Kell antigen could produce serologic conflicts and pregnancy problems in the bearer's partners. Establishing a diagnosis and the causes of Henry VIIIth's ailments after 500 years is practically impossible, while to the question of whether the cause of the King's health problems and his difficulties with producing progeny was syphilis there cannot be just one answer.

Ivan the Terrible (the Formidable)

In exactly the same year in which the life of Henry VIII ended, but in the opposite corner of Europe, a 17-year old youth was crowned Tsar of Russia, and assumed the name

Ivan IV (Fig.4.4). After many years as ruler, he received the additional name of "the Terrible," as translated from the Russian, *groznyj*, but changing its meaning, somewhat. In English, the word *terrible* signifies evil, cruel, or sinister, while in Russian, its true meaning is closer to "inspiring fear" or awesome. Perhaps the most exact equivalent would be "Ivan the Fearsome," or "Ivan the Formidable."

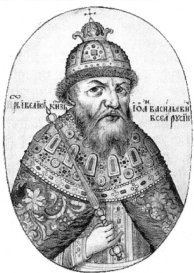

Figure 4.4 Ivan the Terrible

In "Ivan the Formidable" we have a good example of a European ruler suffering from syphilis, but in whom it is easier to prove the presence of this disease than in the case of Henry VIII.

Ivan was born on August 25th, 1530. When he was three years old, his father died, and tiny Ivan received the title of "Great Prince of Moscow." At first, the role of regent was undertaken by his mother, but unfortunately she died or – as some would prefer, was poisoned – five years later. Ivan was brought up at court among unending intrigues and fights between groups of boyars (nobles) competing for power.

When he was thirteen, his best friend was imprisoned, and another was executed. Biographers underscore that, even in his childhood, Ivan had witnessed brutal events, political murders, beatings and outrages. In 1547, Ivan was crowned Tsar of all Russia. Immediately thereafter, there began "auditions" for a wife for the Tsar, for which many hundreds of Russian ladies supposedly applied. The young Tsar decided to break with the then-current tradition of marriage to a daughter of one of the European ruling houses, and instead, to marry a Russian.

A beautiful young girl with great green eyes, Anastasia Romanovna Zakharyina - Yurieva, the daughter of a Russian boyar, became Ivan's wife. The marriage, from its very beginning was considered a success. From the union, six children were born, three daughters and three sons. Of the three boys, only the youngest, Fiodor, survived to inherit the crown from his father. His older brothers, Dimitri and Ivan died tragically. After thirteen years of marriage (his wife reportedly had a calming effect on her husband's violent character), Anastasia got apoplexy, supposedly as a result of quarrels with the boyars, and died. Another version says that she was poisoned, which was said to have been proved by the discovery of arsenic in her remains. Ivan blamed the successful attempt on the Tsarina's life on Princess Eufrozena Chovanska, his uncle's widow.

From the moment of Anastasia's death, there began a period of unprecedented cruelty and bloody fights with the boyars, who were blamed by the Tsar for the death of his wife and disloyalty toward the ruler. It is supposedly during this period that Ivan was infected with syphilis after having sexual relations with a variety of women. In addition to Anastasia, Ivan the Fearsome had seven wives. The Tsar's second wife, was Maria, a woman of great charm, but Ivan quickly grew bored of her. The next chosen was Martha Sobakina, the daughter of a merchant, who died two weeks after the wedding under suspicious circumstances. The fourth wife was Anna Koltovskaya, who, after a three-year bestowal of sexual favors, was dispatched by her husband to a convent. After her were also Anna and Vasilisa. This last one had bad luck, as she was caught with a lover under unambiguous circumstances. The lover was impaled right under her windows, and she was forced to watch the execution. Comparing Ivan's reaction to the infidelity with that of his friend from the Thames, one has to admit that the Tsar behaved like a gentleman, as the only punishment his unfaithful wife met was that of being dispatched o a convent. On this, probably, ended the Tsar's confidence in regard to wives, as the next bride, Maria Dolgoruka was drowned in a lake the day after the wedding. When, on the wedding night, the Tsar came to the conclusion that his new bride was not a virgin, the following morning he put her into a carriage and supposedly, personally goaded the horses with a whip. The speeding vehicle fell into a lake and sank, together with its contents. Ivan again tried to find a wife, this time at foreign courts. He proposed to the sister of the Polish King Sigmund August and to a daughter of Henry VIII, but was refused. Finally, he married another Russian, Maria Nagoya, who gave him a son, Dimitri.

It is difficult to say what particular element of the Tsar's life played the deciding role in pathologizing his later behavior. Was it the result of a difficult childhood and the outrages to which he was a witness and also a victim, or did the loss of his beloved wife, infection with syphilis, or maybe everything taken together, that changed the Tsar into a beast? Ivan IV, in the course of the passage of years, became more and more cruel. His behavior became less and less stable; he had frequent periods of bad moods and baseless attacks of anger. More and more frequently the Tsar's sadistic tendencies became noticeable. It is written of him that that he experienced physical pleasure observing torture and the pain of suffering people. He frequently made performances out of this. At the age of 45, he was a physical wreck, caused by drunkenness and sexual pathology. It was said that he experienced sexual pleasure observing sexual acts carried out by his ruffians. He was said to permit his mercenary soldiers to abduct the wives of his boyars, whom he raped, and then encouraged others to gang rapes of these women. These scenes were conducted, not infrequently, in the sight of their unlucky husbands, which additionally excited the Tsar. In one period of his rule, the Tsar introduced the *Oprichnina*, a group of alternative military police, which to a large extent was responsible for tortures and massacres of the people, and for robbery and rapes. In 1570, on the basis of false accusations, almost the whole population of Novograd (60,000 inhabitants) were tortured and murdered. In these crimes, mostly the *oprichnik*s took part, but the Tsar later suspected them of treason, and condemned them to a cruel death. The height of the madness was the murder of his son and heir to the throne, who stood in defense of a pregnant woman, who had been criticized by the Tsar of wearing clothes that he didn't like. In a fit of rage, Ivan hit his son in the head with his cane, on which was a metal pummel, and thus caused his death. This event, which even he could not get over, only worsened Ivan's mental state, to which were then added the side effects of mercury treatment, which the Tsar had started to take for the treatment of syphilis. This fact is supported by the results of an exhumation that took place in 1960, which showed the presence of this metal in his remains.

Polish Royalty

To the West of Russia is found a country, then a very powerful one, ruled by Wladyslaw-Waza, King of Poland. Near the end of 1645, there arrived in Warsaw, Poland's capital, the betrothed *per procura* of King Wladyslaw, the French princess, Louise Marie Gonzaga. Among the court ladies accompanying the Queen, were many young and beautiful women, all counting on an early marriage with one or another of the rich Polish magnates. Also among them was a little four-year-old girl, Marie Kazimiera, daughter of the Marquis d'Arquiem and Frances de la Chetre (Fig.4.5). Even from her first days in Poland, this little girl became an object of interest, as, at the Warsaw court, there arose gossip to the effect that she could be the illegitimate child of Louise Marie and some French aristocrat. The matter was quickly resolved, because, as historians later confirmed, Marie Kazimiera was, indeed, the "child" of Louise Marie – but a *god*child. It is not known how long little Marysienka (the diminutive by which Marie Kazimiera became known), stayed in Poland. Most likely, she returned to France in 1648 after the death of King Wladyslaw, where she went to the convent school in Nevers for about four years. No later than 1653, she was again seen among the court ladies of Queen Louise Marie, who, in the meantime, managed to get married afresh to the heir of Wladyslaw IV, the next polish king, Jan Kazimierz.

Even as a little girl, Marysienka conquered the hearts of those around her by her cheerful manner and comeliness, while at age twelve she passed as an unusually beautiful girl. According to the opinions of her contemporaries, attention was gained by her regular facial features, a skin of beautiful complexion, luxurious black hair woven into locks, and above all, beautiful eyes, full of fire, yet simultaneously dreamy. (13) The first meeting of the later sweethearts took place in Warsaw during the assembly of the Sejm (Diet) in 1655. At that time, on the occasion of the opening of parliamentary deliberations, numerous celebrations, balls, and festivities were taking place. During one of these balls at the court, the cavalry standard-bearer (and future King John III), Jan Sobieski,(Fig.4.6) met Marysienka for the first time, and, as he wrote later, "fell in love from the first glance." The fact that Sobieski was twelve years older than his chosen one was no impediment to amorous enchantment. Nonetheless, this meeting did not lead to a proposal, despite the mutual attraction that occurred at that time between the future spouses.

Marysienka, as one of the court ladies of Queen Louise Marie, was under the latter's influence, and completely obedient. The Queen, for political purposes, wanted to attract the powerful Polish magnate, Jan Zamoyski, who had great influence among the landed gentry, and a huge estate. Zamoyski, in whose veins flowed the blood of the Mazovian Piast dynasty, was the owner of over 140 villages and nine towns. By offering Marysienka to him, the Queen was counting on binding him and his support to herself and, through him, on influencing the country's gentry in order further to pursue her own policies. At the same time, she was thinking of Marysienka's future, before whom were opening perspectives of an extremely wealthy life, and maybe even a royal crown, as it could not be excluded that Zamoyski could be elected king at some future time. The idea, however, proved to be a terrible one, and this, equally for the court as for young Marie Kazimiera.

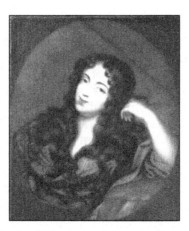

Figure 4.5 Portrait of Marysienka as a Penitent Magdalena

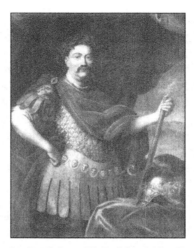

*Figure 4.6 Portrait of Jan III Sobieski in Roman costume
(painted by Daniel Schultz)*

The huge estate and political influence did not compensate for the vices of the magnate, who was known to be an erotomaniac and an alcoholic. Marriage to a young and beautiful woman did not change his habits. Despite the marriage, he still maintained a harem composed of poverty-stricken gentle ladies and illiterate peasant women. As if this were not enough, Marysienka's husband suffered from syphilis (*franca*), with which he probably became infected during some travels to Italy or to France. (14) During the wedding night, the groom got so drunk that he slept next to the bed of his just-wedded wife. This had no great significance for consummation of the marriage, as Zamoyski suffered at this time from *une grand chaud pisse* (gonorrhea), which rendered impossible, or at least greatly hindered, sexual relations. It cannot be excluded that Zamoyski got drunk deliberately in order to shield his young wife from infection. Despite the visible vices of Marysienka's husband, at least during the first part of her marriage, she appeared to be happy. The drunkenness and dissolute way of life of her fifteen-years-older husband did not offend her. It appears that she came to love him, and bore him three daughters. The girls died quickly, with little doubt due to congenital syphilis, although one cannot exclude other causes. The next pregnancy ended in a miscarriage, this time of a boy, who was given the name Jan. Marysienka wrote about this to Sobieski, also a "Jan," with whom she maintained a copious correspondence, devoid, at least at first, of amorous elements. Being a neglected wife – which was not a rarity, particularly in magnates' homes – she unburdened herself of her problems through correspondence to her admirer. The numerous carousings of Sobieski in the company of other women did not interfere with the "love by correspondence," due to the fact that the object of his sighs, although rarely, spent her nights with a husband who reeked of vodka and wine. Sobieski was under pressure from his mother and Queen Louise Marie, who wanted to involve him with a French princess, a relative of the Great de Conde. Nothing came of this, however. Sobieski appeared to have a prescient awareness that Marysienka would some day become his wedded wife, and put off marriage. Both immersed themselves in reading the popular French romances. In the middle of 1661, Sobieski learned that the object of his sighs, with the approval of the Queen, intended to leave for France for a longer while. He arranged to meet with Marysienka in the Carmelite Church in Warsaw, where, secretly before the altar, but without a priest, they pledged never-ending love to each other, which they confirmed by exchanging rings. Sobieski additionally promised not to accept any other woman as his wife. Did they progress to physical contact? This we do not know; we do know, however, that the temperature and frequency of their correspondence, in which the future 'marrieds' began to use code, did increase. The same year, Sobieski's mother died; she had been decidedly against the marriage, and would never have permitted her son's marriage to now-Madame Zamoyska. Finally, Marysienka left for France, but alone.

Zamoyski did not want to leave his companions of the wineglass, and also had to take care of his estate, as he had learned that his wife, with the active help of the Queen, wished to take over the estate of her alcoholic husband. During her stay in France, Marysienka became ill, and began to take the healing waters of Pau for her stomach. Misfortunes multiplied. During her illness, her little daughter died, while a year later, her faithful servant, whom her physicians tried to cure with oral mercury preparations did, also (might this not have been for syphilis?). During her stay at Versailles, despite attempts to appear at court, she was unable to approach Louis XIV, although he managed to seduce one of the ladies accompanying her. This was a clear offense to the ambitious Marysienka. The Sun King, though a known erotomaniac, paid no attention to the beautiful Madam Zamoyska, yet did bed her lady companion!

After returning to Poland, Maria Kazimiera returned to her husband, but began to think of divorce more frequently. Fulfilling her alcoholic husband's caprices clearly began to weigh on her. Simultaneously, pressure grew on Sobieski to accept the position of Marshall and Royal Hetman offered him by the King, something that Queen Louise Marie really wanted. Meanwhile, measures toward a divorce proved unnecessary. A dissipated lifestyle, alcoholism and syphilis did their own thing. Zamoyski died, leaving his enormous estate to his wife.

Initial information about the wedding of Marysienka and Jan Sobieski comes from the report of a Prussian agent directed to the Brandenburg Elector of Frederick Wilhelm. (15) According to this report, the future marrieds were caught during a rendezvous one night by the Queen, who is said to have declared to Sobieski that if he didn't immediately marry Madame Zamoyska, he would be executed. As one can surmise, a priest, who had been waiting just outside the door, had no difficulty in eliciting a *yes* from both sides. As this version sounds almost as though contrived for a romance novel, I will propose another, which says that Sobieski willingly married the woman he had loved for a long time, although maintaining secrecy about the marriage was necessary, based on the need to observe the obligatory mourning period. News of the marriage reached the public, however, and after the passage of three months from the death of Zamoyski, Marysienka and Sobieski wedded again, this time officially, with the joining of the newlyweds celebrated by the papal Nuncio, Antonio Pignatelli, who later became Pope Innocent XII. The wedding celebrations lasted three days, while the new bride was transported to her husband's house by the royal couple, who had also taken part in the wedding ceremonies.

Shortly after the wedding, "some strange allergies, itching over the revolting body," appeared in Sobieski. (16) We do not know whether the cause of this type of ailment was the result of emotions such as a bridegroom may experience on his honeymoon, or were signs of a discrete disease, maybe syphilis? Correspondence between the spouses shortly after the wedding testify to the full fervor of emotions of Jan Sobieski for his wife, and a certain sophistication of their sexual relations already allowed from Renaissance times, but of which one did not speak aloud, based on custom. Many historians stress that the marriage of the Sobieskis was a so-called "marriage of love," which, at that time, was not common among the aristocracy.

After some time, Marysienka became pregnant, and decided to go to Paris to give birth there. She wanted her husband to go with her but his responsibilities as commander-in-chief did not allow Sobieski to leave Poland. They both supposed that their first child would be a girl, remembering Marysienka's first pregnancy by Jan Zamoyski, but this time a surprise awaited them. A boy was born, fat and healthy. He received the name, James, and his godfather was Louis XIV of France, the Sun King. Good fortune did not abandon Sobieski. Not only did he have a son with his long-beloved woman, but he met many favors at court in Warsaw. These were the result of a series of victories gained in the war with the Tatars.

Sobieski became popular among the nobles, and it was hinted that he could be elected King, given gossip about a possible abdication of King Jan Kazimierz. This did not concern him much, as he was lonely for his wife, who was in Paris and solicitously taking care of little James, mindful of the deaths of her children by her first husband.

In May of 1668, while Marysienka was still in Paris, Sobieski developed a fever, pustules appeared on his skin, and he also complained of severe headaches. (17) It is difficult to determine whether these were the signs of secondary syphilis, or of another infectious disease accompanied by a transient rash. Finally, in mid-September, Marysienka returned to Poland together with her son, only to become ill with smallpox six months later. Somehow, she recovered from this without injury, but this raises the question of whether it was, indeed, smallpox, as the latter usually leaves persistent scars after remission. She again became pregnant, but this time, gave birth to stillborn twins. Despite these family tragedies, she took an active part in the political life, and strived toward obtaining the Polish throne for the candidate from France, Prince de Conde. However, Maria Kazimiera's efforts, supported by millions of French *livres* that went for presents for the Electors, were all for naught. The Polish gentry chose Michal Korybut Wisniowiecki, the candidate of the opposition party, for their king.

A threatening civil war in Poland and another pregnancy led Marysienka to another trip to France. On the road between Brussels and Paris, birth pangs began, and she gave birth to a baby daughter, who also soon died. The abandoned and grieving Sobieski wrote that he did not understand why his wife, instead of delighting in the company of her husband, preferred to gaze at his portrait. She, however, was "treating herself at the waters in

Bourbon," and aimed to buy a huge and frightfully expensive property on the Loire. In the end, Sobieski was able to convince his wife to return, and even considered the possibility of leaving for Gdansk to meet her; but, as he wrote, "an ulcer formed in his throat" (in secondary syphilis, there frequently develop changes in the oral cavity and throat), which after a time resolved. Maria Kazimiera, to her husband's joy, finally returned to Poland, and again gave birth to a baby daughter, who, similarly to the previous one, soon died.

Aware of the antipathy of the Polish gentry, who considered her a person scheming on behalf of France, Maria Kazimiera planned to return to her own country, and to settle there for good. Nevertheless, she changed her plans, as the death of King Michal Korybut Wisniowiecki and the victories against the Turks near Chocim, produced a new situation for Sobieski. The road had opened for him to become the King of Poland. Manipulating the votes of the Electors, and taking advantage of his popularity as a victorious leader, and also thanks to the endeavors of his clever wife and French *livres,* Sobieski was proclaimed King on May 21, 1674.

Though the election of Sobieski as King was met with almost universal applause, the coronation of the former Marquise d'Arquien, then Madame Zamoyska, and now Madame Sobieska met with great opposition. In the end, that opposition was broken, and both spouses were officially crowned in Krakow as King and Queen of Poland. The ceremony took place at Wawel Castle, the ancient seat of Polish kings. At the time of her coronation, Marysienka was in her 8th month of pregnancy.

Louis XIV, seeing such great social advancement of his former subject, and wanting to ensure French influence at the Polish court, announced that he intended to adopt Marysienka as his daughter. This was a measure purely for political purposes, as the King was older than his "daughter" by barely three years. This gesture was unusually flattering to the former Miss d'Arquien, who, in the end, accepted the honor of being a relative of French kings. Louis XIV was well aware of the huge influence Marysienka had over her husband, and intended, in this way, to influence politics in Poland. To some extent, his situation was made easier, as Sobieski, being a natural military leader, felt far better on the battlefield then among court intrigues. This division of roles between Marysienka and her husband proved very profitable for Poland, which, in those times, was a European empire. King Sobieski became remembered in Europe mainly for his successful Viennese expedition, also known as rescue of Vienna, in 1683. The Polish army, under his leadership, defeated the huge Turkish army besieging Vienna. Many historians consider the Polish intervention on the outskirts of Vienna to have saved a large part of Christian Europe from Islamization.

In addition to the important victory at Vienna, King Jan Sobieski and his wife are remembered by history as a romantic couple in love with each other, and whose love could not be weakened by numerous family tragedies, among them a major venereal disease, i.e., syphilis. To this day, there is no way to determine from whence the latter came, or who infected whom. According to some historians, the source of the infection was Marysienka's first husband, the erotomaniac and alcoholic, Jan Zamoyski. Others maintain that it was Marysienka who brought syphilis from France. Still others judge it to have been Sobieski, who, in his youthful years supposedly infected himself with syphilis during a stay in France, and whence he also supposedly gained a son out of wedlock with a poorly known woman. It appears that the most likely is the first version, to which would attest the deaths of Marysienka's first three daughters, which she bore during her marriage to Zamoyski. It is most likely that she was then in an early stage of syphilis, which caused intrauterine infection of her offspring. Nonetheless, there is not a 100% certainty of this, as in those days infant mortality, even in royal families, was very high. Marysienka underwent childbirth seventeen times, from which only four children lived to maturity. Her oldest son, James, who was born of the marriage with Sobieski, was not a success. He was physically weak, thin, and deformed, while as to his character and abilities, his parents had many reservations.

Sobieski, particularly in the later period of his life, was frequently ill. Accounts of some of his earlier illnesses could, but do not necessarily correspond to signs of syphilis. During one of his military expeditions in Moldavia in 1684, the King became ill, most probably with malaria. He had attacks of fever every third day that, as I already alluded to, could have had a salutary effect on syphilis. In the 1690s, Sobieski was already very fat, frequently fell asleep immediately after dinner, and had gout. Gout, called the "disease of the rich," also already referred to by myself in regard to the aches of other kings, was the nightmare of those times. It was often caused by drinking alcohol and overeating by the wealthy, particularly of rich meat that raised levels of uric acid in the blood. Frequent attacks of this very painful disease in Sobieski, and also attacks of kidney stones, and – high fevers produced by malaria – resulted in the king's being unbearable in his old age to those around him, and even to his beloved wife, who, it is worth mentioning, was a solicitous and forbearing protectress of her husband. The royal patient was treated consistently with medical knowledge of the time, i.e. by bleeding, rubbing with various medicinal mixtures, and various inventive medicines (we don't know what kind). For several months before Sobieski's death, swelling of the body (hydropsy) was described). Mercury treatments were employed, producing massive salivation, yet after which he was said to have felt better. Unfortunately, the swellings returned, and by correspondence Marysienka turned to the best physicians in Europe for help for her husband. It was decided that he should go to the medical spa in Wiesbaden, but he was already in such a bad state that there was concern that he would not survive the travel. Sobieski died suddenly after an abundant dinner, while the cause of death, according to his physicians, was said to have been a heart attack – although he reportedly had time to make his confession and receive communion! We do not know much about Marysienka's health after the death of her husband. Earlier she had been treated at various spas, often visiting Cieplice in Lower Silesia, where she took mud baths. Reportedly, she lost her teeth quite early, supposedly as the result of mercury treatments, but this is not certain. At that time, the state of dentition, even of monarchs, was terrible. Marysienka Sobieska outlived her husband by twenty years. She died in January 1716 in Blois, France.

The Sobieski marriage registered well in the memories of their fellow countrymen. He was remembered as a good king and victorious leader; she, as a good administrator of the kingdom, and a solicitous wife—and together, as a very good and loving pair. Varsovians remember that the Sobieskis built at least two churches in Warsaw and a beautiful palace in Wilanow, currently one of Warsaw's districts. Even in the seventeenth century, the district currently belonging to the composite City Center was named after Marysienka, while the King's heart was placed to rest in the Royal Chapel of the Capuchin church in Warsaw. The famous couple became the subject of many novels and film scenarios. Few know that their union was poisoned by a disease, which weighed on the family's fortunes in an essential manner.

Writing about the history of the Sobieski family, I cannot rest before recounting my personal memories associated with this surname. A number of years ago, I was nominated to the Board of the International Society for STD Research. There, I met one of the very well known American venereologists, who, during a joint dinner, boasted that he had Polish roots, and that his mother's maiden name was Sobieski. I told him that this was a very well-known name in

Poland, and that King Sobieski is deservedly very well thought of by Poles. He appeared to be very surprised by this, and probably did not know that his mother's maiden name had a royal origin. I joked, then, saying that, if it had not originated with King Sobieski, then Anton, a Professor of Dermatology from Vienna, who was sitting next to us, was a Muslim! Anton corroborated the former fact, and added that near Vienna, on Kahlenberg Hill, there is a chapel dedicated to King Sobieski, founded in thanksgiving for saving Vienna from the Turks. To end, I want to add that, even if my American friend did not know with what the name Sobieski was linked in Poland, I had arrived at the conclusion that his mother knew more on the subject, as attested to by the name she gave him. My American colleague's first name was King!

Louis XIV, XV, and XVI.

I have already alluded to the close ties that the Sobieski family had with the French court and with Louis XIV. That king ruled France longer than any other European leader ruled in those times. As a youth, he was considered an unusually attractive man, although he added to his charm by wearing high-heels and specially made wigs! One need not add that physical attractiveness and a royal title had the result that, from his youngest years, even before his marriage, he was considered "God's gift to women," and the most beautiful ladies at court dreamed of finding themselves in his bed. His marriage to Maria Theresa had no great effect on the customs prevailing at court, and Louis XIV "in his early youth suffered from syphilis, [and] that his physicians made many attempts to cure him." (18) Even the second part of this sentence allows one to assume that it is untrue, as the fact of Louis XIV being a syphilitic would not have been concealable, while there was no possibility of a cure in those times. It is more likely that he was ill with, and was treated for gonorrhea. (19,20) An otherwise putatively fervent Catholic, formally Defender of the Faith, and guardian of morals, he did not observe the sixth commandment, and was unfaithful, not only to his wedded wife, but equally to his official sweethearts, who numbered in the teens. From these unions, he gained at least seventeen children, the majority of whom he acknowledged as his own. One of Louis' first loves was the niece of Cardinal Mazarin, who fulfilled the function of regent when Louis was still a child. Next, he became interested in Henrietta of England, the wife of his brother, Phillipe of Orleans, to whom, as a result of the latter's bisexual tendencies, women were not attracted. Because gossip spread that the King was romantically involved with his brother's wife, Louis, in order to quell the vigilance of those surrounding him, decided officially to adore one of the ladies of her court, the somewhat lame and none too lovely Louise de La Valliers. So what happened? The not very attractive Louise became the multi-year mistress of the King, bearing him four children, of whom a pair died while still in childhood. It is for her that Louis supposedly built Versailles, the magnificent palace complex near Paris.

The next mistress of the King was the Marquise of Montespan, a wealthy woman with three children. Naturally, this did not please her husband, who started to protest loudly, which resulted in his imprisonment in the Bastille. The jealous husband was made fun of in Paris, with the question, "Why is the Marquis of Montespan in the Bastille? And the answer was "For daring to forbid his wife to sleep with the King." When, after a time the Marquis was released from prison and met Louis, the latter asked him why he was dressed in black; the Marquis is said to have replied that it was a symbol of mourning over the loss of his wife, which clearly indicates that the abandoned husband had not come to terms with his fate, and in this way was expressing his protest. In the end, he supposedly reconciled himself to the new situation when he received from the King an estate of considerable value, together with the title of Governor. The romance with the Marquise of Montespan lasted many years, and the fruit of *this* union was seven children. It happened that, besides his wedded wife, Louis XIV simultaneously had yet two more official mistresses. In the course of a military campaign to Normandy, all three ladies followed the commander-in-chief in separate carriages; of these, two were in the last months of pregnancy. Both of them wanted the King to assist in the birth of his heir. I don't know on what the third was counting! The last long-term mistress of the King was the Marquise de Maintenon, with whom he did not have any children, but whom he married monogamously after the death of Queen Maria Therese. For the full picture of Louis XIV, one has to add that this king did not occupy himself exclusively with sex. In France, he is considered one of the more significant monarchs, who made of his country a model for imitation by other European nations. The palace at Versailles, of which he was the builder, became, in those times, an oracle for style and etiquette, while the French language began to replace Latin in international relations. It was under his rule that France colonized today's Canada and a large portion of today's U.S.A. It is thanks to him that the newly discovered lands of central southeastern North America were named Louisiana.

As I already mentioned, the allegation that Louis XIV suffered from syphilis is more than likely untrue – which does not mean that this disease was not 'popular' among the French aristocracy. The well-known chronicler, Saint-Simon wrote the history of Prince Vendome, the illegitimate child of Henry IV of France and Gabriele d'Estrees, who, as an active homosexual became infected with syphilis. (20,21) Prince Vendome had strong leadership talents, and was the main leader of the armies of Louis XIV. Many times he distinguished himself with his bravery and numerous victories on the battlefield. Ill with syphilis, despite distinct advance of the disease, he put off treatment, and even persuasion by the King couldn't induce him, for a long time, to undertake therapy. "He finally took a vacation from the King, and put himself into the hands of the surgeons," in order to 'sweat out' his syphilis." He was said to have stayed three months in the hands of skilled therapists, unfortunately without much success. He returned to court with half a nose, lacking teeth, with a greatly changed face, and with the appearance of a blockhead. Apparently, the King was devastated, and ordered his courtiers not to show disgust at his appearance, so as not to increase his despair. (21) Prince Vendome was not the only case of syphilis described by Saint-Simon. The same chronicler wrote about many instances of syphilis among the courtiers, citing the case of the Marquis de Vaudemont, "whose feet and palms were shedding shapeless flesh and hanging inertly in confusion." (21)

Despite his excessive erotic life, Louis XIV managed to avoid syphilis, although he did not avoid infection, probably with gonorrhea, with which he was ill several times. He lived to 77, of which 72 were as King. He died in 1715 as a result of gangrene, treated with, among other methods, frequent blood-letting, which doubtless only accelerated the death of the patient.

The successor to Louis XIV was his great grandson, also Louis, but number XV. Similarly to his great grandfather, his rule began with a regency, which was conducted by Philip II Duke of Orleans in the name of the underage King. At age thirteen, Louis XV was deemed mature, and assumed the throne, while at age fifteen, he married the daughter of the Polish King, Marie Leszczynska, who was six years older than he. In its early years, the marriage was very agreeable, and Queen Marie bore ten children by Louis. However, with the passage of years, Louis XV also proved to be a womanizer, treating himself to a larger number of lovers than had his great grandfather. Besides cooking (he was an excellent cook) and hunting, chasing women became one of his greatest passions. The list of his intimates is very long, while two of them, the Marquise de Pompadour, earlier Madame Jeanne Antoinette Poisson, and Jeanne Becu, better known as Madame du Barry or Countess de Barry, had a real influence on the politics of France. The Marquise de Pompadour was a patroness of philosophers and artists, writers and painters, while Madame du Barry, the 25-year-old sweetheart of the now ageing King, interfered with, strictly speaking, everything. The King met the future Marquise at a masked ball at which Jeanne Antoinette wore a shepardess costume. Louis was enchanted, and couldn't part from her. After the ball came the first meetings, and so, the beautiful shepherdess became the King's mistress – and that, for many years. This happened despite the expectations of the courtiers, who did not foresee a great future for the union. The King having become dependent on her, the Marquise invited numerous scholars and artists to Versailles (of course, with the monarch's money). Theatrical productions, literary evenings and philosophical meetings were organized. One from the last group was Voltaire, whom she supported financially, although the famous philosopher managed to extract money not just from her. Another of his sponsors was the Russian Tsarina, Catherine II, and the King of Poland, Stanislaus Poniatowski.

Louis' great love for the Marquise did not deter him from entering into d'alliances with other women. The effect of his infidelity was infection with gonorrhea, which he transmitted to the totally unsuspecting Marquise. She endured it bravely, although this did not happen without excuses and apologies. She, nevertheless, came to understand that she could not count on the faithfulness of the King, and to learn to look the other way at his whims. There exists a not universally held opinion that, in proportion to his aging, Louis XV was becoming an ever greater erotomaniac, and began to have a fancy for ever-younger sweethearts. Some assert that there appeared tendencies toward pedophilia in him, as he supposedly met with girls from 9 to 19 years of age. Others, however, say that he became a cypridophobe (one having a morbid fear of prostitutes and venereal diseases), and believed that the younger the lover, the smaller the chance of infection with venereal disease. The Marquise, recognizing her waning attractiveness (she was ill with tuberculosis), and wanting to maintain her influence at court, tolerated the King's caprices, while some maintain that she even organized something in the form of a handy harem, in which stayed frequently replaced young girls, for "serving" the King." This was called Stag Park (*Parc aux Cerfs*), in which, under the guise of a *pension* for destitute girls, were kept young girls for training in the sexual arts. The *institution* is said to have existed for more than thirty-five years, long after the death of its foundress.

After the death of the Marquise, many women wanted to take her place, but the King no longer wanted a constant lover. When Louis was already over 60 years of age, the very young Miss Lange, better known as Madame du Barry, appeared in his life. She was a common prostitute who was discovered for the King by his valet, Monsieur Lebel. It is not known whether, on the basis of the skills of Madame du Barry, of deeper feelings of the King, or maybe simply of age, Louis slowed down the pace of his life. Solicitous Madame du Barry delivered to him from time to time, "for [his] amusement," young girls who had earlier been examined by a physician. As April turned into May in 1774, when the King was occupied in the du Barry home with a young dancer from the Paris opera, the valet awoke du Barry at night, to inform her that the King did not feel well, that he had a high fever, and that red patches had appeared on his face. The summoned Royal physician, La Martinier, ordered that the King be immediately taken to Versailles. When, on the following day, the King looked into a mirror, he saw a swollen face, seeded with pustular pimples. Consultation confirmed chicken pox, which did not auger well for a patient of his age. The King died on May 10, 1774, having lived 64 years, of which 59 were on the throne—and, one might add, a large part of it in bed.

Louis XVI, the grandson of Louis XV, was the complete opposite of his grandfather. Although, like him, he married at age 15, the new royal couple had no progeny for a long time. The King was interested in hunting, the locksmithing, and clock making, while keyholes interested him more than a woman's charms. It turned out that the cause this state of affairs was phimosis, a congenital problem that prevented him from having normal sexual relations. Only surgical intervention at the age of over twenty, allowed him to begin a normal sex life. The historical period in which Louis XVI reign fell was unusually stormy in France's annals. The bad state of the economy and finances, the dissipation of the court, and the helplessness of his ministers led to revolution in 1789. Louis XVI, who was unable to see the danger in time, and his wife, whose behavior was one of the causes of the discontent, paid with their heads. By verdict of the revolutionary tribunal, they were executed by the guillotine.

Napoleon Bonaparte, Rudolf Habsburg, Catherine the Great, and Others

The next French ruler after the period of revolutionary rule was First Consul and later, Emperor, Napoleon Bonaparte. Napoleon, whose erotic life is reminiscent of the earlier Bourbons, suffered from gonorrhea, and that, supposedly, not just once. On the other hand, his sister Pulina and, perhaps, his brother Louis, suffered from syphilis. In 1814, during his stay on the island of Elba, newspapers ill-disposed to Napoleon wrote that he, himself, also had syphilis, and that he had incestuous relations with his sister. More believable is information that his great love and wife, Josephine, later Empress, had many lovers in her younger years, and suffered from gonorrhea, the complications of which, most likely pelvic inflammatory disease or PID, caused her to be sterile. Her inability to bear a descendant for the Emperor cost her the loss of a husband and the crown. Napoleon, in order to ensure a successor, divorced his wife, and married the Habsburg princess, who bore him a son.

A similar situation, except that it took place a hundred years later, happened

to heir to the Austrian throne Archduke Rudolf Habsburg. Rudolf had a mistress from whom he contracted gonorrhea, and next infected his wife. The unhappy wife, Archduchess Stefanie, had complications that caused her to be sterile. That fact became the cause of serious dynastic problems, as the married couple only had a daughter, who could not inherit the throne. Rudolph, himself, did not avoid complications. He developed signs of disseminated gonococcal infection (DGI), with changes affecting his joints, eyes and skin. These last were taken by some, and possibly by the patient himself, as signs of syphilis, but as was later determined, without real foundation (22). Nonetheless, Rudolf, already subject to depression from other causes, came to the conclusion that he was incurably ill. This only worsened his psychologic state, and strengthened his suicidal tendencies. (23) One weekend, he left for the little hunting castle at Mayerling in the company of his new mistress, and there committed suicide. First he shot her, then himself. This story became the topic of many novels and films. The best known of these is the film titled *Mayerling*, in which Omar Sharif played the role of Rudolf, while his mistress, the very young Maria Vetsera, was played by Catherine Deneuve.

Just as Archduke Rudolf might have had only gonorrhea, so his cousin Otto Franz, the son of the Emperor's Franz Joseph brother, had worse bad luck, as he became infected with syphilis, which was the cause of his death (Fig.4.7). Otto was known among women taking advantage of his charms as an unpicky jolly rake, equally toward women from the aristocracy as toward women commoners, and not excluding women of loose habits. His behavior left much to be desired, as the Archduke managed to dance naked in coffeehouses, and once even spilled a bowl of spinach onto a bust of the Emperor – which bordered on being an insult to the latter's majesty. Emperor Franz Joseph, who was a very controlled person, once struck him on the cheek because Otto Franz publicly insulted his own wife, who was pregnant. (25) Another achievement was Otto's jumping over a coffin in a funeral procession when the young Archduke was testing his horse's abilities. It must also be added that his brother, the Archduke Franz Ferdinand, who, after the death of Rudolf, succeeded to the throne, was also blamed for such an act, although he entered history as a result of the attack in Sarajevo, during which he was shot – an event that, as we know, became the immediate cause of the outbreak of the First World War. Otto Franz infected himself with lues in the '90s of the nineteenth century. The disease had a rather stormy course, and Archduke Otto died in1906 after long and severe sufferings. In his last years, one of his mistresses, Louise Robinson, who was called "Sister Martha," took care of him, while his own wife no longer wanted to have anything to do with him. Nonetheless, before infecting himself with syphilis, Otto Franz managed to father a son, Karl, who grew up to be a handsome and intelligent young man; after the death of Franz Joseph, he became the last Austro-Hungarian Emperor. As we know, after the end of World War I, Austria became a republic, and "Emperor" Karl settled on the island of Madeira, where he died of pneumonia at the age of 34. The ex-emperor must have been a person of exceptionally winning character, as, even until today, he is favorably remembered by the inhabitants of the island. The monarch was buried in Funchal, in the chapel of the church of *Our Lady of Monte*, situated on a rise from which stretches a view of the town and its surrounding Atlantic Ocean that is beyond beautiful.

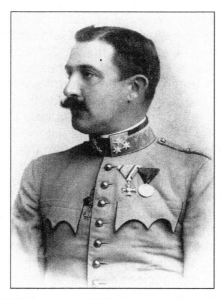

Figure 4.7 Archduke Otto Franz of Austria (1899)

Up to this point, I have written almost exclusively about the vices of the male monarchs suffering with syphilis or other venereal diseases. Not wanting to be judged a misogynist, I want to finish this chapter by relating the case of a certain eighteenth century female ruler, whose erotic life was equally colorful to that of male rulers of that epoch. This woman was a German, who became the Tsarina of Russia, one of the greatest in the history of that nation.

Sophie Friederike Auguste – for that were her names – appeared in Saint Petersburg at the court of the Russian Tsars, as the betrothed of the successor to the throne, the nephew of the Tsarina Elizabeth. Sophie was the daughter of Prince Christian August von Anhalt-Zerbst-Dornburg from Szczecin (Stettin) and his wife, Joanna Elizabeth Hostein-Gottorp. This once bashful and modest young lady became, after some years, one of the most powerful monarchs in Europe, the co-foundress of a great empire, which for several centuries became an essential player, not just in European politics. Currently, few remember her German origins, as she entered history as Catherine II, or Catherine the Great (Fig.4.8). This name she took as she converted to the Orthodox Church, and married the future Tsar Peter III.

Even during the engagement period, the young couple did not burn with affection. Later, it was said that the lack of harmony between them was the result of Peter's sexual indifference, caused by the same problem that afflicted Louis XVI, i.e., congenital phimosis. Peter III was not physically attractive, while, in addition, during the engagement period, he became ill with smallpox, which left him with permanent facial scars. In the course of the illness, there occurred periods of healing, then newly recurring rashes, (26) – which is not very typical of smallpox, and which could actually have been signs of secondary syphilis. The outcomes of Catherine's first pregnancies, as well as the appearance of their son – if, indeed, Pavel (Paul) was Peter's son – could indicate infection with that disease. Very soon after the wedding – some asserted that even before the wedding – Peter, as well as Catherine had been unfaithful to one another. The best known of Peter's many sweethearts was Elizabeth Vorontsova, while the list of Catherine's lovers only begins with Sergei Saltykov, accused of Catherine's first two pregnancies, and some say the third, also. Catherine's first pregnancy ended in a miscarriage in her second month; although the second lasted longer, it ended the same way. The third, however, ended successfully. Catherine gave birth to a boy, who, though very weak and sickly, became the legal successor to the throne. While the majority of historians point to Saltykov as the father of the child, by a singular coincidence, the boy resembled Catherine's husband, Peter III, in appearance, even more. Paul's face (Fig.4.9) has many of the features of one ill with congenital syphilis: saddle nose and flat face, flat forehead and chin, the whole reminding one of a bulldog. (27). I will add personally that drawing conclusions based only on facial appearance, and without other characteristics of the disease, which would require examination of the child, can be misleading. The fact that two previous pregnancies ended in miscarriage could indicate that Catherine could have been infected with syphilis, but by whom? By her husband, or by Saltykov – as the latter is included among those at higher risk "because of his libertine views and the fact that he was of the military?" (27) In the case of congenital syphilis, there exists something called "Diddy's Law of Decrease," or, by another eponym, "Kassowitz' Law," which say that a mother ill with syphilis during the first trimester will miscarry or will give birth to dead offspring, whereas each subsequent pregnancy is less likely to be affected by a syphilis infection, until the birth of a child free of the disease. Catherine's fourth pregnancy was the fruit of her love for Stanislaw Poniatowski, later to become King of Poland. The result was a seemingly healthy girl, Anne, but who died before reaching her second birthday. Catherine was to bear healthy children again, at least twice, although historians claim that there were about nine pregnancies in total.

After the previous Tsarina Elizabeth's death, Peter was crowned as Tsar of All Russia, and became Peter III. His rule lasted but a short time. He was an untalented and unloved ruler for, among other things, his pro-Prussian sympathies. Six months after the coronation, Catherine was at the head of the revolution, the leaders of which were the brothers Orlov. One of these, Gregory, had been Catherine's lover for a long time. After deposing Peter III, Catherine was proclaimed Empress of Russia, while her husband disappeared from the political scene, murdered in prison by one of the Orlov brothers. From this time forward, Catherine was to rule Russia for the next 34 years. Her rule occurred during the *Age of Reason*, or the *Enlightenment*. She was interested in literature and art, and promoted the education of women. She invited to Russia, not only renowned philosophers and scholars, but also writers, artists, and well-known actors. She built hospitals, and was a pioneer for vaccination against smallpox. She ruled with a heavy hand, brutally and effectively; the guilty she punished severely and without wavering. Simultaneously, she was unusually forbearing for her own weaknesses, particularly those concerning her erotic life, while her generosity and good heart in regard to her lovers was probably unmatched in all of Europe. As summed up by historians, in the course of her rule, Catherine spent the sky-high sum of close to 100 million rubles for the support of her lovers, on presents, rewards, and similar expenses. (28)

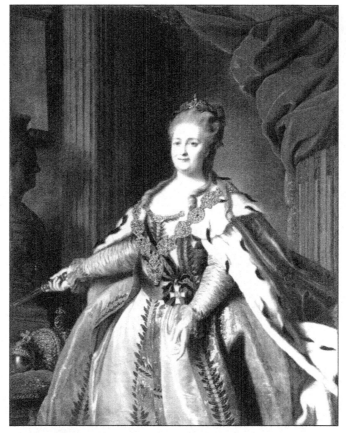

Figure 4.8 Portrait of Catherine II of Russia (1780s)

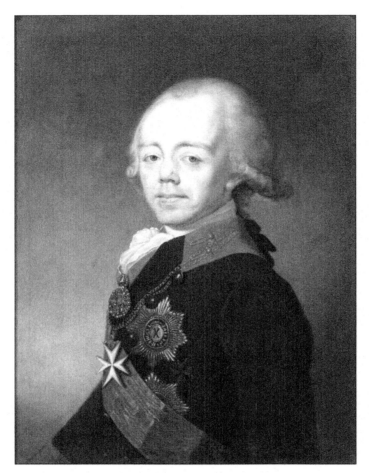

Figure 4.9 Portrait of Russian Emperor Paul I (by Stepan Shchukin)

In his work, published in *Genitourinary Medicine* (1991), R.S. Morton numbers twelve of the Tsarina's lovers. Some maintain that there were many more. Many of her unions with men lasted years. Probably her longest functioning lover was Grigorij Potemkin, who occupied her bed for many years, and even after moving out of the Tsarina's bedroom, remained her loyal friend, as well as the conduit for his successors. He was not only a lover, but also confidante and adviser in national affairs. Potemkin discharged all of his roles unusually solidly, while, in general, he was very careful and accurate in choosing new lovers for the Tsarina. He was steered not only by the physical attractiveness of a candidate, but also by his intellectual qualities, so that Catherine would not be bored with his company. There developed a type of ritual method of recruiting lovers and their testing. Candidates were usually young officers, handsome and well built. There was no shortage of volunteers. Being chosen meant promotion with the speed of lightning, and a high social status. The more enterprising young men would put into their thin and skin-tight breeches thoughtful inserts, which would embellish their manhood. When the initial choice had been made, the candidate for lover underwent a medical examination by Dr. John Rogerson with the aim of excluding venereal diseases or other problems that could have an influence on his sexual prowess. The last step in the recruitment was a test conducted by a so-called *alcove lady*, who not only verified the fitness of the candidate "for service," but, in case of need tutored the young man in the sexual act, and informed him of what the Tsarina liked and what she disliked. The candidate, thus prepared, was led into a special room, next to the Tsarina's bedroom, in which a packet of banknotes, containing around 100,000 rubles, awaited him. This was supposedly the standard fee for a "freshly-baked" candidate.

The preparation connected with fulfilling the role of a lover for Catherine's testifies that the Tsarina was aware of the dangers of venereal diseases, which some biographers take as evidence that she had been venereally ill earlier, and was afraid of a repetition of infection. Still another supposed proof for confirming this thesis, was the activism of the Tsarina in the area of organizing help for those with venereal diseases. She was the initiator of one of the first hospitals in Europe dedicated to venereal diseases in Saint Petersburg.

Despite such precautions having as their goal the elimination of venereally ill lovers, Catherine was not able to avoid infection. One such lover who served in the role for two years, proved himself unfaithful, and infected the Tsarina with an "ugly disease," most likely gonorrhea. (29) He was Ivan Korsakov, one of the ancestors of the well-known Russian composers, Rimsky-Korsakov. After passing the procedure described earlier, including examination by Dr. Rogers, Korsakov became one of the Tsarina's lovers. It must be assumed that he solidly acquitted himself of his duties, as he rose very quickly from a low-ranking officer to major general, while, on his chest, many medals appeared. Having certain musical talents, he, himself, accompanied the Tsarina with a violin, and also accompanied her during concerts of other musicians at the court. He also tested his strengths in literature, and even started to complete a library, which was supposed to make him into a writer. Catherine, enchanted by the eloquence and charm of this favorite, did not see his artificiality, and heaped a variety of favors and expensive presents on him. Unfortunately, she made a mistake, as he turned out to be an ingrate. Not only did he infect the Tsarina with the "ugly disease," but dared to fall in love with Countess Bruce, with whom he was caught in an unequivocal situation. Rumors flew that behind the whole affair stood Gregorij Potemkin, who wanted to rid himself of his mortal enemy, Field Marshall Rumiantsev, whose sister was Countess Bruce. It appeared that for such a blunder, Korsakov would be sent to Siberia – and what else? And nothing! Korsakov and the Countess were asked to leave the court, and the pair lived in a palace near Moscow offered them by Catherine. The Tsarina could not forget the intoxicating moments she spent in Korsakov's arms, and apparently invited him over several more times until the moment when the next favorite, Aleksander Lanskoj, a 22-

year-old youth discovered by the solicitous Potemkin, appeared. (29, 30)

As she aged (Catherine was already 55), the Tsarina began to like younger lovers. After the death of Lanskoj, whose service in the Tsarina's bed cost the national treasury many millions of rubles, subsequent lovers—Yermolov, Mamonov, and the brothers Zubov—were each in their early twenties. An inclination to ever-younger lovers, occurring in aging monarchs is not exclusively a female trait. I will remind the reader of the behavior of France's Louis XV, who, the older he got, the more often he selected young girls.

Catherine II died at age 67 as the result of a stroke, although there is no lack of descriptions of more fantastic causes for her death. (31) One of these says the Tsarina died in the bathroom, by sitting on a commode in which was mounted a dagger. About others, I will not write, as relating them would exceed the bounds of good taste.

CHAPTER 5

SYPHILIS AND THE ARTS

From the first days of the pandemic until the beginnings of the 20th century, syphilis affected the lives of millions of people. The disease not only shortened life, but rendered it a torture, a daily struggle, with increasing suffering and advancing invalidism. Yet, having to deal with patients with syphilis intensified attempts to cure it, particularly in the first centuries of the epidemic, during which treatments were worse than the disease. One can only wonder that, despite the dearth of evidence of effectiveness of therapies, so many people endured them.

Syphilis is a generalized disease of the whole person, and even in its early stages comes to involve almost all organs, not excluding the central nervous system, including the brain. Treated early, it does not produce any of the more serious changes, and now belongs to diseases that are completely curable. Things looked different even a hundred years ago, not to mention in an earlier period in history, when a dearth of more effective medications resulted in this disease leading to serious disability and death. It is difficult for today's dermatologists to imagine how extensive, frequently disfiguring and deforming were the changes resulting from third-stage (tertiary) syphilis even just a hundred years ago. Every time I am in Paris, I try to visit St. Louis Hospital (L'hopital St. Louis), where is found perhaps the largest collection in the world of so-called *moulages* (*moulage,* Fr. = casting, molding) representing the skin changes that appeared in those ill from lues even from before the juncture of the nineteenth and twentieth centuries.

I recommend this to all medical residents in dermatology and venereology, so that they can trace the evolution of the terrible disease that syphilis once was, but which now, even though inaccurately, passes for an almost banal illness.

Late syphilis occurs only rarely at present, because those ill, who don't even know their disease, "treat themselves unconsciously" to some extent, taking antibiotics prescribed them as a result of different bacterial diseases. Paradoxically, it can be said that the common overuse of antibiotics (taken, for example, in instances of mild colds) has had the effect that many cases of lues have been cured (suppressed?) during its early stage.

During my medical studies, and later in the course of a residency in the department of dermatology and venereology, I had the opportunity to take care of a number of patients with tertiary syphilis. My experience from the 1970's and 1980's are nevertheless different from those described several centuries earlier. Claude Quetel, in his excellent book on the history of syphilis, writes that at the end of the sixteenth century:

> [Spanish authors] hinted at the idea that, although syphilis is an enemy of the flesh, [it] is a friend of the spirit, and that the primary chancre [ulcer] produces pale, melancholy individuals more suitable to the Republic than red-faced ones, gluttons and drunkards beyond imagination, in a word sparkling with health."
> (1)

Using other words, sixteenth century Spaniards asserted that the disease favored the development of the soul, although not of the body. In a later period, at the end of the nineteenth century, when it was already known that general paresis (GP) was a manifestation of late syphilis, it was considered that, although in the majority of cases, GP "from the beginning, weakens the mental faculties, maybe in certain instances assuming an 'expansive' form, manifesting itself by an enhancement of intellectual and affective processes."(2) Leon Daudet, the French publicist and companion of the acknowledged syphilologist, Edmond Fournier, wrote "the microbe of [this] terrible disease is "equally good a whip that awakens genius and talent, heroism and soul, as a general palsy." (3) Daudet, whose father became infected with syphilis in his youth and who suffered for many years with *tabes dorsalis* – a sign of tertiary syphilis – believed that lues could be a cause of genius, or that it was a hereditary disease:

> At one moment stimulating and exciting, at another paralyzing, piercing and tormenting the cells of the marrow and brain, the master of hyperaemia (excess blood), psychoses, hemorrhages, great discoveries and sclerosis, of hereditary [treponematosis], strengthened by [the] crosses … [borne by] … syphilitic families it played, plays, and will play a role similar to that played in antiquity by fate [destiny]. (3) [He considered that] "the greater part of degenerations, the majority of the consequences associated with alcoholism could be attributed to the spiral [bacterium]. The spirochete was the same from the point of view of drive and agility as the producer of life, connected through it in many ways by hereditary transfer, leading it simultaneously to a dramatic intensiveness of life, to infertility, which is its opposite, and to most difficult plagues.(3)

The idea of a stimulating action on human mental powers by the pale treponeme gradually lost supporters, although even in the second half of the nineteenth century, there was no lack of adherents. The well-known French writer, poet and journalist, Anatole France, an admirer of Friedrich Nietzsche – who is known to have suffered from general paresis – maintained that "*la paralyse general fait seule les grands hommes*" (general paresis only makes great men). He looked upon syphilitic insanity as providing the drive and restless energy so necessary for the advancement of the human race." (4) In the course of time, belief in the heritability of syphilis, and positive opinions about its advantages, were forgotten, and in the tw[entieth] century, no one would say, for example, that the exceptionally talented politician Winston Churchill gave credit for his career, or maybe his artistic talents (he was a talented painter), to the lues from which his father, Lord Randolph Churchill suffered, and died at the age of 46.(5)

My own observations on patients with late syphilis differ from those reported by adherents to the theory attributing a stimulatory action of lues on human mental powers. None of my patients became more congenial as a result of the disease; on the contrary, in almost all of them we observed a decline of intelligence, depending on the degree of its advancement. It may be that this was due to the fact that none of those under my care was a prominent composer, poet or painter. My patients were average people, who learned about their disease rather late, and, despite the fact that after treatment they were cured of syphilis itself, they suffered as a result of its sequelae, such as *tabes dorsalis* or general paresis. Many of them, at the time of admission to the hospital had skin changes typical of late syphilis, such as gummas, disease of the circulatory system, or neurologic and psychiatric changes. Some of these ailments yielded quickly to treatment, while others required long, specialized care. None of my patients was a prominent person, although some believed that they were a "second Messiah," or a "prophet foretelling the end of the world," while one, a professional taxi driver, declared that he was the First Secretary of the Communist party, and asked that he be addressed as "Mr. First Secretary!" Of course, these were patients with general paresis, having delusions of grandeur, who were later taken care of by my psychiatric colleagues. Similarly, patients with neurologic changes required many months of rehabilitation, while patients with circulatory system changes required cardiovascular surgeons.

Looking at the syphilis epidemic from its beginnings until the present, one can readily say that this disease was never a stimulant of the intellect or a source of talent. Its actions were exactly the opposite. The disease caused a dulling of the mind and shortened the lives of talented people. Among those ill with lues were many prominent people, geniuses in their own way, who did not owe their talents to the disease, but to the contrary, rather than developing them, wasted time with their hopeless battle with it. Probably, no one can definitively appraise the losses to our culture and art resulting from syphilis. We will never know how many operas, symphonies and concerts were never written only because the composer, instead of writing music, had to apply mercury ointments, or take recourse to morphine because of the pain. We will never know how many splendid stories were never written, nor masterpieces painted because the author had attacks of panic, or the painter could not pick up his brush as a result of paralysis of the hand?

To illustrate the loss that culture and art suffered as a result of syphilis, I chose well-known artists living during the nin[eteenth] century who suffered from, and died of lues. I picked out those most famous ones, whose works are commonly known, who because of their fame obtained/received biographies permitting the recognition of their attainments and habits, showing their weaknesses and also revealing details from their private lives. I will remind the reader that syphilis has always been an embarrassing/shameful disease that disgraced the infected person, while information on its subject results in sparse details, even in biographies, and then those details were not always based on convincing proofs. Another problem is the question of correct diagnosis since in the nineteenth century lues was not always differentiated immediately from other diseases transmitted by the sexual route, which resulted in many well-known artists receiving the label of *syphilitic*, and which, according to today's criteria, most likely they were not. Some biographies contain very detailed accounts of the last years, months, and even hours from the life of the ill ones, showing how terrible a disease lues was before the introduction of effective medications to its treatment. Many of the artists described suffered from other diseases that had nothing to do with syphilis, and it will be difficult today to define which of them produced the greater devastation of their health or were the direct cause of their death.

In order to avoid boring the reader with descriptions of the disease and its accompanying sufferings, I widened the information provided about well-known syphilitics and about details of their private lives, by presenting their silhouettes against the background of the period in which they lived, historical events in which they took part, or were just witnesses. Their private lives were often complicated, and their erotic lives often characterized by risky behavior that exposed them to infection. I also allowed myself to memorialize their greatest artistic accomplishments, which will allow one to grasp the extent of the losses we have suffered as a result of their illnesses and early deaths. The individuals presented here constitute a modest extract from the list of artists who suffered from syphilis, not to mention other famous people touched by this disease, but about whom I cannot write because of the limitations and nature of this publication.

CHAPTER 5a

MUSICIANS

FRANZ (FRANCIS) SCHUBERT (1797-1828)

Franz (Francis) Schubert was born in Vienna on January 3rd, 1797. He was the twelfth of fourteen children of Franz Theodore Schubert, a teacher and owner of a school in one of the districts of Vienna. (Fig.5a.1) The composer's mother, Elizabeth Vietz was from Silesia who before her marriage, was a servant, and later took care of her home and her children.

At age five, young Francis began his studies at his father's school. At the same time, his father began to teach him how to play the violin, and his older brother, Ignatius, the piano. Francis learned to play the organ from Michael Holzer, the organist at the local parish church. It must be added that the whole Schubert family was very musical, and often played together. They formed something like a string quartet, in which the elder Franz played the cello, the two brothers played violin, and young Francis, the (alto) viola. As a teenager, Schubert took part in a competition for a position in the Imperial Boys' Choir, membership in which provided free education and board in the *Stadtkonvikt Imperial Seminary*. One of the judges and later teacher of young Schubert, was Antonio Salieri, the famous court composer and rival of Mozart. The new school provided the student with not only a wider contact with music (taking part in concerts, visits to the opera, etc.), but also assured a certain social advance, as students at the school included children "from influential families," i.e. sons of aristocrats, higher-rank officers, and court staff. At school, Francis was a good student, and his musical talents were recognized quite early. He was soon named Concert Master of the school orchestra, which was run by student colleagues eight years older than he, and by his later friend, Joseph von Spaun. (1)

In 1813, after five years at the *Stadtkonvikt*, Schubert left the school, and entered the Teachers' College, at which, a year later, he passed the examination entitling him to assume a position of teacher. During this time, he continued to take lessons from Salieri; these continued until he was nineteen years old. Schubert was grateful to Salieri for those years of teaching, and many times he underlined how grateful he was to that splendid musician.

The work of a teacher in the school, which was run by his father, left Schubert with much free time. In just one year, when he was eighteen years old, he composed two symphonies, four operas, two Masses, and about 150 songs, not counting several smaller piano compositions. (2) Schubert had an uncommon facility for composition. Spaun, his school friend, related that the song entitled "Der Erlkonig" (The Elf King) – one of the best known of Schubert's songs – was composed in the course of one afternoon. (3) The same Spaun tried to interest Goethe – one of the greatest of the German poets of the time – in Schubert's songs that were composed to a variety of poems, but the great poet paid no attention, returning the material to the sender.

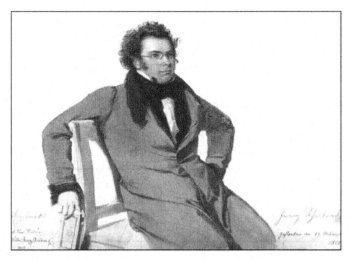

Figure 10a.1 Portrait of Franz Schubert (1825) by Wilhelm August Rieder

Most of Schubert's companions asserted that Schubert was very amorous. His first love, when he was eighteen, Therese Grob, was not as pretty as she was graceful, and had a beautiful voice. Schubert composed several songs for her, among others, *Salve Regina* and *Tantum Ergo.* He wanted to get married, but as an impoverished teacher and a still not overly well-known musician, he was not seen favorably as a future son-in-law. Also, at this time, the government issued regulations, requiring a future husband to demonstrate assured sources of income sufficient for supporting a wife. Schubert was unable to meet these requirements, and so, the graceful soprano became the wife of a baker several years later. (4)

In autumn of 1816, Schubert definitively finished his teaching career, and undertook composition. He received profitable orders for composing larger works, and for the first time felt that he could make a living from this undertaking. Besides composing, he also gave music lessons. For a while, he was the teacher of the children of Count Esterhazy, a relative of the Prince of the same name, who also employed Joseph Haydn. He moved to the country, to Zseliz (currently Zeliezovce in Slovakia), where the Count had a small estate. Teaching music didn't take much time, and Schubert could devote a lot to composing. We do not know how much of this time he was devoting to a chambermaid named Pepi, with whom he had a romance. (5) It was also during this time, apparently, that he composed his famous *Marche Militaire*, one of his better-known compositions. In late autumn 1818, the entire company returned to Vienna, where Schubert continued the musical education of the Count's children. He rented a room, in which he lived together with a friend, the poet Johann Mayerhofer, a homosexual; this gave birth to many speculations regarding Schubert's sexual orientation. Schubert also lived for a time with Franz von Schober, a law student, who came from Malmo in Sweden, and whose father was on the city council of Vienna. Many friends maintained that von Schober had a bad influence on the composer. Their mutual bad luck was soon to be convincing. The following year Schubert went on vacation with the baritone, Michael Vogel, with whom he was on friendly terms, to the latter's family locality, Steyr. The men resided in a house belonging to a professional miner, who played the cello. He ordered a piano quintet from Schubert, suggesting that, as a theme, he should utilize the melody, *Die Forelle* (The Trout). This quintet, also named "Quintet in A-major (The Trout)," is one of the best-recognized compositions by Schubert. Also during this time, he composed a piano sonata in A-major for the daughter of the local iron dealer, which would appear to testify that he could not pass by a pretty girl with indifference. (6)

The makeup of friends surrounding the composer was subject to frequent change. There nevertheless arose a certain social ritual, which continued, regardless of the group's composition. The friends met two-three times a week to listen to music, mostly by Schubert, or to discuss literature and the latest happenings in politics. Sometimes sporting competitions were organized, gymnastics performed, and trips out of town arranged. The games ordinarily finished with a night of revelry at some inn or beer hall (7). These affairs, called *Schubertiades* continued for many years, even when Schubert was already seriously ill.

The circumstances of Schubert's becoming infected with syphilis are not known. The fact that he, as well as his friend, von Schober, were being treated for the disease at the same time, could indicate that they contracted it during a mutual merry bout, possibly from the same female partner, but this is not at all certain. Many biographers suppose that Schubert was infected with syphilis at the end of 1822, when he was 25. Initially, the fact of his infection was kept secret; however, after some time, it became the subject of correspondence between friends, and also is found in the records of his physician, Dr. Bernhard, (8) with whom Schubert became friends, and to whom he dedicated a series of songs. Nowhere, however, is the word *syphilis* found.

Personally, I have some reservation as to the actual time of infection, as, apparently, Schubert did not take part in any social gatherings in December of 1822. One can speculate that during this time, he was either already under treatment and did not leave the house, or had visible skin changes (a rash?), especially on the face and extremities, as these are commonly seen in secondary lues, and which appear more or less at 2-4 months after infection. In one of his letters, it is said that Schubert stopped wearing a wig, and that his hair was re-growing, which could be evidence that several weeks earlier he had completed mercury treatment as that can lead to hair changes. (9) Another cause of hair loss could be the lues itself, during the course of which can appear so-called *moth-eaten alopecia*, an irregular balding reminiscent of a fur eaten by moths. This type of balding appears in the second stage of syphilis, usually about a half-year after infection.

(10). Either way, it appears that the composer of "The Trout," could have been infected in early autumn of 1822. The time period during which infection occurred is connected to the fate of one of Schubert's symphonies, namely the *Unfinished Symphony*, which suggests that it was started before he became ill, and the composer no longer had the heart to finish it. (11)

On February 28, 1823, Schubert wrote to his publisher that "the circumstances of my health do not allow me to leave the house." (12) In October or November, he spent several weeks on the ward of the General Hospital of Vienna, doubtless due to treatment, which probably did not help much, as the patient still wore a wig at year's end, and had problems with his left arm. The latter interfered with his piano playing, and, additionally, he was unable to sing, due to some changes in his throat and oral cavity. There is no way today to determine whether these troubles were connected to the development of the illness, or whether they were side effects of mercury treatment.

It appears that in the following year, Schubert experienced a significant improvement in the state of his health. He followed his doctors' orders, which means that he often was outdoors, and exercised. In summer, he again left for Zseliz at the invitation of Count Esterhazy, who without a doubt had no idea of the state of health of his children's music teacher! It was a widely known secret that music teachers were famous for seducing their female students, particularly when these were at an age when young women are attracted to somewhat older men. Pepi, with whom Schubert had an earlier romance, stayed in Vienna, and the composer awoke the (probably platonic) emotions of the young Countess Caroline. He dedicated one of his more beautiful Fantasies, "Fantasy for four hands in F-minor," to her. (13) It is a very impressive creation, full of mystery, yearning, and, possibly, sentiment, which Schubert could not utter aloud.

From the time of becoming ill with syphilis, periods of depression and critical self-perception became interwoven with periods of good health and intensive compositional work. In the summer of 1825, Schubert once again left for Steyer with Vogel. There, they visited several friends, with whom they again arranged "Schubertiades." During one of the trips, they stopped in the small town of Gmunden, beautifully situated on the picturesque Traun Lake. Among the treasures of the local church, is found a porcelain statue of the Blessed Virgin Mary, known as the Virgin in a Cape. It was here, that Schubert composed the melody, "Ave Maria," of world renown – originally to the words of a verse by Walter Scott, titled "Ellen's Song." And it was here that was born the idea for the Symphony in C-major, called *The Great*.

This was one of the better periods during his illness. After returning to Vienna, the *Schubertiades* were renewed, ending, often at 2 or 3 a.m. Nevertheless, Schubert tried to compensate for the re-appearance of despondency and a depressive state, by games with his friends, frequent visits to coffeehouses and seductions of women. He worked hard, composing many of his masterpieces. He completed his great *Symphony in C-major* (his tenth) and a cycle of songs given the title, *Winter Travels*, composed operas, all despite feeling none too well. He drank too much, suffered attacks of aggression. He complained of headaches and dizziness, and also rushes of blood to the head. The New Year, 1828, he greeted with his friends at a reception, while in March, he gave a public concert that brought him a considerable income. This was not without significance, as for some time he was treated by Dr. Ernest Rinny, one of the best physicians in Vienna, and medical adviser to the Emperor, whose honoraria were not among the lowest. Unfortunately, Medicine of the time was almost helpless in regard to syphilis, something to which the recommendations that Schubert received from his doctor testify, i.e. "fresh air and exercise." (14)

In September 1828, Schubert moved to the house of his brother, Ferdinand, who rented a large apartment in a new district, bordering on green meadows at the outskirts of Vienna. Despite almost pastoral surroundings, he didn't feel well. He complained of severe headaches and dizziness, (15). A month later he went with his brother and several friends to a tavern named "Under the Red Cross" for a fish dinner, after which he felt ill. From that time new problems arose with his stomach. He vomited everything he ate and lost weight. From the middle of November, he was practically confined to bed. Greatly weakened, he managed only the short distance to his armchair and back. (16, 17) He fell into a coma, and died on the 19th of November 1828. Francis Schubert was buried in the cemetery in Wahring, but at the turn of the century he was transferred to the Central Cemetery in Vienna, where he was laid to rest in a section designated for composers, next to Beethoven, Brahms, Strauss, and Hugo Wolf.

Despite the fact that for almost six years, Schubert was ill with lues, the cause of his death has not been definitively determined. For a long time, it was maintained that death was due to typhoid fever, (18) and although one cannot rule that out, the numerous mercury treatments that were administered for syphilis, could have damaged his liver, stomach or kidneys. He lived only thirty-one years. Would he have lived longer were it not for syphilis?

GAETANO DONIZETTI (1797-1848)

Gaetano Donizetti, composer of Italian Romanticism, came from Bergamo, a beautiful town in the Italian Alps, situated near the Swiss border. At the time of composer's birth, Bergamo was a part of Lombardy, which then found itself under the domination of the Habsburgs. He was younger than Francis Schubert by almost ten months. (Fig. 5a.2)

Gaetano came from an impoverished family; he was the fifth of six children of a seamstress and a modest pawnshop employee. Already in his early youth, he had to have shown a lot of musical talent, as he was accepted to the newly organized School of Music, organized by Johann Simon Mayr, a well-known composer of Bavarian origin. Mayr very quickly recognized Donizetti's talent, became his mentor, and sent him for further studies to Bologna.

Donizetti composed his first operas at age twenty, but his first opera, *Enrico de Burgogna* (1818), was not well received. On the other hand, his next one, *Zoraida di Granata,* achieved enormous success, and Donizetti was given the title of "main pretender to the throne of Rossini," and it was arranged for him to be Composer and Director of *Teatro Nuovo*, later, the Royal Theatre in Naples. (19) In the 1820s, Donizetti was directing other composers' works, writing his own, and teaching at the Neapolitan Conservatory. He worked intensively, so that in the course of the next twenty creative years, he composed more than fifty operas, and many of them are still performed today.

Until the present, it has not been determined when or from whom Donizetti became infected with syphilis. Some claim that this took place during his stay in Bologna, others that it happened in Naples shortly before his marriage. In June of 1828, Donizetti married Virginia Vaselli, the sister of his friend of many years, Anthony Vaselli, a physician practicing in Rome. It appears that the composer might knew nothing about his illness when marrying, which soon it became apparent as it weighed in tragically on the family fortunes and later life and career of Donizetti himself.

The 1830s were the most creative ones for the composer. It was this period, which produced his best-known works. His first great success was the opera, *Anna Bolena* (Anne Boleyn), performed in 1830, and very quickly attained to premieres in Paris and London. Before long, the next scenic hit of Donizetti, *L'elisir d'amore* (The Elixir of Love) appeared; this is a comic opera, which, today, is one of the most-frequently performed of this composer's operas. His next was *Lucrezia Borgia*, which did not please Schumann, who called its music, "music for marionettes." (20)

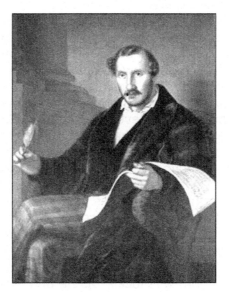

Figure 5.a.2 Gaetano Donizetti - Portrait by Giuseppe Rillosi

In 1835, in Naples, was shown what was later to be the most frequently performed of Italian operas, *Lucia di Lammermoor*. The famous scene of frenzy, or the sextet from the second act, evokes the delight of listeners and storms of applause for the performers until the present. In the same year, another famous Italian composer, Rossini invited Donizetti to Paris, where was born the thought of a permanent move to that city. Paris was then the unquestionable cultural capital of Europe, and provided greater possibilities of development for the talented composer.

The years of professional triumph were simultaneously a period of difficult experiences and family tragedies for the composer. In the course of a short, barely nine-year marriage, three children were born to the Donizettis, of which none lived longer than two weeks. The first son was premature, and lived just a short while; the newborn was deformed, and had episodic convulsions. (21) The next two births were likewise premature, and also quickly ended in death. It was not difficult to surmise that the cause of these tragedies could be syphilis, with which Donizetti might have infected his wife. Virginia died after the third birth, and although biographers write that she may have died as a result of smallpox, scarlet fever or cholera, (22) one cannot close one's eyes to the fact that lues could have contributed to her early death. One can easily imagine the reactions of the father and the husband. Donizetti was heartbroken, and as has been written, never completely recovered. (22)

A year after the death of his wife, Donizetti moved to Paris, where, thanks to the success of his operas, he expected to earn more money. This had happened to his mentor, Gioachino Rossini, the composer of *The Barber of Seville*. Here, I will add that Rossini also suffered from venereal disease, but was luckier as he only had gonorrhea. He was infected at age twenty when he was still living in Italy. This disease, which, even untreated, can remit by itself after the passage of time, became in Rossini's case, the curse of his life, and tormented him even into his old age. (23) He experienced complications, rarely encountered today, that are related to a narrowing of the urethra, causing him problems with urination, as well as frequent infections of the urinary tract. He underwent multiple catheterizations, which only worsened the state of the lower portions of his urinary tract. In addition to this, the famous composer suffered from psoriasis, with changes on the scrotum, which should not have, but apparently caused severe itching. He was treated according to the state of the art of the Medicine of those times, which recommended rest, warm baths, trips to the spas, and leeches! (24)

Donizetti, on the other hand, did not undertake treatment, or maybe there only may be no evidence for it, as it is difficult to believe that after the deaths of his wife and three children, he did not know that he was ill with lues. The composer was at the height of his fame, while the culmination point of his career occurred in 1843, in the *Theatre Italien* in Paris, with the comic opera, *Don Pasquale*. About this time he was appointed to the position of *Kapelmeister* in Vienna, and divided his time between the latter and Paris. Among his credits he already had 70 operas, but, unfortunately around this time the disease started to make itself known more clearly. Even earlier, in his correspondence with friends and family, he had complained about constant headaches and stomach cramps, but these were not necessarily ailments directly related to syphilitic infection. Only after finishing *Lucia di Lamermoor* did he begin to complain of violent headaches and neck pains, convulsive episodes, fevers, mental disorientation, personality changes and depressions (21). More frequently in his letters, there appear references to something being wrong with him, and feeling as though someone was constantly hitting him in the head with a hammer. He wrote that he had disturbances in consciousness, during which he was unable to distinguish between reality and illness visions. From 1845, as a result of his worsening state of health, he had to resign from several lucrative proposals.

During one of his trips to Vienna, Donizetti's mental state decidedly worsened, and it was noted that his behavior became "marked with intensive eroticism." He engaged prostitutes from the park on the Prater (it appeared that he liked two at a time) and cultivated this habit after returning to Paris. In his letters, there began to appear numerous obscenities. (25) In January of the following year, alarmed at Donizetti's deteriorating health, his nephew Andreas asked for a consultation with three physicians, including the famous Parisian venereologist, Phillipe Ricord. The group decided that the composer was not capable of logical thought and independent decision-making and that he should be placed in a hospital for the mentally ill in Ivry near Paris. On the pretext that he was leaving for Vienna, he was transported to the hospital, where he was detained, explaining that the carriage in which the group was travelling had broken down, and that they would have to wait for repairs; then, that they had to stay longer, as his servant had been stopped by the police due to a robbery. After a while, it began to appear to Donizetti that it was he, himself, who had been arrested for robbery, and he sent plaintive letters requesting help. (21) The contents of the letters attest to the fact that at times he was aware of his situation, whereas at others, he again fell into insanity. When his nephew next visited him, he proposed afresh that he would take his uncle to Italy; however, the prefect of the Parisian police did not grant him permission to leave the hospital. When Andreas returned eight months later, he confirmed that the composer had changed into little more than a vegetable. Only after seventeen months of obligatory stay at the hospital did the Ivry police permit the patient to be taken by friends to Paris, on the condition that the house in which he would live would be watched by the police. (26) (Fig. 5a.3. Next, after much pressure from family and friends in the Parisian police, as well as involvement by Austrian authorities in the action, Donizetti was allowed to leave for Italy. At the end of September 1847, he again found himself in Bergamo, the place from where he came. Reports about his health from this period confirm the hopeless state of health of the composer, who was paralyzed, psychotic, and lacking the ability to communicate with his surroundings. He frequently had a fever, perspired, had serious difficulty with swallowing, and was incontinent of both urine and feces. He had uncontrollable muscular pains and cramps. Gaetano Donizetti died April 8, 1848 at the age of barely 50. The results of an autopsy confirmed the diagnosis of syphilis of the central nervous system, (21) with characteristics of *taboparalysis.*

In one of the works dealing with Donizetti's illness and creativity, the authors posed the question of whether the mental derangement that the composer exhibited could have had an influence on the type of music composed by him, and particularly on the musical illustrations for scenes of insanity in such operas as *Anna Bolena* or *Lucia di Lamermoor.* They suggested that "perhaps because of the composer's sensitivities and his own neurological illness, he may have been particularly attuned to know, understand and translate into melody the disorganization, delirium and torment of severe mental illness." (21)

This appears to me to be of little likelihood. Both *Anna Bolena* (1830) and *Lucia di Lamermoor* (1835) were composed at a time when the composer was mentally competent, although after the premiere of *Lucia di Lamermoor* allusions to "mental disorientation" and "personality change" appeared in his letters. As a venereologist, I cannot remember any patient with tertiary syphilis whose illness might have stimulated him to creative work, or even to *any* work. To the contrary, serious neuropsychiatric symptoms were usually the beginning of the end of their professional activity. Let us remember that, at the time when Donizetti composed music to scenes of insanity, he was already very familiar with the illness that destroyed his family and might took those nearest to him from this earth. One should also remember that the composer must have recognized that no one other than he himself could be responsible of these tragedies. It is almost certain that this so-painfully experienced artist understood the sufferings of others, a fact that could have translated itself into the type of music that illustrated the sufferings of his heroines.

It is the irony of fate that the artist created music for scenes of insanity, which he later experienced himself. In Donizetti's time, many operas appeared whose librettos contained scenes of madness, as that was the mode then. Bellini's *Il Pirata* (1827) and *I Puritani* (1835), Giuseppe Verdi's *Nabucco* (1842), or Meyerbeer's *Dinorah* (1859) all contain music for scenes depicting madness on the stage. The public loved this. Prima donnas performing arias of this type gathered applause and homage, and opera theater ticket offices were filled with the financial proceeds.

I wanted to bring attention to yet another problem that in my opinion is important. The average person does not recognize the degree of suffering experienced by mentally ill people. Talking about it does not always reach the hearer's imagination. There are people for whom words have little meaning; they do not move them, nor do they evoke understanding or sympathy. On the other hand, music, or words plus music, can accomplish this. This quote is so true: "Music penetrates deeper into the psyche than words alone, music modeled to words in opera can convey a particularly powerful sense of mental derangement, with its mingling of pain and flights of fantasy, reality and delusions horror and pathos." (21) Although, from the times of Donizetti, the public's attitude toward the mentally ill has undergone a tremendous evolution, these illnesses are still degrading for the patient, and they are treated worse than, or, in the best instances, just differently from those suffering from other illnesses.

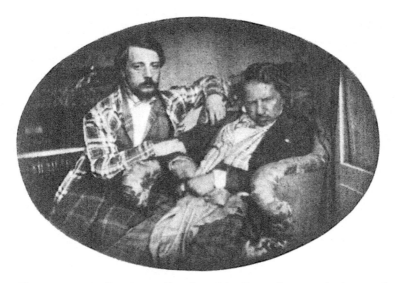

Figure 5a. 3. Gaetano Donizetti in the advanced stage of tabo-paralysis caused by syphilis. Daguerrotype showing composer (right) with his nephew in Paris, August 1847

If the musical menu of Donizetti's operas can evoke understanding of and sympathy for people with psychiatric disorders, even to a small degree, this will be a probably unintended, yet still great victory of the composer, who was himself the victim of such an illness.

ROBERT SCHUMANN (1810-1856)

Robert Schumann (Fig.5a.4), one of the better-known composers of the German romantic epoch, came from Zwickau, a not very large town in Saxony, located close to the frontier with the Czech Republic. In communist times, Zwikau was known for its factory for the "Trabant," a small car that reigned on the highways of the DDR (*Deutsche Demokratische Republik*). The Trabants were relatively inexpensive, having a body made of artificial material (plastic); their owners had to be careful not to park in areas where there were rats or other animals, as they could consume, in the course of a single night, a large part of a fender or other part of the car's body. Zwikau is also famous for a house standing near the town square, the birthplace of the famous composer.

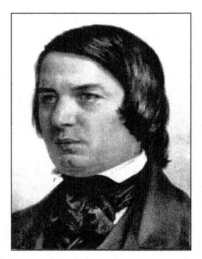

Figure 5a.4 Portrait of Robert Schumann (before 1856)
Author: Adolph Menzel

Robert Schumann's father, August, was the proprietor of a grocery shop and later of a small publishing house, in which he published the books of various authors, including his own. Robert's mother came from a medical family – her father was a surgeon. Schumann's education in the art of the piano began at age seven and when he was eight years old, he composed his first works. Four years later, he already was the author of a larger creation for voice and orchestra. Besides playing the piano, Schumann played the viola and the flute, sang well, and wrote poetry. When he was sixteen, his father died, leaving Robert a considerable inheritance; this remained under the direction of a trustee until he attained majority. Despite his distinct musical talents, Schumann's mother wanted him to have a more serious profession, and persuaded her son to become a lawyer. He began his studies in Leipzig, later moving to Heidelberg, but he did not finish law. To the consternation of his mother and his guardians, Robert decided to devote himself to music. He rented a piano and began to compose. He travelled a bit in southern Germany, as well as to Switzerland and Italy. He stopped in Milan, where, in La Scala, he listened to and watched Rossini's operas, (27) then after returning to Germany together with his professor of law – an enthusiastic musician – he took part in weekly receptions at which singing and playing took place.

His love for music did not prevent young Schumann from taking part in revelries, orgies, and drinking to excess. He had romances with two young women, Nanni and Liddy, was fond of the daughter of a certain chemist from Augsburg, and then became enamored with the wife of a certain physician from Colditz. Reportedly he also practiced youthful homosexuality with friends and roommates. (28) At age nineteen, he lived through the "most dissolute week of his life, staggering from tavern to tavern getting drunk to unconsciousness, so that he had to be taken home." (29) It appears that this type of extravagance was nothing extraordinary in the case of a rich young man. Apparently, a dissolute life, frequent changes of women, and other sexual excesses, alcohol and narcotics, fit into the canon of artistic behavior, and even was supposed to awaken creative inventiveness! (30)

In the autumn of 1830, at age twenty, Schumann began music lessons from the outstanding piano teacher, Frederick Wieck. After an introductory audition, Wieck wrote to Schumann's mother that, in three years, he could make of her son one of the most splendid pianists of his time. (31)

These words testify to Wieck's great acknowledgment of the talents of his student, as well as the great magnanimity of the teacher, who, knowing the carousing style of Schumann's life and his inclinations toward alcohol and women, as well as his advanced age for a student, nevertheless agreed to become his teacher.

Schumann took up residence in Wieck's house, and after several months started to romance a girl by the name of Christel, who either was a student like Robert, or just worked for the Wiecks (32). In May of the following year, in a diary written by Schumann, there appears the notation that a sore had appeared on the author's penis, becoming very painful with the passage of time. The alarmed lovers turned for help to a friend of Schumann's, Christian Glock, who had recently finished his medical studies, and who recommended soaking the part in narcissus water (probably an extract of *Narcissus* flowers). We do not know whether the treatment helped, but we do know that it was unpleasant, as Schumann bitterly complained that it burned him! (33)

Shortly thereafter, other symptoms appeared; as Schumann described in a letter to his mother, these resembled cholera. He had abdominal pain and headaches; he had chest pain, memory losses and feelings of constant rage. Despite pleas by Glock to refrain from sexual relations, he continued sleeping with Christel, although, as he wrote, he did so with a certain degree of fear and far less pleasure. (33) Schumann again began drinking heavily, and, as he confided to his diary, felt an urge for self-destruction. After a certain time, his physical ailments remitted, but Robert's mental state did not improve much. In September 1831 he wrote to his brother of tormenting anxiety and wanting to "blow out his brains." (34) Although an earlier infection with syphilis cannot be excluded, it would appear that Christel was the probable source of infection, considering the fact that, after relations with her, Robert had signs that could correspond to a primary chancre of syphilis.

The fact that the ulceration described by Schumann was painful (the typical primary chancre is painless) does not necessarily exclude syphilis, as a primary chancre, if secondarily infected, can be painful, and that, very much so. Nevertheless other venereal diseases, in which changes on the penis can be painful, cannot be excluded; these include infection with genital herpes, or soft chancre (chancroid). Or, taking into account another fact, namely that Schumann was a person prone to over-exaltation, as one can readily note, could have magnified his experience so that the small amount of pain that sometimes accompanies a primary chancre in syphilis could have been magnified, or was described in an exaggerated manner by the patient.

Suggestions that Schumann could have been infected by his older sister sound like pure fantasy. Infection by nonsexual means, such as by using a common towel or by drinking from the same glass were – and remain – unusually rare, and belong to favored responses of people who, asked about the source of infection, don't want to reveal their contacts. Older by fourteen years, his sister Emily, committed suicide as a result of depression caused by a chronic skin disease, which also involved the area around her genito-urinary organs, and "threw its poisons onto the most precious parts of her body." (35) The fact that the illness involved the sexual organs would suggest that it could have been lues. However, as a dermatologist, I can name a dozen or more skin diseases (including common psoriasis), which, in addition to their typical locations can also involve the skin of the genital and anal areas. I have seen many patients with generalized skin changes who suffered from itching, burning, or dry skin, and whose symptoms led to the verge of depression. I am speaking of the situation currently, when we prescribe medicines that are incomparably more efficacious than those of Schumann's time. I can easily imagine a young woman, whose disfiguring skin changes, additionally causing pain or persistent itching, including in the genital area, could lead to suicide. If one assumes that Robert was not the only person in his family subject to psychotic tendencies, the suicide of a young woman as a result of a chronic, generalized skin disease seems to me to be totally credible.

Other suggestions, such as problems with a finger on Robert's right hand being a complication of the initial sign of syphilis in this location sound equally improbable. Even if one were to assume that he "put his finger where he shouldn't have," and infected himself with syphilis in this manner, the typical initial sign remits, even without treatment, and without leaving a scar, not to mention any long-lasting lameness. Problems with the finger, which put a finish to Schumann's dreams of becoming a piano virtuoso, were most likely the result of physical exercises of the palm, which were called "finger torture" by Wieck. During his teacher's absences, Schumann took advantage of a mechanical apparatus that was supposed to spread out the arrangement of the hand, and to strengthen the fingers. Mechanisms of this type were then in common use, and famous pianists used them. Apparently Schumann himself constructed such an apparatus – the consequences of which were deplorable.

The contusion of his hand finished his career as a pianist. All that remained for him was composing or a career as a violinist, inasmuch as this instrument required the use of only his left hand. Still another suggestion is that Schumann's problem with his fingers was a side effect of mercury treatment, (36) but for that there is no convincing evidence.

In the summer of 1833, Schumann availed himself of the advice of Dr. Franz Hartmann, a physician from Leipzig engaged in the homeopathic treatment of those ill with syphilis. Hartmann assured the composer that his medicines would not only relieve him of lues, but would also improve the state of his right hand. Though skeptical about the methods, Schumann agreed to take a rather small amount of powder – most probably arsenic – and to adhere to a diet without coffee or wine, and only a small amount of beer. (37)

One can ask a question why after two years beyond infection (if, indeed the infection had occurred then), Schumann began treatment for syphilis. Could it be that signs of secondary syphilis had appeared?

In addition to hints about the occurrence of occasional fevers (and who hasn't had such?), we have no information about the appearance of any other signs or symptoms associated with the disease. Generally, this was not a good period in the composer's life. During the same year in which Schumann was being treated for syphilis, his sister-in-law, Rozalia, with whom he was on friendly terms, and to whom he confided about his fears, died. Rozalia's young son, to whom Robert was godfather, also died, while his brother, Julius Schumann, was in the last stages of tuberculosis. In addition to all this, Schumann's career as a piano virtuoso was definitively finished, while his career as a composer was distinctly limping. One night, after Rozalia's death, he had a nervous breakdown, suddenly felt that he would go mad, and almost jumped out of a window. He was in a deep depression, and from that time began to suffer from a morbid fear of heights (*acrophobia*). (38)

Besides music, Schumann was interested in journalism, mainly musical journalism. In 1834, together with some colleagues, he started to publish a musical journal, among whose editors was his music teacher, Frederick Wieck. The periodical appeared twice weekly, and was independent of musical publishers. The same year, Schumann almost got married. He wanted to become engaged to a student of Wieck's, the very young Ernestine von Fricken, the adopted daughter of some pretended Baron. When it turned out that she was the illegitimate daughter of, not the Baron, but of a relative of his, and also had no dowry, "love" was extinguished. The next object of Schumann's interest was Clara Wieck, the 16-year-old daughter of his teacher (Fig 5a.5). When her father realized that his talented and beloved daughter had fallen in love with Schumann, he fell into a panic, and sent her to Dresden. The lovers managed to avoid the proscriptions of her grim father and maintained secret contact with each other. They determined to marry despite her father's opposition; however, Clara was a minor, and they had to wait until she attained the age of majority before wedding. In the end, they were happily married!

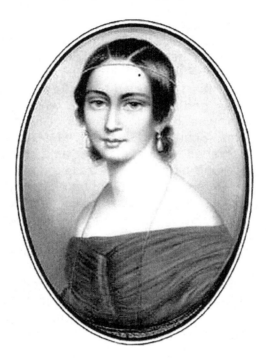

Figure 5a.5 Portrait of Clara Schumann (1838) Author Andreas Staub

Schumann worked intensively, composing piano music and vocal creations, while his first symphony in B-major, the *Spring Symphony*, was performed for the first time in March 1841, under the baton of the Schumann's friend, great German composer Felix Mendelsohn. Robert's marriage continued without any major clashes, and in the course of thirteen years, produced eight children. It is worth noting that all the children were healthy, with the exception of one boy, who died of unknown causes in his infancy. The fact of the birth of eight healthy children neither confirms nor excludes Robert's earlier diagnosis of lues, because, after several years, sufferers stop being infectious. This would be supported by the good health of Clara, and a lack of any information whatsoever that she had been treated for syphilis. According to reports, even though Clara's births were greeted with joy, her later pregnancies were greeted with anxiety and written about as "a new anxiety and fearful anticipation." (39) This type of description could suggest that the married couple were concerned about the health of their newborn children. I would remind the reader that, in the middle of the nineteenth century, it was the prevailing view that an ill father, regardless of whether the mother was ill or not, could transfer his illness to the child. It is also possible that the concern was about Clara herself, for whom pregnancy or birth could have, for whatever reason, constituted a danger.

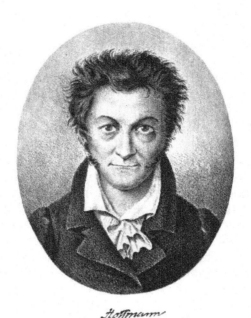

Figure 5a.6 Self portrait of E.T.A. Hoffmann (before 1822)

In the first period of his activity as a composer, until 1840, Schumann composed works intended for the piano almost exclusively. One of the better known of these is *Kreisleriana*, a creation with a large content of emotionalism, composed as an illustration of the literary authorship of E. T. A. Hoffman (Fig.5a.6). Ernst Hoffman, versatile in talent, was the author of tales of fantasy, wrote poetry, and was a talented artistic draftsman, caricaturist, and composer. Although popular in the nineteenth century, he is remembered today mainly as the result of Jacques Offenbach's operetta, *The Tales of Hoffmann*, but even more so due to the very impressive barcarole of this operetta, which even persons not especially interested in classical music recognize. Few people know that the author of the story for the famous ballet of Peter

Tchaikovsky, *The Nutcracker,* was actually Ernst Hoffmann, and that Leo Delibe's ballet, *Coppelia,* was based on one of his tales.

I interrupted my narrative about Schumann to pause at Hoffmann, not without reason. The popular nineteenth century author was married to a Polish woman, and lived and worked for the Prussian administration then occupying western Polish lands. Another reason I am writing about him in this book is syphilis, from which Hoffmann suffered and died at the age of 46. He became infected probably in Berlin, in 1807, and, despite treatment, most likely with mercury, several years before his death signs and symptoms of *tabes dorsalis* appeared. In 1821, Hoffmann had serious problems with walking, and a year later, he became completely paralyzed. Until the end, he was intellectually sound, and his last works he dictated to his wife and secretary. Ernst Hoffman died in June 1822.

Returning to Schumann, the 1840s were a period of intense work, equally for Robert as for Clara. In January 1844, both left for a *turnee* to Russia, where Clara, among others, performed for the Tsarina in Moscow. Professional successes were disturbed with increasing frequency by Robert's worsening health. After moving to Dresden in the fall of 1844, his mental state worsened considerably. Clara noted that "Robert didn't sleep through the night even once, his imagination offering the most horrible pictures, and early morning would find him bathed in tears ... so that he abandoned all hope for himself." (40) Schuman complained about "growing weak, dizziness and headaches, ringing in the ears, while every sound changed into music." (41) His hypochondria worsened. He feared infection, particularly with cholera, but despite his fear of diseases did not follow his doctors' recommendations. In autumn of 1849, there appeared a chance of obtaining the position of director of the Dusseldorf orchestra, of which Schumann availed himself eagerly, as Clara wanted to take him away from Dresden, in which there was no position worthy of his talents. In the new surroundings, Robert appeared to regain a new creative strength. He composed many works—among others, a third Symphony in E-major, called the *Rhine Symphony*, and a viola concerto. With the position of director, however, there were problems. Schumann was never a good director, and contacts with a large company of people, considering his labile mental state, exposed him to frequent conflicts. In 1852, he again began to hear voices. Speech disturbances appeared. The concert in September of that year almost led him to a nervous breakdown. (42) (This incident was immortalized in a 1947 film, entitled *Schumann's Song of Love*, in which the role of Clara was played by Catherine Hepburn). Schumann turned to religious music, composing an oratorio on the life of Luther, a Mass and a Requiem. He became interested in the spiritualism movement that was unusually fashionable at the time.

In mid-1863, Schumann underwent a strange paralysis, which a physician attributed to rheumatism, and a month later, lost his voice. Serious troubles began at work, and it was suggested to Schumann that he assign the direction of the more important concerts to his assistant. In February of the following year, he began to have "such violent auditory hallucinations that he couldn't close his eyes all night. Sometimes he heard single notes, at other times a full orchestra. Occasionally the music was more beautiful, and played on more exquisite instruments than had ever sounded on earth, while sometimes there was a cacophony of voices of hyenas and demons." (43) Robert asked his wife to leave him if he were to hurt her, and one night he rose from his bed in order to write music that angels had sent him. On February 27, 1854, he tried to commit suicide by jumping into the river, but was saved by the captain of a passing steamer. Several days later, on the advice of his family, and at Schumann's request, he was admitted to the psychiatric hospital at Endenich (currently a district in Bonn). The director and owner of this institution was a Dr. Richarz, who ran the hospital on a high level. In it there were barely fourteen patients (the cost was very high), and the ill were treated in a highly civilized manner, i.e. avoiding tying up patients or using straightjackets whenever it was possible to avoid them. Treatment included baths in alternating very cold and very hot water. The *internal* body, on the other hand, was cleansed by bloodletting and feeding patients foods difficult to digest, while simultaneously giving them laxative agents. (44)

I want to remind the reader at this point that, in the middle of the nineteenth century, few patients believed that syphilis could be the cause of insanity or psychiatric illness. There was no shortage of shrewd observers who noted that among a certain group of those ill with syphilis, or that, after a dozen years or more following infection, mental and neurological changes would occur. Only at the end of the nineteenth century did Alfred Fournier begin to promote the concept that general paresis and *tabes dorsalis* could be a sequel to syphilitic infection, and that "the nervous system, as a whole, could be a victim of third stage syphilis." (45) The correctness of Fournier's hypothesis was proved by two discoveries: In 1907, Plaut confirmed that the Bordet-Wasserman serologic reagent, which began to be used then, gave positive results equally in the blood as in the cerebrospinal fluid of general paretics, and six years later, Nogushi and Moore discovered the presence of treponemes in the cerebral cortex of those suffering from syphilis. (44a, 45)

Returning to Schumann, it was easy to conclude that the methods used in the hospital by Dr. Richarz didn't have much effect on the mental state of the patient. Short periods of remission alternated with worsening psychiatric symptoms. Dr. Richarz did not want Clara to visit her husband, explaining this by a fear that such meetings could increase the excitability of the patient, and even could end with an attempt at suicide. Even her letters were stopped, so that Schumann asked Johannes Brahms, the famous composer and a long-time friend, who was a visitor at one point, whether his wife had died. Clara, despite the fact that she was very busy, was interested in her husband's state, and it pained her that she was unable to visit. She worked hard, taught piano, and spent much time organizing concerts or musical *turnees*. One of these involved visits to Liverpool and Manchester, in England, and in Dublin, Ireland, where she gave almost thirty public and private concerts. (46) One cannot but be surprised at her hard work. She had to support seven children and had large bills to pay for her husband's stay in the hospital. Schumann's mental state continued to deteriorate. Convulsive episodes tormented him, and he had occasional tremors, suffered from auditory hallucinations or talked to himself. He would walk around his room without purpose, or fall to his knees, wringing his hands. He was often violent and loud, and yelled or spoke incoherently. (46, 47) Nonetheless, there were periods when he was calmer and thought sensibly. His connection with the external world and the source of information about his wife and family was Brahms, whose assistance to the patient and his family was difficult to overstate.

In April of 1856, after visiting him in the hospital, Brahms wrote that Schumann had changed a great deal. The patient recognized him, and was very happy with the visit, but Brahms couldn't understand a single word spoken by Schumann. The latter spoke almost without ceasing, but it was an unrecognizable stammering. (48) Clara was informed about her husband's deteriorating state, and allowed a final visit; the description brings tears to ones eyes. (48) Robert Schumann died July 29, 1866.

For many years, it was not recognized that Schumann's mental illness was a sequel to luetic infection. Dr. Richarz's notes were not published until 1991, over a hundred years after the composer's death. Until that time, it was judged that the cause of that death was other conditions. One of them was supposed to have been poisoning with the mercury used in the treatment of his syphilis. The labile character, suicide attempt, periods of intensive creativity alternating with depressive states, all these signs leaned toward a diagnosis of bipolar disorder, schizophrenia or other mental illness. (49) During the autopsy of Schumann's remains, however, a yellow, gelatinous tumor was discovered at the base of the brain. We do not know the results of the histologic testing of the tumor. It could have been one of the brain tumors, but it could also have been a gumma. Gummas were a frequent sign of third-stage syphilis. They appeared in the skin, the periosteum, frequently in the brain, and less often in other organs. It is very probable that the tumor found during autopsy of Schumann's brain was a gumma, a sign of late syphilis. (50) In addition to the tumor, "atrophy of the brain, thickening of the leptomeninges ... and their adherence to the cerebral cortex in several places" were noted; such changes are often seen in persons dying with general paresis.

BEDRICH SMETANA (1824-1884)

Bedrich Smetana is known as the father of Czech music. Many musical authorities do not recognize the "nationality of music;" nonetheless, it is not difficult to disagree with this opinion (Fig. 5a.7). When I listen to the works of Grieg or Sibelius, their music conjures up for me landscapes of Norwegian fjords or Finnish forests and lakes. When I hear Chopin, I remember walks in the park of Zelazowa Wola, (Chopin's birthplace), and see the plains of the Mazowsze landscapes in Poland. Everyone who listens to a performance of Tchaikovsky's *Piano Concerto in B-minor* will associate its first chords with a view of the *Sobor Vasyla Blazennego*, St. Basil's Cathedral on Red square in Moscow, whereas someone listening to Copeland's composition of

"Rodeo," undoubtedly – and defenselessly – associates it with Texas.

This is so, also, with Smetana's symphonic poem, "Ma Vlast" (My Fatherland), whose beginning (played by flutes) brings to mind the sough of a mountain stream, and upon listening further, we float along the Vltava River in the middle of the Czech landscape.

In the case of Bedrich Smetana, there also appears a certain element of patriotism, since during the time in which he lived and created the Czech nation did not exist, as its lands were included in the Austro-Hungarian Empire. Composing national music at a certain period, he did so knowingly on a wave of patriotic sentiments, or even nationalistic feelings, carrying over his investment to the so-called "People's Spring," when in 1848, the people of the Habsburg Empire demanded more national and personal freedom.

In similarity to the majority of musicians about whom I have written up to this point, so also Smetana was infected with music almost from childhood. Playing the violin he learned from his father, and performed in public for the first time at age six. Bedrich appeared in Prague at age fifteen, as a student of the Prague Academic Grammar School, where he found his way into an environment of youth with a national patriotic mindset. Education in school did not interest him much, and he often was a truant. On the other hand, he regularly went to concerts, and joined an amateur string quartet. He also tried to compose. His father, the manager of a brewery, did not see a career in music for his son and transferred him from Prague to *Nove Mesto*, where his cousins lived. There, young Bedrich became romantically involved with his cousin daughter, Louisa, the fruit of which was the composition of a polka, (Louisa's Polka), and Smetana's transfer to Pilsen, another Czech town, and one known for its excellent beer. Smetana spent three years there, finished middle school, while yielding to romances with many young women, of which one, Katherina Kolarova, later became his wife. Young Bedrich was in love with her up to his ears, and wrote in his diary, "When I am not with her, I feel as though I am sitting on hot coals, and cannot experience peace."

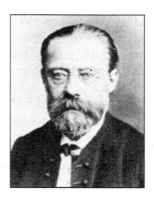

Figure 5a.7 Bedrich Smetana (before 1880)

In 1843, Smetana returned to Prague, and began musical studies in the Prague Music Institute, for which he paid with his own money, earned by giving music lessons. One of his employers was Count Thun, at whose estate he met the Robert and Clara Schumanns. He presented them his latest composition, "Sonata in G-minor," anticipating their delight, but it was received without any great enthusiasm. In 1848, the period of "the People's Spring," found him in Prague, where he took part in revolutionary incidents on the side of Czech patriots. Smetana, a Czech patriot, did not speak their language, yet, nonetheless, composed several patriotic musical works. The same year, Smetana opened his own school of music, the Piano Institute, at first with not a great number of students. Shortly thereafter, he married Katherina, his beloved from Pilsen, and moved his school to a building that was the property of Katherina's parents. The school grew greatly, and had a good reputation, thanks to, among other reasons, frequent visits by Franz Liszt, with whom

Smetana had become friends. Despite many successes, including those of composition, Smetana became disenchanted with Prague, and, in 1856, left for Sweden. He was employed as piano teacher by the wife of a rich businessman from Goteborg. He gave frequent recitals and concerts, and there enjoyed the local social life. He became popular, and many ladies wanted to take lessons from him, so that he complained that it was "difficult for him to keep pace with such a demand." (51) One female student whom he did not refuse, a young married woman, Frojda Benecke, soon became his muse and mistress. It was in her honor that he composed a transcription of two of Schubert's songs from the cycle, *Die Schone Mullerin*. Smetana composed a great deal, and frequently traveled to Prague. During one of these trips, his wife, who had long been ill with tuberculosis, died. Bedrich had four daughters with her, of which three had died in childhood. A year later, Smetana married again, to Bettina Ferdinandova, younger than he by sixteen years, and with whom he returned to Goteborg. His popularity in Goteborg rose and in the spring of 1861, he gave a concert in Stockholm where he was applauded by the Swedish Royal Family. Despite his successes in Sweden, Smetana returned to Prague, encouraged by numerous patriotic events. He began an intensive study of the Czech language, wanting to give proof of his completely belonging to that nation. During this time, many compositions of a "nationalist character" appeared, while the composer himself received an ever-greater acknowledgement from his fellow countrymen. He won the competition for a Czech patriotic opera, having entered his *"Braniboři v Čechách"* ("The Brandenburgers in Bohemia"). Smetana conducted the performance of this work in the so-called Provisional Theater, which was to become the venue for performances of Czech national productions. Smetana sought the directorship of the Prague Conservatory, but unsuccessfully, although, in autumn of 1866, he was nominated director of the Provisional Theater.

In May 1866, the premier of his best-known opera, *Prodaná nevěsta* (The Bartered Bride), was performed. This is a comic opera about cheerful life in the Czech nation, in which there appear: a beautiful damsel, the farmer's son, the village idiot, a circus troupe, and a chorus singing about good Czech beer. This was agreeable, though nationalistic, something that the composer intended. In addition to the operas already mentioned, Smetana composed another two: *Dalibor*, and, in 1872, *Libuse*, one of the most ambitious of his compositions, the premiere of which was withheld until 1881, the date of the opening of the National Theater in Prague.

Up to this point in Smetana's biography, there was no real information about the state of his health, until, in 1874, he noted in his diary, on April 30, that he had an ulcer (he did not write where), while in July of the same year (2-3 months from the appearance of the ulcer), that he had a throat infection and a rash. Next, there appears information about blockage of his ear, hearing problems and dizziness. In September, Smetana wrote to his superior about "the cruel fate," that he had met. He was hearing sounds of varying tones, and said that he had "a roar in his ears, as though he were standing next to a great waterfall." (52) He was already practically deaf in his right ear, and in October he no longer heard in either ear.

Personal conflicts with important people in the musical life of Prague and problems with his hearing forced Smetana to resign from the Provisional Theater. This affected his financial situation, which was saved by benefit concerts organized by his friends and former mistress, Frojda Benecke. He composed a great deal, but complained "Deafness would have been relatively tolerable, were it only quiet inside my head." (53) From this period come many of his loud operas, well-known string quartets, and vocal and piano compositions. It is also when the cycle of symphonic poems entitled, "Ma Vlast" (My Homeland), appeared, creations that, even for a poorly discriminating or less sophisticated listener, evoke the Czech nation and Smetana's name. It is also in this period that the "String Quartet in E-minor" was composed; it begins with music resembling an intruding roar in one's ears!

The composer sought treatment, both at home and abroad, but unfortunately, without any great effect. Smetana was close to a breakdown, and, as he noted in his diary in January, 1875, "If my disease is not curable, I would rather be freed from such a life." (53a) During short periods of remission, he tried to compose, but works begun gave way to interruptions, due to the worsening state of his health. In October 1883, in the course of a banquet, he behaved inappropriately, causing a loss of self-confidence and boycotting by his friends. Four months later, he stopped reasoning logically and periodically became violent. Next, there appeared depression, insomnia and hallucinations, followed by dizziness, muscle cramps, and speech disturbances. In April of the same year, his family, unable to take care of him at home, confined him to a psychiatric hospital in Prague, where Bedrich Smetana died in May 1884.

The circumstances of Smetana's infection with syphilis are not known. It appears almost certain that the ulcer described by him in 1874 was a primary chancre, while the throat changes and rash were evidence of the disease's progressing to its secondary stage (secondary syphilis). In this second stage, there can appear symptoms of ear involvement; these are commonly bilateral, although they may occur in one after the other ear in a short period of time. Accompanying them there is often rapidly progressive loss of hearing, and a significant decrease in bone conduction of sound. Quite characteristic is ear pain at night. With today's methods of treatment, these symptoms remit very quickly. Unfortunately, in Smetana's time, such effective treatment was not known.

Symptoms of general paresis after four-five years from infection may confirm a luetic etiology. It appears that the cause of illness and death in Smetana's case provokes no diagnostic reservations, a conclusion which is supported by the results of his autopsy, published by a German neurologist, Dr. Ernst Levin, in 1972, as well as by the results of tests on material obtained after exhumation, performed in the tw^{entieth} century, which corroborated a diagnosis of syphilis. As is common in such cases, there was no shortage of skeptics, who had alternative opinions, despite the fact that, shortly after his death, the composer's family admitted that the disease, which developed in Smetana after 1873 was caused by a syphilitic infection.

HUGO WOLF (1860-1903)

Hugo Wolf was born four years after Schumann's death. As a composer, he is known for his authorship of lyrical songs, grouped in cycles, and depending on the poets to whose works he composed the music (Fig.5a.8) In his early creative period, he imitated the works of Schubert and Schumann, with whom he also shared a common disease. He was an ardent critic of the creativity of Brahms, the same Brahms who took care of Schumann during his illness, and later of Schuman's wife and his family for many years.

Wolf was born in Gradec in Slovenia, then a province of Austro-Hungary. The greater part of his life, however, was spent in Vienna. Even in childhood, he studied the violin and piano, and subsequently continued his musical education at the Vienna Conservatory. In school, he had never-ending problems, devolving either from a lack of interest in the subjects taught, or as a result of bad behavior. At the conservatory, he befriended Gustave Mahler. Wolf and Mahler shared an apartment, not rarely sleeping in a single bed, and often having to share the proverbial bread crust. On occasion, as a result of a shortage of funds, they had to sleep under the bare

sky. (54) In contrast to Mahler, Wolf did not finish his musical studies, as he was dismissed from the conservatory due to breach of discipline. After dismissal, Wolf taught music and composed, and, because he had talent and a personal charm, easily won over people, who then helped him.

One of his sponsors was the father of Vally Franck—the young woman with whom he fell in love, and to whom he was engaged for close to three years. They broke up just before Wolf's 21st birthday, and the causes of the end of their informal union could have been many. If one can believe the accounts of Alma Mahler, Gustave's wife, Wolf became infected with syphilis at age seventeen during a visit to the bordello that was funded by his friend Adalbert, who was a pianist. (55) This is supposed to have been the year before he met Vally, and may have been concealed from her, only later coming to light. Another cause may have been the unstable character of the composer, suggesting, according to some biographers, bipolar disorder, which makes long-term life with such a person difficult to endure.

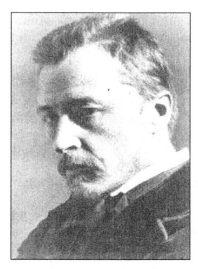

Figure 5a.8 Hugo Wolf (1860-1903)

Regardless of the causes, the fact is that the young couple broke up, and Hugo returned to his family for a short time. For a while, he worked as second director (second *Kappelmeister*) in Salzburg, but didn't distinguish himself in anything, and, after less than a year returned to Vienna in order to teach music. He again composed songs, but it was noted that his choice of the texts to which he composed his music was different: they now expressed suffering, a sense of sinfulness, and sorrow. This could be consistent with suppositions that Wolf was overwhelmed with sorrow caused perhaps by his recent breakup with his beloved, or the awareness that the disease from which he suffered could be the beginning of his end. Other cause could be depression if his mental condition was due to bipolar disorder. At about this time, he tested his skills as a music critic. In his opinions about the creativeness of other composers, he could be mocking and severe, which did not gain him friends. About Brahms he said, "He is only an imitator, and attributed only one quality to him – skillful professionalism." (56) Wolf maintained that Brahms' entire set of works was a splendid variation on the creative theme of Beethoven, Mendelsohn and Schumann. One can readily conceive that the ridiculed and insulted musicians did not feel that they owed him anything! Brahms spitefully wrote that "thanks to the creativity of Wolf, modern song-writing attained its limits". (57) The aggressive tone of Wolf's articles gave him the nickname "Wild Wolf."

I have already mentioned that during his earlier, creative phase, Wolf imitated Schubert and Schumann, but that his real, yet never-attained, example was Richard Wagner. Wolf greatly mourned the death of his master, and in February, 1883 composed one of his best-known songs, *"Zur Ruh zur Ruh"* ("To Peace, to Peace"), which is like an elegy in Wagner's honor. Besides Wagner, he greatly treasured composer's father-in-law, Franz Liszt, who, for his part, expressed himself very flatteringly about the creativity of Wolf, and encouraged him to compose greater musical works, such as symphonies or operas. Wolf composed a string quartet in D-major, a symphonic creation of Penthesillea, and one of the better known of his creations, the "Italian Serenade," which began as a string quartet, but was later transformed into an orchestral version. Wolf also composed two operas, *Der Corregidor*, and *Manuel Venegas*. The latter, he couldn't finish as a result of a nervous breakdown. The libretto of *Der Corregidor* is about a marriage triangle, reminiscent of his own experience, when he fell in love with Melanie Kochert, the wife of a friend. The husband eventually found out about the long-lasting romance of his wife with Wolf, but, did not divorce her, and even helped Wolf during his later, difficult moments.

In September 1897, as a result of delusions, in which he imagined himself to be the director of the Viennese Opera, Wolf wanted to dismiss Mahler. The same evening, he became aggressive, and attacked the hotel concierge. After this incident, and using subterfuge, Hugo was placed into an insane asylum, where for a time, he was afflicted by a variety of hallucinations. After remission of symptoms, he was discharged from the hospital, but was no longer capable of independent existence, nor of any creative work. Wolf recognized this fact, and in October tried to commit suicide. He threw himself into the river, but after a few moments, the cold waters of the Danube revived him, and, changing his mind about suicide, he swam to the riverbank. This episode again landed him in a hospital for the mentally ill. During glimmers of normalcy, Wolf tried to play the piano, but, despite periods of remission, his mental state worsened, month by month. From September 1901 he was continuously bed-ridden. Hugo Wolf died February 22, 1903.

Wolf's last love, Melanie Kochert, visited him in the hospital, and took care of him to the end. Her former marital life with her husband ceased to be tenable, and pangs of conscience or Wolf's death induced her to follow in the footsteps of her lover. Melanie committed suicide three years later.

What the cause of the mental illness and death of the composer was is difficult to determine with certainty. From early youth, he was a person of labile character, with features of bipolar psychosis. Taking into account his earlier infection with syphilis, his last years could indicate that symptoms of general paresis had developed, and that these could have been the beginning of the end for the composer.

FREDERICK DELIUS (1862-1934)

The history of the disease of Frederick Delius is an example of how various forms of third-stage syphilis influence the life and creativity of prominent artists. In the cases of Schumann, Wolf or Donizetti, the illness definitively finished the period of their creative work. Delius, fortunately, did not suffer from general paresis, and, despite a serious disability, managed to work creatively almost until his death, thanks to the help of his wife and sacrifices of his friends.

Frederick Delius is, together with Elgar, Williams and Britten, one of the most prominent British composers of the nineteenth and twentieth centuries. He was born in Bradford, England, the son of a wealthy wool merchant of German origin (Fig.5a.9). Even as a young boy, he played the violin and piano, and was very interested in music. During his studies at the International College in Isleworth, Delius did not apply himself especially to them, spending the majority of his time at concerts and the London opera. His father, for whom Frederick's career as a musician was totally disagreeable, tried to employ him in his own firm, sending him to his businesses in France, Germany and Sweden. When he had already completely lost hope that his son would develop into a proper merchant, he sent him in 1884 to the United States, where Delius was to manage an orange plantation in Florida. According to another version, it is said that the initiative for going to Florida was Frederick's own, who, watching the performance of a Negro concert group in England, became interested in this type of music, and wanted to learn more on the subject. After arriving in Solano Grove, not far from Jacksonville, Delius, instead of occupying himself with the cultivation of oranges, began to learn music from Thomas Ward, an organist from Brooklyn, who had come to Florida to improve the state of his health, which had been weakened by tuberculosis.

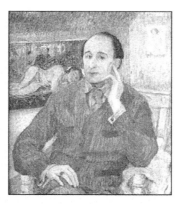

Figure 5a.9 Portrait of Frederick Delius (1912) painted by his wife Jelka Rosen

Listening to Negro music coming from the steamboats coursing along the St. John's River, and observing nature in Florida, Delius, who was later named a musical impressionist, was gathering material for his later compositions. Apparently, in addition to Negro melodies, he was charmed by a certain black-skinned beauty, (*Zwei braune Augen,* Two Black Eyes) with whom he is supposed to have had a child. There are also suggestions, that during his time in Florida, he could have become infected with syphilis. The credibility of these revelations is questionable, while their author, Percy Grainger, is accused of easy credulity. Apparently, he took too literally the stories of Delius, who was famous for making up various tales that were not always true. (58) After leaving Florida and a short stay in Virginia, Delius returned to Europe. His father reconciled himself with the thought that "nothing will come of my son," and financed a half-year's course of study at the conservatory in Leipzig, Germany. It was in Leipzig that Delius met Edward Grieg, the famous Norwegian composer, who, after listening to the former, declared to Delius' father that a splendid musical future was opening up before his son.

In 1888, Delius moved to Paris, where he spent the next 8 years. He immediately found his way into the Parisian Bohemia, to which belonged mainly writers and painters, who displayed their works in the so-called Salon of Independents. There, Delius befriended the Swedish dramatist, August Strindberg, the Norwegian painter Edward Munch, and the French impressionist painter, Paul Gaugin. The environment in which he now found himself was characterized by great sexual freedom, the sequel to which was a large number of syphilitics among them, for instance, Paul Gaugin, Eduard Manet and Henri Toulouse-Lautrec. Delius easily adapted himself to the mores of his new friends, because as his biographer, Diana McVeagh wrote, "He was found to be attractive, warm-hearted, spontaneous and amorous." (59) It would appear that it was in just this period that Delius contracted syphilis, which became the cause of his disabilities in later years.

Being in this artistic environment, Delius befriended the sculptor, August Rodin, known for his courageous sculptures and drawings saturated with eroticism. He also met his future wife, Helene Rosen, known as Jelka. Jelka was a paintress and friend of Rodin, younger than Frederick by four years. She very quickly became interested in the young composer, who was not indifferent to her charms. Bringing them closer was also a mutual interest in the works of Frederick Nietzsche, the German philosopher, who spent his last years in a psychiatric hospital as a result of general paresis caused by syphilis. After a short period of separation, caused by Delius' voyage to America (supposedly he was trying to find his earlier love and child), Delius moved into a house in Grez, near Paris, bought for him by Jelka. Mr. and Mrs. Delius lived there, with a short interruption during the war period, to the ends of their lives. Frederick was not a good husband. Capricious and demanding, he had frequent romances outside the marriage, which were tolerated with leniency by his wife, who, especially in the first years of their conjugal life, financially supported her husband.

Delius did not have good relations with the French musicians, and a large part of his creativity during this period was displayed in Germany and England. Thus, premieres of his better-known works, such as *Koanga*, a piano concerto in C-minor, and *Appalachia*, a choral-orchestral variation, based on Negro musical themes he heard in Florida, also took place in Germany. "The Sea Drift," a cantata to the words of the poet Walt Whitman had its premiere in 1906 in Essen, Germany, while the opera, *A Village Romeo and Juliet*, premiered in Berlin the following year.

In the beginning phase of Delius' creativity, one recognizes the influences of Grieg, Wagner, Chopin and Tchaikovsky. By his later years, he had developed his own style, unlike that of anyone else's. Similarly to his painter friends, he was an impressionist to the extent that, in music, he drew his inspiration from nature; he painted with sounds.

A great promoter of Delius' music in England was the well-known British director, Thomas Beecham. Being the manager of the New Symphony Orchestra, and director of the Royal Opera House, Beecham introduced Delius' compositions into repertoires of concerts performed by himself. It was he who organized a six-day festival dedicated to the creativity of Frederick Delius in 1929, when the composer was already seriously ill. Taking part was Delius, himself, unfortunately having to be brought for this occasion in an invalid or bath chair. Present at the festival was Neville Cardus, music critic for the *Manchester Guardian* newspaper, who described Delius as a "physical wreck, yet there was nothing pitiable about him... his face was strong and disdainful, every line graven on it by intrepid living." (59a)

After the end of the First World War, the Deliuses returned to France, and again took up residence in Grez. Unfortunately, the disease progressed, and symptoms attesting to the take-over of the central nervous system by lues, in the form of *tabes dorsalis*, appeared. Treatments in several locations in Europe produced no results and strained the family budget. In 1922, Delius was no longer able to move about without the help of two canes, while in the course of the next six years, the disease led to complete paralysis of the extremities and to blindness, though preserving his intellectual functions in not too bad a state. Friends and admirers of the composer supported him financially. One of the young lovers of Delius' creativity, when learning that the sick composer was still striving to compose by dictating the musical notes to his wife, offered his services *gratis*. He was Eric Fenby, a subsequent author of many publications about Delius, and an ardent lover and promoter of his music. With the help of Fenby, many new compositions and revisions of earlier creations appeared. The effects of their joint work, are such creations as: "Cynara" (to the words of Ernest Dowson), "A Song of Summer," the prelude "Irmellin," and "The Idyll;" the last was a revision of an earlier opera by Delius, *"Margot la Rouge"* ("Margot the Red"), and many others. This strange compositional collaboration lasted four years, and was not easy for either party. The composer was impatient and criticized the young man, saying that he did not grasp and understand his intentions quickly enough. (60) This impatience doubtless irritated Fenby, as did the caprices of the sick man. The work, which they undertook was uncommonly exhausting, but was carried out relatively efficiently, despite the advanced illness of its major executor.

As Fenby wrote: "The complexity of thinking in so many strands, often all at once; the problem of orchestral and vocal balance; the wider area of possible misunderstandings...resulted in that, after every such session, both were completely exhausted. (61) I underline that this is what the young man wrote of his collaboration with the composer in the latter's last stage of syphilis.

The story of Fenby's collaboration with Delius attained a screening as the film, *The Song of Summer*, by Ken Russel, filmed by British Broadcasting Corporation (BBC) television in 1968. It shows the difficult relationship between the composer and his young assistant, showing that Delius, who, though completely paralyzed and blind, managed to work creatively (Fig.5a.10).

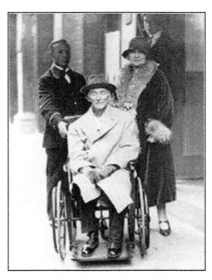

Figure 5a.10 Portrait of Frederick Delius in wheelchair due to tabes dorsalis caused by syphilis

The creativity of Frederick Delius is not as well-known and liked as that of other musicians of this period; it never became fashionable. As Fenby writes, "The music of Delius is not an acquired taste. One either likes it the moment one first hears it, or the sound of it is once and forever distasteful to one. It is an art which will never enjoy an appeal to many, but one which will always be loved, and dearly be loved, by the few." (62) Personally, I belong to those few. I encourage you to listen to it.

SCOTT JOPLIN (1868-1917)

Scott Joplin, an African-American composer, was born in Eastern Texas between June 1867 and January 1868; the exact date is not known (63-65) (Fig.5a.11). His father was a farm laborer, while his mother worked as a domestic.

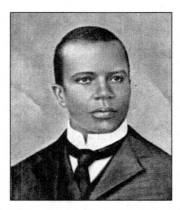

Figure 5a 11 Photograph of Scott Joplin (ca 1900)

Scott, who was the second of six children of Giles Joplin and Florence Givens, represented the first post-slavery generation of African-Americans. A few years after Scott's birth, the family settled in Texarkana, where his father got a job as a laborer for the railroad, and his mother did laundry and cleaning to supplement their modest income. (66)

The Joplin family was a musical one. Giles played the violin, while his mother played the banjo, and sang. At the age of seven, Scott began playing the piano in the house of the white family where his mother washed clothes. He began to play the piano on his own, but soon his obvious talent was noticed by a local music teacher, Julius Weiss, a Jewish immigrant from Germany. Impressed by the talented young black boy, Weiss taught him free of charge for several years. (67) It was he who introduced Scott to folk and classical music, including operas, playing for him, and teaching him about the great European composers. Julius Weiss helped Scott's mother to buy a used piano, which enabled the young boy to play whenever he wished. Weiss also stimulated and encouraged his pupil to become a composer. In later years, Joplin didn't forget Weiss' role in his career, and helped his former teacher financially until he died.

In the 1880s, Scott Joplin lived for a time in Sedalia, Missouri, and attended Lincoln High School in the black neighborhood (68). Some sources tell us that he went on to St. Louis to begin his career in music in a city that was to become an important center of ragtime. In 1891, Joplin returned to Texarkana, and started working as an itinerant musician with a minstrel troupe, a popular form of entertainment in those days. There were very few opportunities for a black man starting a career in music to obtain a permanent job other than in churches, dance halls or brothels. Joplin traveled around the Midwest and South with different musical troupes, playing pre-ragtime music, mainly in various red-light districts.

In 1893, during the World Fair in Chicago, Joplin performed for the visitors, playing in the saloons, cafes and brothels of the Tenderloin District. In Chicago, Joplin organized his first musical group, which allowed him to select and arrange music for the band to play. It is believed that Chicago's World Fair, attended by 27 million people, had a profound effect on the popularity of ragtime music, which, a few years later, became a national craze across the country.

After the Fair, Scott Joplin returned to Missouri, and joined a cornet band in Sedalia. Shortly thereafter, he formed his own group of musicians, with whom he traveled around, performing at various events. He also played the piano at two social clubs in Sedalia, the "Maple Leaf Club" and the "Black 400 Club," both attended by "respectable black gentlemen." It is believed that his most famous composition, "The Maple Leaf Rag," published in 1899, was named after the Sedalia club, but there is no direct evidence in support of such a link. During his work in Sedalia, Joplin taught piano to several students, including future ragtime composers, such as Brun Campbell and Scott Hayden. (69)

Joplin's first two compositions, two songs, titled "Please Say You Will," and "A Picture of Her Face," were published in 1895 in Syracuse, N.Y., while in 1898, he published six new pieces, including his first rag composition, "Original Rags." There is no doubt that rag music, especially his signature tune, "The Maple Leaf Rag," boosted Joplin's popularity, and made him one of the top performers of ragtime music, which was becoming more and more popular.

Shortly after publication of "The Maple Leaf Rag," Joplin composed "The Ragtime Dance," a kind of ballet, which showed the type of dancing in Sedalia's Maple Leaf and Black 400 Clubs. The dance was staged at Wood's Opera House in Sedalia in November of 1899, and was performed by young Sedalians from the Black 400 Club. A few years later, Joplin undertook even more ambitious projects, namely two operas, *A Guest of Honor* and *Treemonisha*. The first of these was staged in several States, but had no luck. During the tour, somebody associated with the opera company created by Joplin stole the box-office money, and Joplin couldn't meet the payroll nor pay all the bills. It was said that the score of the opera was lost, and probably destroyed, due to the default on payment of the company's boarding house bills. (70) *Treemonisha*, his second opera, was also a failure. Its libretto told the story of a black American woman who was educated (taught to read) by a white woman, and who subsequently became a leader of the local community, leading her town's people out of ignorance and superstition to racial equality. The heroine is persecuted for her convictions and is about to be thrown into a wasp's nest, but finally is saved by her friend. The story emphasized the importance of education in the fight against racism. Joplin was the author of both the libretto and the musical score, and it is clear that part of it was a tribute to his own mother, whose hard work, persistence and constant encouragement allowed Joplin to pursue his musical career. The opera was an amalgamation of a European opera production (some say it has elements of Richard Wagner) and African American folk tales. *Treemonisha*, staged for the first time in New York, was a financial failure. Poorly staged, it went unnoticed, nearly causing its author to have a nervous breakdown. (71)

Joplin's operas, at least initially, were great disappointments; however, his light compositions, especially those done in the increasingly popular ragtime style, achieved recognition. While still in St. Louis at the beginning of the new century, Joplin composed several of his best-known works, such as "The Entertainer," "March Majestic," and the afore-mentioned "Ragtime Band." Other well-received works include "Cascades," written for the Chicago Fair, "The Sycamore," "The Favorite," and "The Chrysanthemum," dedicated to his second wife. Together with Louis Chauvin, Joplin composed "Heliotrope Bouguet," one of his most charming rags. The style of music that he composed was very popular in those days, and was played in almost every nightclub, bar and dance hall across the country. It is important to note that Joplin, who was by [then][already a well-known composer, added his name to that of Chauvin in order to help his younger colleague financially, who was a drug addict and was dying of syphilis. (72)

The new style in popular music became unusually widespread in the U.S.A. at the beginning of the last century. Works in the Ragtime style were performed in almost every meeting hall and dance club, and also in nightclubs and bars. Ragtime was played either by live pianists or recorded on paper rolls for mechanical pianos.

Joplin's artistic life, which was a mixture of successes and failures, was very similar to his private live: a mixture of happiness and tragedy. Joplin was married three times. His first wife was Belle, the widow of Scott Hayden's older brother. (73) They had a baby daughter who died only a few months after birth. The cause of her death remains a mystery and, one may ask the question of whether the newly born baby could have suffered from congenital syphilis. It was a well-known fact that Scott Joplin had syphilis, which he most likely contracted while working in the red-light districts of Sedalia, Chicago, or anywhere else. Regardless of the death of their first offspring, the relationship with Belle was difficult, as she had no interest in music.

During one of his visits to Arkansas, Joplin met a 19-year-old woman, Freddie Alexander, and fell in love. After a short period of separation from Belle, he finally divorced her, and returned to Little Rock to marry Freddie in June 1904. The newlywed couple returned to Sedalia, where Scott continued his concerts and composing. Unfortunately, their happiness didn't last long. One day, Freddie caught a cold that developed into pneumonia, which was very often an incurable disease in those days. She died of complications, barely ten weeks after the wedding day. (74) Joplin's first composition after her death was "Bethema," recognized as one of the most beautiful ragtime waltzes.

Later, while in New York, where Joplin was working on his opera, *Treemonisha*, he met Lottie Stokes, whom he married in either sometime between 1907-10. (75) One of his biographers, Vera Brodsky Lawrence, suggested that Joplin was aware of the consequences of late syphilis and the state of his health, and, therefore, worked feverishly to orchestrate his opera, "consciously racing against time," trying to complete it before it was too late.

Although there are no samples of audio recordings of Joplin's playing the piano, there are seven piano rolls that give us some idea of his musical style, at least as used with mechanical pianos. All were made in 1916, and many of them reveal signs of neurologic problems related to syphilis. Joplin's biographer Edward A. Berlin theorized that already in

St. Louis, Joplin experienced a disordered movement of his fingers, as well as tremors and slurred speech, (76) the signs indicating *tabes dorsalis* or tabo-paralysis. One of the rolls, on which Joplin played his signature tune, "The Maple Leaf Rag," was described as shocking ... disorganized and distressing to hear. (76a)

In 1916, Joplin suffered what was described as a "nervous breakdown," and in January 1917, he was admitted to a mental institution in New York, the Manhattan State Hospital. He died three months later (of dementia), at the age of 49. From then on, he was practically forgotten as a man and musician, as jazz replaced ragtime as the popular music until the latter's revival in the 1970s. In the meantime, some jazz musicians included ragtime in their works of "traditional jazz," but the real revival exploded in the 1970s, when Joplin's music inspired the director of the film, *The Sting*, to use it in the score. Music in *The Sting* included Joplin's classics, such as "Pineapple Rag," "The Entertainer," "The Easy Woman," and "Solace." This very popular movie, in which leading roles were played by Paul Newman and Robert Redford, won many awards, including the one for best music. Since the success of *The Sting*, Joplin's music became very popular, and was included into the repertoire of famous piano performances and renowned orchestras, for instance the Boston Pops. Even *Treemonisha* was staged in a full opera production by the Houston Grand Opera, with world famous sopranos Carmen Balthrop, alternating with Kathleen Battle as the title character. Today, Scott Joplin is recognized as a talented composer who was able to merge white European classical forms with African-American rhythms and harmony. Not without reason, he was named the *American Schubert*, by one of his biographers, for his talent in composing small musical forms – and, perhaps, the same fate shared with Schubert—syphilis, which ruined both of their lives.

WOLFGANG A. MOZART (1756-1791); LUDWIG van BEETHOVEN (1770-1827)

Writing about famous composers in the context of syphilis, one cannot fail to mention Mozart and Beethoven. Both composers have been the subject of innumerable biographies and works, concerning not only their creativity, but also their private lives. In many of these can be found details about the intimate lives of the composers, together with commentaries about diseases that touched them, not excluding syphilis.

I will start with Wolfgang Amadeus Mozart, about whom it will be easier for me to prove that accounts of his being ill with syphilis are the product of pure fantasy. Information on Mozart's supposed syphilis is derived from gossip, and even more specifically, gossip in which one originator states that the composer fell victim to poisoning with mercuric chloride, the sublimate used in those days in the treatment of lues. This information appeared in 1963 in a book authored by German physician, Dieter Kerner, under the title, *Krankheiten grosser Musiker,* or Illnesses of the Great Musicians. (78) One of them says that Mozart was being poisoned with mercury, not only by the composer Antonio Salieri, who was jealous of Mozart's talent, but also by Gottfried van Swieten, the son of Gerhard van Swieten, known to us from the chapter on the treatment of syphilis, and discoverer of the famous Liquor for the disease. (79) Those who saw Milosz Forman's excellent film from the 1980s under the title of *Amadeus* certainly remember the figure of Baron Gottfried van Swieten, lover of Mozart's music, who, in one scene of the film, shields Mozart when criticized by the director of the Imperial opera.

The authors of the aforementioned book suggest that Mozart was covertly given sublimate of mercury during the concerts, which were performed regularly in the home of Baron von Swieten. One can pose the question, was the

176

Baron treating Mozart by doing so, or was he trying to poison him? The whole story is preposterous, because the Baron could not treat Mozart, as he was not a physician, nor try to poison him, as he was his friend and protector. It was none other than Gottfried van Swieten who helped finance Mozart's family and after his death took care of his funeral.

Another hypothesis provided concerning the cause of Mozart's death says that it was an *unintended* poisoning with mercury. The famous composer was supposed to have taken it for syphilis, which he brought upon himself in the bad company of the theater's director, Emanuel Schikander.

> Mozart acquired, or believed acquired syphilis during a liaison that occurred in the summer of 1791. (His wife was pregnant and in Spa at that time and Mozart and Schikander were partying in the company of other ladies). By the fall, as the signs became apparent to him, he began to treat himself with the remedy of the day – Van Swieten's liquor, developed by Gerhard van Swieten just a few decades earlier. (79a)

It is probably true that Schikander was a debaucher, and it could be that he was ill with syphilis, but that has nothing to do with Mozart. Emanuel Schikander, the author of the libretto, *The Magic Flute*, and performer of the principal role, did work with Mozart, and was friends with him, but this does not mean that they had to be ill with the same disease.

Mozart had enough problems with his health on his own. At age sixteen during travel to Italy, he became infected with the virus of hepatitis; after his return, he felt very weak and his skin had a yellowish tint. (80) He had frequent angina, periodontal abscesses, and scarlet fever. It is most likely that it was these infections, produced mainly by hemolytic streptococci that give rise to rheumatic fever (rheumatic inflammation of the joints and heart) that according the opinion of most examiners shortened the life of the genius composer. It is said that another cause of his death could have been renal failure and uremia, inasmuch as, shortly before his death he fell into a coma.

In Mozart's time, because of the low level of home sanitation, and of a generally low level of hygiene in society, rheumatic fever was encountered thirty times more frequently than now, while its course was far more severe. (81) Even in his youth, Mozart had attacks of this disease, while the one which led to his death was the fourth in a row. For fifteen days before his death, Mozart had a fever and painful swellings of the hands and feet, causing him to be unable to move, while a rash appeared on his skin. Mozart's wife and her sister, sewed special nightshirts for him to be warm because due to the swellings he could not turn around in bed. Physicians who were summoned employed measures typical for fevers at the time, i.e. cold compresses, emetics, and bloodletting, which doubtless speeded the composer's death.

It is interesting that one of the physicians wrote that, during Mozart's last illness, "The disease simultaneously attacked many other inhabitants of Vienna, manifesting in a portion of these the same symptoms, and ending in the same way as Mozart's death." (82) It has been assumed that this could have been an epidemic of influenza, but one cannot exclude even other diseases. Recently a new concept has appeared, saying that Mozart could have died from trichinosis. That illness is usually caused by eating undercooked pork infested by a parasitic worm, *Trichina spiralis*. The signs are almost the same as those observed in Mozart's case, while its presence in others ill in Vienna at the time could indicate some form of mass infection from infected pork.

I believe that we will never learn what the truth is, as no autopsies were performed on Mozart's remains, while there is no possibility of exhumation, as Mozart was buried in a common grave, which, in addition, was used many times by others after him.

Beethoven's is a rather different story. Whereas in Mozart's case, one can state with considerable certainty that there was no credible evidence to the effect that he had syphilis, in Beethoven's case, the situation is not quite so clear. The author of one of the best books about Beethoven, George R. Marek, wrote in *Beethoven, Biography of a Genius* that "for every ten investigators contending that Beethoven did not have syphilis, there are another ten who maintain that he did. (83)

As for myself, until not so long ago, I belonged to a third group – those to whom it did not matter! However, now that I am writing about syphilis among musicians, I cannot avoid taking a side in this matter. After analyzing much evidence, or pseudo-evidence, and looking over a range of biographies and citations from declarations on the subject, and after comparing this information with a handbook of syphilology, plus my own experiences in this area, I came to the conclusion that there simply is not enough evidence to confirm that Beethoven was ill with syphilis. To the favorite arguments of the adherents of the hypothesis that Beethoven had lues belong excerpts from correspondence and statements of friends, but, above all, the results of post-mortem examination of his auditory organs. *Grove's Dictionary of Music and Musicians* states "All the symptoms were most likely caused by syphilitic infection in an early period of his life." Another source says:

> This diagnosis, for which I am indebted to the courtesy of my friend, Dr. Lauder Bruton, is supported by two discovered prescriptions, about which I learned from Mr. Thayer, after the writing of the words mentioned, while he, in turn learned about them from Dr. Bertolini. (84)

The first edition of *Grove's Dictionary* appeared in 1878, and as its author was known as a very upright man, it was accepted that deafness and some other health problems that Beethoven had were the result of infection with lues. In the autopsy report concerning changes in the auditory apparatus, the words "most likely" were used, whereas the diagnosis was given on the basis of a macroscopic evaluation of the appearance of this apparatus, without histopathologic testing, which would have been more convincing. Information on the subject of the two so-called prescriptions comes from a third or even fourth-hand source, and cannot be verified in any way. Those prescriptions, possibly for mercury ointment or cream have been lost, while Dr. Bertolini's notes and correspondence with his patient were purportedly lost by their owner during a cholera epidemic. Dr. Bertolini was said to have been convinced that he was going to die, and destroyed all of Beethoven's medical history in order to avoid compromising him. (84, 85) At this point, one would want to ask Dr. Bertolini whether he destroyed *all* of his patients' records, or was concerned exclusively about the reputation of Beethoven.

In regard to prescriptions for an ointment or cream containing mercury, it is worth remembering that mercury in medicine has been prescribed since time immemorial. Even in the tw[entieth] century, mercury ointment was used in treating infestations with pubic lice, as well as in some skin diseases of bacterial and even allergic etiology. Besides, even if such prescriptions by some miracle were re-discovered, they could not be used as proof of syphilis. Who will deny that mercury preparations might not have been prescribed for the composer for pubic lice, which he might have contracted during contact with some so called "rotten fortress?" [*vide infra*]. If Beethoven was, in fact, treated with mercury as a result of syphilis, he would have had to use it for a long time, which, as we know is associated with very sorry signs and symptoms that would have been visible to those around him.

Remember that Schubert wore a wig after mercury therapy, and didn't leave the house for a long time. Even if one were to accept that Beethoven took already known oral mercury preparations – and van Swieten's Liquor could have particularly suited him from the standpoint of its high alcohol concentration – then a generally recognized, multi-week treatment of someone could not have passed unnoticed due to the unpleasant breath odor and disagreeable body odor that appeared after a prolonged use of the medicine. (86)

In 1910, the laryngologist/otologist, Dr. Leon Jacobson, published an article, in which he asserted that Beethoven could have suffered from syphilis, although he did not state that this was the cause of his deafness. He also pointed to the swelling on the right side of Beethoven's skull as a sequel to luetic infection. It is visible on photographs of skull casts obtained during an exhumation, and also on a mask of the composer, made while he was still alive. (87) Another physician, Dr. Theodore von Frimmel, contends "the loss of hearing could have been only one of the symptoms, but that the disease itself has a different name." (88) Probably, he had syphilis in mind, but if so, why did he waver?

It is true that in syphilis, damage to the auditory apparatus can occur. One should add, however, that besides damage to the auditory nerve, damage to the vestibular nerve commonly occurs at the same time. Signs and symptoms of damage to these nerves can appear simultaneously, or sequentially. Normally, first dizziness, ocular nystagmus vomiting and balance problems occur, then hearing deficiencies appear. The characteristic signs of an "attack" on the hearing apparatus by the syphilitic process, include (a) serious derangement of bone conduction of sound, (b) a particularly notable diminution of the perception of low tones, and (c) a selective loss of hearing of only some tones (*scotoma auditiva* or auditory scotoma). (89)

The clinical picture of Beethoven's deafness does not correspond to this typical picture of syphilis. Beethoven did not complain of derangements of balance, dizziness or nystagmus, which could have attested to damage of the vestibular nerve, while bone conduction of sounds remained the longest lasting of mechanisms allowing him to hear them. The stepwise and generally indolent process of loss of hearing experienced by Beethoven is equally inconsistent with the picture of luetic damage to the auditory nerve, which normally causes a sudden and rapidly progressive loss of hearing, as happened in the case of Bedrich Smetana. In syphilis, there normally are changes in both ears, while in Beethoven's case, first his left ear was attacked, then after a time, his right. I agree in this case with the opinions of Drs. Schweisheimer and Neumayer that the most likely cause of the composer's loss of hearing, the start of which appeared in 1795, was typhus. (90, 91)

Another etiology considered for Beethoven's loss of hearing is otosclerosis, but against this hypothesis stand the autopsy results, in which the characteristic stiffening of the auditory ossicles (bones) in that disease were not reported. Nevertheless, it cannot be excluded entirely, as many signs and/or symptoms observed in Beethoven are consistent with otosclerosis.

Anatomical abnormalities of Beethoven's skull described by Dr. Jackson, such as the thickening of its parietal bone, is an error in the plaster casting done during exhumation, while the thickening of the parietal bone seen in the mask made while Beethoven was still alive comes from the whiskers behind his ear. (92)

Some of the facts from the life of the composer and fragments of his correspondence are interpreted as corroboration that Beethoven had syphilis, although probably in none of these is the disease named. (93, 94) This is surely nothing extraordinary, as in all of the literature relating to famous people who were ill with syphilis, naming it is avoided.

In all of the pertinent biographies, it is stressed that Beethoven did not like the wife of his own brother, the mother of a boy toward whom he wanted to be a protector. He warned the young man to avoid temptations that lay in wait from every side in Vienna, and criticized the boy's mother for conducting herself immorally. (95, 96) Unfortunately, he did not always conform to principles that he, himself, loudly proclaimed. From letters to his friend, Nicholas Zmeskall, one can conclude that the composer utilized the services of prostitutes – women, whom he described by the name of "rotten fortresses." He was simultaneously romantic and sentimental, and, as his physician, Andreas Bertolini, wrote, "Beethoven was uninterruptedly involved with some amorous experience." (96, 97) In a biography by George R. Marek, Beethoven is said to have carried on correspondence that could be named "amorous" with at least 10 named women. This testifies that he was able to be romantically in love frequently. Unfortunately, the majority of women for whom he longed came from well-known families, often aristocratic ones, for whom an open romance with Beethoven would have been socially compromising. Remember, that we are speaking of times in which there was a strict class separation, and a marriage of a countess with a music teacher was quite unthinkable.

Beethoven's first youthful love was Eleonor von Breuning. Next named is the singer Magdalen Willman, whom he met while still in Bonn. In the 1890s, he proposed, but the offer of marriage was rejected, as he was not handsome enough for her, and also of an unbalanced character. (98) Next was Countess Josephine Brunsvik, the wife of Count Deym, after whose death Beethoven tried once again, but the idea of marriage was unrealistic, based on class differences. The next candidate for Mrs. Beethoven was Countess Giuletta Guicciardi, to whom he dedicated the "Moonlight Sonata," but despite that, Giulletta preferred to marry another aristocrat. Then, when he was already 40, he proposed to 18-year-old

Therese Malfatti, the niece of his physician, but nothing came of it. He also fell in love with many "proper women," among which was the "legendary beloved," about whom legends circulate to this day.

Romantic feelings for women of higher circles were disturbed by desires of the flesh. Beethoven confided to his friend Karol Holz, "that the necessary requirements of the flesh tempt [me] to something that is contrary to that of the better part of [my] nature." (96) These types of declarations could lead one to believe that the composer of the "Triple Concerto" took advantage of the services of prostitutes on occasion – which was very risky behavior, considering the frequency of syphilis and other venereal diseases in those times, particularly among women following the prostitute's profession. Did he contract any diseases from them? One cannot exclude that it was so, but it did not have to be syphilis right away, as it could equally well have been another disease transmitted by the sexual route, of which, in the environment of Viennese prostitutes, there certainly was no shortage.

We know that Beethoven was interested in venereal diseases. This is attested to by a note from 1819, in which it is said that he intended to buy a book by L.V. Legunan, *L'art de connaitre et de guerir toutes les contagions veneriennes* (The Art of Knowing and Fighting All the Venereal Contagions). Somebody noted that this could imply that he lost confidence in physicians, and wanted to undertake the care of his health by himself. It is more likely that he wanted to have it for the education of his nephew, of whom he was taking care, and wanted to protect him from this type of danger. (99)

All the biographers of the composer of the *Ninth Symphony* draw attention to his frail health. In letters to friends, Beethoven constantly mentions stubborn colics, stomach pains and diarrhea, accompanied by fever. These ailments, with various breaks, continued for many years, and in 1823, to them were added ocular ailments. The same combination of symptoms repeats itself the following year, when Beethoven wrote that his light intolerance was so bad that he "had to bind his eyes for the night, and to be thrifty with them." (100)

The causes of these symptoms are interpreted in various ways that are not consistent with the natural course of syphilitic infection, not excluding secondary syphilis. (101) During the second stage of syphilis, in addition to various types of skin rashes, lesions on the oral mucous membranes and the throat, loss of hair, and *leukoderma, a* patchy depigmentation of skin, all characteristic of lues. Non-specific changes, such as fever, swelling of the joints, ocular changes, or even diarrhea can also occur; however, this stage does not last longer than two years. The composer's health problems, noted earlier, appeared at least several years after the conjectured infection with syphilis, which adherents of this theory ascribe to the end of the '90s of the eighteenth century. I wanted to underscore at this point that anyone ill with syphilis, just as any other mortal, has the right to have a fever, such as from a viral infection; headaches, as from a migraine; inflammation of the joints from rheumatic causes; or diarrhea, as a result of food poisoning. In a word, one could attribute everything to syphilis, "the great imitator."

Modern physicians name several diseases that according to the signs and symptoms described could have afflicted Beethoven for many years before his death. Included are chronic pancreatic inflammation (based on prolonged alcohol abuse), irritable colon, Bang's disease (a form of brucellosis) and Crohn's disease, among others. For myself, I could throw in several additional diagnoses to this constellation, including Reiter's syndrome, and concurrent bacterial infections of the bowel, but do not wish to extend the list too far. The most likely, and, in my opinion, the best diagnosis appears to be *enterocolitis regionalis Crohn* (Crohn's disease). This is a chronic disease of the large intestine, probably of autoimmunologic cause. Changes can occur in any segment of the intestinal tract, but most often involve the terminal segment of the colon. It commonly appears in the third decade of life, rarely earlier, and is characterized by recurrent pain. To typical symptoms belong abdominal aches, fever, and frequent diarrhea. Recurrences are often accompanied by ocular changes – inflammation of the conjunctiva and of the iris, causing extra sensitivity to light, ocular pain and headaches. Against this diagnosis, however, are the findings at the composer's autopsy, during which no post-inflammatory changes in the small or large intestines were noted.

Without delving into further speculations on the subject of diagnosing the illnesses tormenting Beethoven for ten years before his death, I will move on to the immediate cause of that death. The majority of authors agree that the composer died of cirrhosis of the liver, the sequel of which was abdominal hydrops, which appeared in the last days before death. Cirrhosis of the liver can have many causes, but the most common is prolonged alcohol abuse. Although one cannot call Beethoven a chronic alcoholic, he belonged, without any doubt, to those people who abuse alcohol, particularly wine. Other causes of cirrhosis of the liver could be Crohn's disease or a virus-caused hepatic inflammation, from which Beethoven may have suffered for seven years before his death. (102) Viral hepatitis can be caused by infection with Hepatitis A virus, transmitted by the oral route, or by hepatitis B or C viruses, which are primarily blood-borne or even sexually-transmitted. Hepatitis caused by HAV (hepatitis A virus) is rarely a cause of cirrhosis of the liver, something that cannot be said about type B jaundice caused by HBV (hepatitis B virus). In Beethoven's case, we may be dealing with a synergistic effect of several agents, viral inflammation of the liver caused by hepatitis B or C viruses, intertwined with chronic Crohn's disease and alcohol-related liver damage.

In concluding considerations regarding the health of Beethoven, I will have good news for both groups of investigators: those who maintain that Beethoven's health was ruined by syphilis, and those who are of a different opinion. Hepatitis caused by type B or C viruses can also be considered venereal diseases, but not always. The composer could have been infected by them through the sexual route, taking advantage of the services of a prostitute, who had recently menstruated. He could also have infected himself by some other means, which will surely console the opponents of a "venereal theory," for instance, while shaving in a barber shop at a time when blood got drawn accidentally while using unsterilized instruments. Hepatitis B currently occurs more often among homosexuals, but of this, until now, Beethoven has not been accused – although I am not certain whether I am mistaken or not! (103).

CHAPTER 5b

POETS and WRITERS

ALFRED DE MUSSET (1810-1857)

Alfred de Musset, poet, dramatist and author, came from the moderately wealthy French aristocracy (Fig.5b.1). After finishing the exclusive Collège Henri IV in Paris, he attempted studying law, but quickly became discouraged. Next, he signed up for medicine, but here, also, didn't last very long, as a result of the disgust he felt toward assignments in the anatomy laboratory. For a while, he studied music, took English lessons, and for half a year, would go to the Louvre to study drawing and painting. Finally, he came to the conclusion that his calling was literary creation, and determined to become a writer. At the age of seventeen, thanks to the sponsorship of a renowned writer, he was accepted to the Parisian literary salon, *Cenacle*, and two years later published his first collection of poems, titled *Tales of Spain and Italy*.

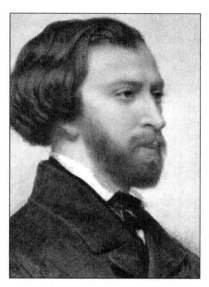

Figure 5b.1 Portrait of Alfred de Musset painted by Charles Landelle

Even before reaching age 20, de Musset was a well-known and liked person. He dressed modishly, liked strong drink, and was successful with women. Not long afterwards, he became the object of social sensation and the subject of much gossip resulting from his romance with a well-known lady writer, with the *nom de plume*, George Sand, who was older than he by six years. (1) This romance lasted from 1833 to 1835, while his stormy ventures were recorded in Musset's autobiographical novel, *The Confessions of a Child of the Century*, which, in 1999 became a screenplay. The film entitled *Children of the Century* tells the love story of two talented people, a story of violent emotions full of passion, mutual devotion and sacrifice, but also of betrayal and infidelity. Both hero and heroine already had a certain past. Vocational successes and defeats were not unknown to them, nor were longer or shorter d'alliances with different partners. George Sand was a well-known and popular writer, and had behind her an unsuccessful marriage with Baron Dudevant, with whom she had two children. A public *secret* was the fact that, after divorce from her husband, she had numerous lovers. She had the reputation of being eccentric, dressed as a man, smoked tobacco, and had a companion actress, Marie Dorval, with whom the relationship was probably something more than just friendship. George Sand, whose real name was Amantine Aurore Dudevant, *nee* Dupin, apparently inherited genes that predestined her for excessive eroticism, as she was the great, great-granddaughter of Polish King August II the Strong, who supposedly fathered over 200 out-of-wedlock children!

Alfred de Musset himself was no angel either. He lost his virginity as a teenager, had numerous mistresses, was a frequent guest at bordellos, used alcohol to excess, and treated himself to opium. It is most likely in this period that he contracted syphilis, which, in his later years could have been the cause of his early death. In the film that I mentioned, there are many scenes from his trip to Venice with George Sand. These relate the numerous quarrels between the lovers about Alfred playing in the bordellos, taking part in orgies with Venetian prostitutes, even while George Sand was ill or had to work. The authoress did not remain in his debt, consoling herself by romancing her doctor, Pietro Pagello, who later was to save de Musset on many occasions. De Musset not only abused alcohol, but also used opium. On one occasion, during a drunken night, he overdosed on narcotics, and found himself, as determined by Dr. Pagello, in a pre-agonal state. The doctor let his blood, which treatment resulted in the patient's revival, although he continued to behave like a madcap for a long time.

After this incident, the lovers parted. De Musset returned to France, while George Sand remained in Venice, entertained by the aforementioned doctor. After a while, she, also, returned to Paris, where she next fell in love with the renowned Polish composer, Fryderyk Chopin, with whom she lived for over ten years. They parted fewer than two years before the composer's death, from tuberculosis, in 1849. The authoress, despite numerous problems, was blessed with the health of a horse; she apparently did not become infected with any venereal disease (I was not able to find anything on this subject) nor even tuberculosis, despite living under one roof for many years with Chopin, who was ill with the latter. She died in 1876 at the age of seventy-one.

De Musset, after parting with George Sand, returned to Paris, recovered, and continued his literary work, for which he was rewarded in 1845 with the Order of the Legion of Honor (a high French distinction), and, seven years later, by membership in the French Academy, an association consisting of prominent persons from the world of literature and art. Unfortunately, he neither stopped drinking nor using opium, which resulted in his causing disturbances frequently. In the *Journal* of the de Goncourt brothers, dated August 1, 1856 – that is, not less than a year before his death – is found an account of one row brought about by the poet, which ended in a challenge to a duel.

On a certain evening, [de] Musset, in the foyer of the French Theater, drunk as usual ... Augustine Brohan (an actress of the theater) addressed him: "My dear Mr. [de] Musset, by what right do you brag that you slept with me? - Me, indeed! [he responded] If I am to brag, then it would be that I did not sleep with you!" Broham stood as though dumbfounded. [de] Musset verbally abused her, and so loudly that Houssaye (a writer and critic) intervened: Sir, I will not allow you to insult the lady in my presence. I am at your service. Capital, capital! But you are not going to tell me that you will fight for this mare! You are looking to brawl with me, Sir, because you are a poor author, because there is no way to read your work! As you wish! ... Such a wonder! At your orders! Whenever you wish!" (2)

Apparently, this did not lead to an actual duel, but the scene described shows the customs of the literary world, as well as de Musset's behavior near the end of his life. The uncivil behavior of a drunken de Musset is not in any way evidence that Augustine Brohan was *not* his mistress. The de Goncourt brothers suggest that one of the comedies written by de Musset arose in her house, where the actress tenderly took care of the writer.

Augustine Brohan was not the only woman with whom de Musset was involved at this time. Shortly after breaking up with George Sand in 1837, Alfred became engaged to a young woman from an influential family, Miss Aimee D'Alton, but both quickly came to the conclusion that their feelings had no chance for the future. Another of de Musset's loves was the 40-year-old famous actress from the *Comedie Francaise*, Allan-Despreaux, known as Mile, who also performed in St. Petersburg in Russia. Yet another well-known mistress was Louise Colet, an authoress and aspiring poetess, the former mistress of Gustave Flaubert.

In completing the portrait of de Musset, one has to add that, besides poetry and literature, opium, absinthe, and women, the poet was a skilled chess player. He was a member of an elite circle of chess players, who met regularly in the Parisian coffee house, *Café de la Regence*, where de Musset went almost every day. On one day in 1848, when the Revolution had broken out, he was so involved with the chessboard that he did not notice the gunfire outside his window (3). Alfred de Musset entered history not only as a talented poet, dramatist and lover of George Sand, but also as a patient, from whose illness came a particular medical term, called *de Musset's sign* (4). He most likely became infected in his youth with syphilis, which in his later years, became the cause of his heart disease, specifically, a cause of the appearance of an aneurysm of the aorta. Aortic aneurysm and its insufficiency was one of the more common manifestations of late syphilis of the cardiovascular system. A person ill with this problem nods the head rhythmically, in synchrony with the heartbeat. This sign is seen not only in cases of aortic aneurysm due to syphilis, but also in other diseases causing damage to the aorta, for instance rheumatic fever.

And so, the last name of an unsuccessful medical student finds itself in a medical dictionary! (4) Alfred de Musset died in his sleep at age 47, while the cause of his death was most probably heart failure, as a sequel to infection with syphilis.

CHARLES BAUDELAIRE (1821-1867)

Charles Baudelaire is one of the best known and appreciated French poets of the nineteenth century (Fig.5b.2). In addition to poetry, he was involved as an art critic and translator, particularly the works of Edgar Allan Poe. He was born in Paris. At the age of six, Charles lost his father and his mother remarried a professional army major, Jacque Autpick. The young Baudelaire jealously loved his mother. Psychiatrists maintain that this type of childhood trauma—the loss of a father and remarriage of the mother—can affect later behavior and character, as it did Baudelaire.

At age eight, Charles was placed in a boarding school in Lyons, where his parents lived for a while. He did not like the school very much, and the young man also suffered as the result of separation from his mother. In 1836, the family moved to Paris, where Baudelaire became a student of the Parisian Lycee Louis le Grand. He was very interested in romantic literature, and became engrossed in reading the works of Victor Hugo and the novels of Saint-Beuve; other subjects interested him far less. He was removed from the school as a result of bad behavior, and took his exams as an extern, having a private tutor. After finishing his high-school studies, Baudelaire entered law school, a direction frequently taken by persons who didn't really know what they wanted to do in life. Baudelaire certainly belonged to these, as he did not feel called to any type of work, and would most have liked to remain supported by his mother.

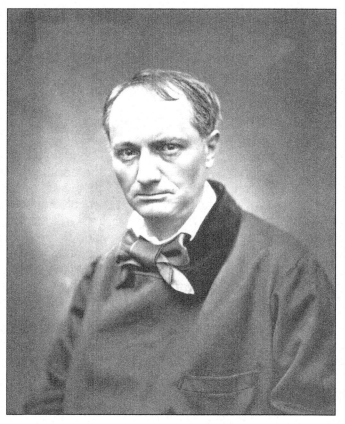

Figure 5b.2 Portrait of Charles Baudelaire (ca 1862) painted by Etienne Carjat

Even as a student, Baudelaire liked to play. He dressed very modishly (he was considered a dandy) and often incurred debt. He frequented Parisian bordellos, where he most probably became infected, first with gonorrhea, then with syphilis. On the advice of his older brother, Alphonse, he contacted a pharmacist who took care of venereal diseases on the matter, and took some type of medication. For a time, he maintained a constant contact with a prostitute by the name of Sara, and very often stayed with his brother as a result of a shortage of means for living. His stepfather, who wanted Baudelaire to become a diplomat, himself an ambassador, did not approve of his stepson's life, but provided a small monthly sum for his upkeep, which the young man squandered in a few days, mainly on clothes, alcohol and women. Not many people knew that Beaudelaire had contracted syphilis; the first information we have on the subject comes from a letter that he wrote to his mother in 1861. (5, 6)

Hoping that Charles would break with his lifestyle, surroundings and companions that depraved him, his parents decided to finance a trip to Calcutta for him, under the protection of a friend who was the captain of a ship sailing to India. The sea voyage and visiting foreign ports had no great effect on the young man, who now decided that he would be a writer, so the captain under whose protection Baudelaire travelled sent him home. The financial means invested in the trip by his parents did not go entirely for naught as the poet used his impressions from the travels in his later literary creations.

After returning to Paris, Baudelaire occupied himself with writing. He met with friends, to whom he presented samples of his writings. Unfortunately, he also returned to the lifestyle, which displeased his parents, particularly his step-father. At age twenty-one, the young man inherited a considerable fortune from his father. He managed to squander half in the course of two years, leaving him with debts he accrued on his own. His family intervened and a court judgment was obtained to allow the appointment of a curator to manage the remaining inheritance, pay off his debts, and give the poet a small monthly pension. At about this time, a Miss Jeanne Duval became interested in him (or maybe he in her); she was the former mistress of a well-known caricaturist and photographer, Baudelaire's friend, Nadar, whose real name was Felix Tournachon.

About Jeanne Duval it is written that she was an actress-dancer born in Haiti, the daughter of a French woman (supposedly a prostitute from Nantes) and a black man. (7) Baudelaire met her when he was twenty-one and their bond, while having its tempestuous moments, lasted over twenty years. The poet called her the *Mistress of Mistresses*, for him the symbol of sexuality and the alarming beauty of creole women. Edouard Manet, the painter, and the poet's friend (also a syphilitic) painted a portrait of Jeanne entitled, *Baudelaire's Mistress, Reclining* (Fig.5b.3). Baudelaire dedicated a number of his works to Jeanne, financed her whims, and protected her even after their breakup. Baudelaire's mother considered Miss Duval to be the source of all evil for her son, and that she exploited him both emotionally and financially. One of the poet's biographers described Jeanne as "an insatiable prostitute, a leech, experienced in providing all types of sexual delights ... She easily guessed his needs and erotic inclinations, and knew how to satisfy them." (8)

As did Baudelaire, so, also, Jeanne Duval suffered from syphilis, which was most probably the cause of her death, although there are two versions regarding that. One says that Jeanne died in 1862, that is, 5 years before Baudelaire, while another, says that her former lover, Nadar, saw her for the last time in 1870, when she was moving about on crutches. The latter could bear attest that she outlived Baudelaire, but had problems with walking, perhaps caused by syphilitic derangement of the nervous system (*tabes dorsalis*?).

In the course of his acquaintance with Jeanne, Baudelaire found himself in a state of deep depression in

1845, caused by, among other things, his financial difficulties. He wrote a farewell letter and last will and testament, which he left for his mistress. "The misery associated with going to bed and awakening have become beyond endurance. I am killing myself, because I have become of no value for others, and dangerous to myself." (9) Baudelaire attempted unsuccessfully to kill himself with a knife, but fortunately was saved. The attempted suicide improved his relationship to his family, but only with his mother, and his relationship with his stepfather remained cool.

One of the first and best-known of Baudelaire's creations was a poetic collection entitled *Le Fleurs du Mal* (The Flowers of Evil), published in 1857, although some poems contained in it appeared somewhat earlier. As maintained by some aficionados, several of the poems in this collection arose under the influence of Edgar Alan Poe and of the poetry of late romanticism. They are supposed to be a testimony to the spiritual tearing apart of a poet quarreling with his surroundings and yearning to escape from everyday life, and are like a protest against the official opinions of the epoch. (10) It is also felt that Jeanne Duval was the source of inspiration for a certain fragment of the collection, entitled *Venus Noire* (The Black Venus).

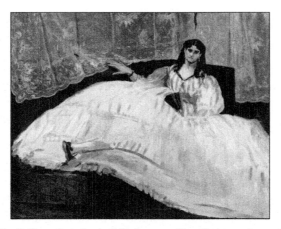

*Figure 5b.3 Baudelaire's Mistress, Reclining. Jeanne Duval
as painted by Edouard Manet (1862)*

From the very beginning, *Les Fleurs du Mal* became the
object of attacks from the side of protectors of morals, and
similarly to Flaubert's *Madame Bovary*, and one of the
publications of the de Goncourt brothers, were investigated
by the Ministry of Internal Affairs. (11) Baudelaire, his
publisher and printer, were all found guilty of the legal verdict
of insulting morality. It was further ordered that six poems, in
which the poet wrote about lesbian love, be removed. It must
be admitted, however, that, after a time, the monetary
penalty imposed on the author was reduced, while after
almost a hundred years, in 1949, the poet was rehabilitated.
Shortly after publishing *Les Fleur du Mal*, partly as a result of
the legal process and objections to the publication of immoral
writings, the author became a well-known person. His work
was met with sympathy from many independent writers,
while Gustave Flaubert and Victor Hugo both wrote
enthusiastically laudatory letters to him. In addition to *Les
Fleurs du Mal*, Baudelaire was the author of a collection of
poems in prose, *Le Spleen de Paris,* and skits about
literature and art. Well-known composers created music for
his poems, one of these being Claude Debussy, who in 1890

composed the music to six poems by the poet. Even contemporary composers utilize Baudelaire's poetry in their works.

At the end of the 1850s and 1860s, despite a worsening of his health, the poet was still productive. He wrote new poems, translated those of Thomas de Quincy, and wrote a critique of the creativity of Flaubert, Balzac, and other French writers. Two new women appeared in his life: the actress, Maria Daubrun, and the artists' friend, Apolonia Sabatier (actually Apollonie-Algae Savatier}, to whom he dedicated several of his works. In correspondence with his mother, Baudelaire complained of having a lack of confidence in his own strength, and wrote of signs of neurosis:

> I believe I am sick, and a sick man, even if the sickness is imagined, is a sick man. What else could be these perpetual fears, these palpitations and this breathlessness, especially during sleep. . . . I have cultivated my hysteria with enjoyment and terror. I always have vertigo now, and today, 23 January 1862, I have experienced an unusual warning: I felt pass over me" the wind of the wing of madness. (12,13)

In the 1860s, Beaudelaire's health problems were exacerbated, and some of them could be attributed to advancing syphilis. He complained of problems with his eyes (which made reading impossible), stomach problems lasting months, bouts of fever, particularly at night, bouts of pain and as he wrote, "absolute abdication of willpower." (14) Periods of remission were intertwined with vertigo, stomach pains, nausea and vomiting, on occasion lasting weeks. The ill poet tried to treat himself, taking opium, digitalis, valerian, ether and laudanum. He overused opium, which could have been weaker in its effect as a result of his earlier abuse of this substance.

At the beginning of 1866, Beaudelaire arrived in Belgium, where he had gone with the hope of selling his author's rights to some of his publications. After a long wait at the post office, he got wet, chilled, and caught cold. He developed a strong migraine and the following day was seriously ill, writhing on the floor and vomiting. The doctor that was called concluded that this was an attack of hysteria, and recommended a diet, while forbidding the use of alcohol, which, in Baudelaire, caused an unsurprising indignation. (15) In February of the same year, he wrote to a friend about his health problems, "which [have] lasted 20 months." He wrote of headaches, rheumatic pains, numerous falls, vomiting bile, and strange sensations in his brain, (16) which are reminiscent of the beginnings of general paresis. In March, after a night of heavy drinking, he awoke partially paralyzed. Two days later, it was determined that this was a hemiplegia. Madame Hugo, who visited him, told her husband, "Baudelaire is finished ...The illness has almost entirely destroyed his brain; they despair of the invalid." (17)

At first, the poet was placed in a nursing home run by the Sisters of Charity, but, after a certain time, his mother took him from there, and brought him to France. There, his friends could visit him, among them Edouard Manet. The famous painter visited Baudelaire together with his wife, who played, on the piano, fragments of Wagner's creations, a composer whom the paralyzed poet liked very much.

At the junction between April and May, Baudelaire's mental state worsened considerably. A friend of the poet, Asselineau, wanted him to sign a certain bill; the poet halted his pen in the air, as though trying to remember what his own name was. Asselineau offered him a copy of one of his books, hoping that the author would remember his own name. Baudelaire loosely traced the name of the author, and slowly signed the document. On another occasion, when his nurse was combing his hair and beard, he saw his reflection in the mirror, and graciously bowed, not fully realizing that he was bowing to himself. (18) Baudelaire died on August 31, 1867, in the presence of his mother; the official cause of death was apoplexy.

In Baudelaire's case, it would be difficult to determine to what degree the cause of the poet's illness was syphilis, and to what extent other problems, particularly abuse of alcohol and opium, were at play. A number of signs could indicate the beginning stages of general paresis; nevertheless, there are several that could also indicate meningovascular syphilis. In addition, we have to deal with signs indicating other diseases, for example, high blood pressure, stomach ulcer, rheumatism, heart disease, and serious migraine. Which of these conditions was the most likely cause of the poet's death remains an open question.

GUSTAVE FLAUBERT (1821-1886)

Gustave Flaubert, the French storywriter and one of the pioneers of realism in literature, was born in Rouen in Northern France (Fig.5b.4). He came from a medical family, his father being the chief surgeon of the hospital in Rouen, which status Gustave's older brother inherited. His mother was also the daughter of a physician.

Before Gustave became a writer, he attempted the study of law in Paris, but nothing came of it. Paris, as a city, did not appeal to him, while instead of his law studies, the local brothels interested him more. At the same time, health problems appeared, and these put an end to Flaubert's legal career, forcing him to return to Rouen. His father bought him a house situated close to his own so that he could more easily take care of his son. The disease that changed Flaubert's life was epilepsy, a first attack of which occurred in January 1844. (19, 20) Not all agree with this diagnosis, maintaining that, shortly after his arrival in Paris, Flaubert may have become infected with syphilis, and that the epileptic attacks were symptoms of the effects of the disease on the central nervous system. His father and brother treated

Gustave in accord with existing medical principles of that time, by letting blood and instituting a diet. (21, 22, 23)

Shortly after Flaubert's first attack, others appeared, these resulting in more bloodletting and a more stringent diet. He was not allowed to drink alcohol, and leeches were applied. The clinical picture of the seizures appears to be typical of classical epilepsy. Although, on the basis of the reports alone, other causes of the illness cannot be excluded. In early lues, epilepsy-like (epileptoid) attacks can appear, indicating involvement of the central nervous system, in particular of the meninges and the vascular tree of the brain. One then speaks of meningovascular syphilis, of which one of the signs is seizures reminiscent of epilepsy. Attacks of this type usually appear after two-three years following infection and are accompanied by other signs such as irritability, constant feelings of fatigue, and difficulty in concentration. These last also accompany classical epileptic seizures, which does not make differentiation any easier. In meningo-vascular syphilis, there also appear, somewhat later, neurologic signs, such as unequal pupils, stiff, jerky movements, Argyll-Robertson (unequal) pupils, or signs indicating damage to the cranial nerves. To the best of my knowledge, none of these, other than fatigability and, possibly, irritability, were observed in Flaubert – and they also accompany ordinary attacks of epilepsy, not to mention other diseases.

Regardless of whether Flaubert's epilepsy was actually related to syphilis or not, within several months from the first seizure, he was handed over to mercury treatment on the basis of a skin rash, which could have been a sign of secondary lues. Inasmuch as his neurologic state improved, Flaubert returned to Paris, with the intent of continuing his studies. Unfortunately, the seizures returned, occurring almost daily, which caused the unfinished attorney to return to Rouen. Flaubert settled in Croisset, a bit beyond the boundary of Rouen, where he lived, with some absences, to the end of his life. Thus ended Flaubert's law career, and his career as an author began, bringing him worldwide recognition.

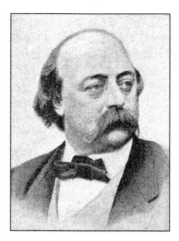

Figure 5b.4 Portrait of Gustave Flaubert (by Felix Nadar)

Before the first significant literary works of Flaubert appeared, he began a trip, together with a friend, Maxime du Camp, also the son of a physician, in order to improve his health, as it was said. The trip lasted a year and a half, and the gentlemen visited Egypt, Syria, Turkey, Greece and Italy. Flaubert's mother maintained that her son undertook the trip for reasons of health, but some less-charitable friends said that the future author did it "out of boredom and for image ... in order to have something to write about, and to obtain the adulation of the inhabitants of Rouen." (24)

In the course of his travels, Flaubert wrote letters to family and friends. In his correspondence with family, he described the raw nature of the Near East, the beauty of the historical monuments visited, and the customs of the inhabitants. In letters to his friends, however, specifically to Louis Bouilhet, poet and dramatist, Flaubert boasted of his

203

erotic achievements, and, associated with these, his health problems. In a letter to Bouilhet dated November 24, 1850, written in Constantinople, (Istanbul), Gustave wrote:

> You have to know, dear Sir, that in Beirut (I noticed them in Rhodes, the Isle of the Dragon), I had seven chancres, which finally merged into two, then one. In this state, I rode horseback from Marmaris to Smyrna. Every evening and morning, I changed the dressing on my wretched penis. Finally, it healed, and in two or three days, scarred. I will be careful of this. I suspect that I received this present from a certain Maronite[1], but it could be from a young Turkish lass. Turk or Christian, what's the difference?" (25, 26)

Flaubert later wrote that Maxime noticed, despite the fact that they have not had intercourse already for six weeks, double abrasions of the foreskin, "which looks to me like a double/two-headed chancre. If that is so, it would already be a third infection with lues from the time of our departure. There is nothing better than travel for improving your health!" (25) Three months later, he wrote to Bouilhet:

> In regard to myself, the chancres about which I was so afraid, have healed. The hardened swelling on my member, I have still, although it has a tendency to disappear. Another thing is disappearing, that, much faster, is my hair. You will see me with a skullcap. I will be as bald as a office clerk, as a dried-up notary, everything that is most troublesome in premature aging the fact of early old age.

---

[1] Maronite – a member of the Eastern-rite Catholic Church that was established in the XVIII[h] century on the territory now including Lebanon and Syria.

He wrote further, "as a result of mercury treatment, my teeth will go. 'My piano keys are leaving me.'" Next, he commented on the rash on the skin in of lower abdomen and a weakening of his sex drive. (26) When he arrived in Rome, problems appeared with one of his testicles and a painful neuralgia of the face. Some of these ailments could have been associated with intensive mercury treatment, although problems with his testicle could have had a different etiology, for example gonorrhea, which, in Flaubert's time was a common cause of inflammation of the epididymis (*epididymitis*).

Many authors believe that it was in Beirut that Flaubert became infected with syphilis. (27) If this were really so, then all suggestions that Flaubert was ill with syphilis in Paris would be without foundation. I already wrote about the appearance of intercurrent infectious immunity (premunition) in syphilis, an inability to re-infect oneself with this disease by a person already once infected. It is said that effective treatment weakens this immunity, although it doesn't eliminate it entirely. There have been several reports of instances of multiple infections with syphilis, but this is rare, and dependent on the effectiveness of the therapy, (28) which, in the case of mercury treatment, is almost nil. One should not be surprised that Flaubert attributed both his own ailments, and those experienced by his friend, Maxime, to syphilis. In those times, almost all ulcerations that appeared on sexual organs were attributed to that disease. The fact that Maxime became infected with syphilis, and that, three times, appears to be of low probability, unless the first ulceration was the primary chancre, while the latter two were a papular rash or *condyloma lata.* These are flat growths that are a sign of secondary syphilis, and which, additionally infected can appear as small erosions or ulcerations.

Another cause of the lesions observed by Flaubert and Maxime du Camp could have been chancroid. August Ducrey discovered the bacteria causing soft chancre only in

1889; these were named *Haemophilus ducreyi* in honor of their discoverer. This latter disease is transmitted by the sexual route, similarly to syphilis, and is characterized by the presence of *painful* ulcerations on the sexual organs; however, from the clinical point of view, the lesions are different from the primary chancre of syphilis, which is mostly painless. Unfortunately, Flaubert's descriptions are not clinically precise, yet it is difficult to blame him for not paying attention to details of little importance from the point of view of the patient. On the other hand, neither a later rash nor balding fit the clinical picture of chancroid – they do not appear in that disease. (29)

Without indulging in difficult-to-distinguish speculations about when Flaubert became infected with syphilis, we can accept that he did suffer from it and was treated for it, and that it identified itself by its symptoms in his later years.

Citing fragments of his correspondence with friends, I wanted to bring attention to the totally lackadaisical approach Flaubert had to his disease. From today's perspective, it appears grimly comical, but the poet wasn't the only patient who reacted in this way. Many famous syphilitics took such a posture (see de Maupassant), although they were, in fact, well aware of the seriousness of the situation. In one of his letters, Flaubert wrote:

> So, you laughed, you old [lout], you perfidious guest, at my small sword. Now know that, for the time being [at least], it is healed. There remains a small hardening, but this is the scar of a hero. It adds poetry to it. One can see that it survived, that it had gone through misfortune. Its appearance makes one think of loss and curses, which should cause anyone who thinks about it, to like it. (26)

Flaubert is disarmingly sincere in descriptions of his sexual exploits, sometimes easily exceeding the bounds of good taste. His descriptions of contacts with a famous courtesan in Egypt, accounts of contacts with underage male prostitutes, an attempt at relations with a 16-year-old prostitute – which was not successful, when the girl asked to see the writer's genitals, and was afraid of becoming infected with a venereal disease – all indicate that the author was a "realist," not only in literature. As can be seen, he had no reservations when it came to satisfying his erotic wants, and saw no need to maintain any greater discreetness in these matters.

Taking advantage of sex-for-pay does not mean that Flaubert did not have relationships with, let us call them, "proper" women, although he never married. His first longer-lasting relationship was with the poetess, Louise Colet, which began as early as 1846. Flaubert met Louise in the studio of the sculptor James Pradier in Paris, where he went with the aim of ordering a bust of his recently deceased sister. He was then twenty-five years of age, while Louise was thirty-six. This was during a period when he lived celibately; some maintain that that was due to his lues, while others want to believe that it was due to his desire to devote himself completely to literary creation. Until that time, and not counting seduction at age nineteen by a certain aging female hotel owner in Marseille, (30) he did not live in a steady relationship with any woman, limiting his erotic life to occasional visits to bordellos.

When they first met, Louise was the wife of Hippolyte Collet, a flutist from the Paris conservatory, and had a daughter, who was the fruit of her romance with Victor Cousin, with whose help she ran a literary salon in Paris. She was considered a beauty, though a somewhat strange one, having both feminine and masculine characteristics. She looked and behaved like a seductive woman, while simultaneously "walked like a dragoon, and spoke with a hoarse voice." Apparently, the combination of such characteristics unusually excited Flaubert. Their first meeting in the studio of James Pradier (who, it is believed, not just sculpted Louise), resulted in Gustave and Louise spending a mutual night in a hotel – although, supposedly, Flaubert did not then perform as expected. (31) (After a long period of sexual abstinence, men often experience problems, the most common of which is premature ejaculation). Louise treated this with complete understanding, for which Flaubert was very grateful. The following days, which they spent together worked out very well, as testified to by a letter dated August 6th, 1846, in which Flaubert wrote:

> You are the only woman with whom I fell in love and whom I possessed. Until this moment, desires aroused by one woman, I calmed in others. You forced me to contradict my principles, my heart, and even, perhaps, my nature, which, itself unfulfilled, seeks that which is not fulfilled. (32)

After several days and nights, which the mutually enchanted lovers spent together, Flaubert left for Rouen. Both must have realized that their relationship was facing a rather uncertain future. Louise was not free, having a husband, a daughter and *permanent* lover; Flaubert, for his part, had a mother, who could not imagine life without her beloved son, and who would do everything to prevent a relationship with a woman of not the best of reputations.

Flaubert was in a huge quandary, and wrote that "I feel exhausted and empty, as though after a long orgy, and can neither read nor write, nor think that [my] love sadden[s] [you]." (33) In the course of eight years, a supposed total of twenty confirmed meetings were kept secret from Madame Flaubert. Gustave and Louise's relationship at this time can be judged to have been largely confined to correspondence since as a result of his mother letters from Louise wandered to Flaubert through Maxime du Camp, who served as a contact box. To the extent that Flaubert reconciled himself to such a situation, so Louise, who was not only a beautiful, but also, an ambitious woman, wanted something more. She insisted that Flaubert rent an apartment in Paris so that they could regularly see each other, from which proposition Flaubert wiggled effectively, hiding behind his work. In March of 1848, Louise notified Flaubert that she was pregnant, judging, perhaps, that this information would bring him closer to her. Apparently she was not aware of Flaubert's views on fatherhood, set forth in one of his works, entitled, "November," in which he wrote that "one who commits murder commits a lesser crime than one who fathers a child[!]" (34) It turned out that the source of the pregnancy was someone else, and Louise underwent an abortion, about which she informed Flaubert by letter. Flaubert broke up with her and didn't say anything for a long time; he also did not write any letters to her during his long travels in the Near East. Louise, on the other hand, remained interested in her lover, asking about him among mutual friends, and trying to mend the relationship – which did not interfere with her seeking consolation in the arms of other men! In 1851, she decided on a visit to Croisset, where she encountered a rough dismissal. Despite the cooling of relations, the former lovers exchanged letters with one another, ridding themselves of their individual problems connected mostly with literary creativity. There is no doubt that Louise admired Flaubert as a writer, something that he did not return in kind. In the meantime, both of them had their own erotic lives. Louise started a romance with Alfred de Musset and with Alfred de Vigney. Flaubert, on the other hand, romanced the beautiful wife of the sculptor, Prodier (supposedly half the men in Paris slept with her), and together with his friend, Bouilhet, sought to satisfy the well-known actress, Beatrix Person.

Contacts with Louise ended in 1854, after a quarrel, during which his former mistress kicked Flaubert in the leg, and from which time are dated her spiteful remarks about the authorship of *Madame Bovary*, as well as the placement of his person in the story entitled, *Lui* (Him), in which she presents Flaubert as a "miserly dwarfish Origen act for act." (35)

Another woman, with whom Flaubert was involved for many years, not excluding his first love, Eliza Schlesinger, was Miss Juliet Herbert. Their relationship, which lasted a quarter century, began in 1854, when Miss Herbert replaced waspish Miss Hutton in her position as the English governess of Caro, Flaubert's niece. Juliet was twenty-five, well educated, pretty, and spoke good French. In a short time, she earned the respect of Madame Flaubert, and found a place in the heart of her 8-year-old pupil – and in the hearts of others. In a letter written in May 1885 to Bouilhet, Flaubert wrote:

> When I noticed what an effect our governess has had on you; at table, I deliberately slide my eyes over the gentle slope of her bosom. I am certain that she sees this. Not without cause is [her face] flooded with a blush five to six times during a meal. (36)

Juliet had to have been more beautiful and smarter than Louise Colet, but, first of all, was more faithful. Unfortunately, no correspondence between them has survived. Most likely it was destroyed by mutual agreement. Juliet taught English, not only to Flaubert's niece, but also to him. The lessons often took place in the evenings when everyone was already asleep, and in a letter to Bouilhet, the poet confessed that the governess excited him tremendously saying, "on the stairs I control myself forcefully not to grab her by her little tail." (36) Flaubert was able to appreciate not only the curves of Miss Herbert's body, but also her intelligence and linguistic abilities. Together, they translated Byron's "Prisoner of Chillon" into French, and, later, *Madame Bovary* into English. Unfortunately, for unclear reasons the latter work was not finished until 1892; this book did not appear in England until 1892, and then in a translation by Eleonor Marx, the daughter of Karl Marx, the author of *Das Kapital*, and the guru of later communists.

Juliet Herbert's stay in the Flaubert household ended in the spring of 1897, at the completion of Caro's home education. This did not mean breaking contact with the family, as Miss Herbert came many times to France for vacations, staying with the Flauberts.

Familiar relations with a former governess were not then as common as currently, and one can presume that Miss Herbert, under the pretext of visiting Madame Flaubert and her former pupil, also visited Flaubert with the aim of mutual work, as described above. She often stayed at an apartment in Paris rented by Flaubert's mother, which was situated under the apartment rented simultaneously by her son. Contacts between Gustave and Juliette were kept secret, even from friends. We know that Flaubert traveled to London many times, where he met with Juliette, also in a rented apartment. He also visited her mother and sister. During the 1870s, and over the course of the 20 years from when they became acquainted, Juliette visited Flaubert in Paris at least five times. About these meetings, no one was informed, while, when he was leaving the house, Flaubert tried to provide himself with an alibi, explaining that he had some important matters to take care of in town, or told his friends that he was going somewhere else, whereas he would go to Paris for a meeting with Juliet. In letters to his friend, Edmond Laporte, written during this time, he mentioned something about incredible sexual exploits, or made some comment of the type, "Everyone thinks that I am in Saint Gretien, whereas I really am in Paris, where I am dusting off my weapon." (37) I wonder what kind of "weapon" Flaubert used for several years before his death, considering his barely cured syphilis and the multiple mercury treatments, which are not conducive to general good health. As one can see, he didn't do badly, although he could have been only bragging, when he wrote to Laporte about his sexual activities, and asked Turgeniev not to be surprised about his prolonged stay in Paris, as he was there as a result of *Veneris causa*. The last meeting of Juliet and Gustave took place a year before the writer's death, and probably also concluded successfully, as he recounted to Laporte. (37) Juliet outlived her lover by over 20 years; she died in London in November 1909.

Flaubert's most famous novel is *Madame Bovary*. Its preparation took the writer five years. The book was printed in parts in 1856 in the columns of *Revue de Paris*, whose founder and publisher was the author's friend, Maxime du Camp. Because it contained, according to the morals police, a fragment offending morality, both gentlemen went before a magistrate. The prosecutor demanded two years in prison, but the verdict was acquittal. (38) *Madame Bovary* is a realistic-psychologic account. It speaks of a woman, not in love with her husband without requite, and who seeks escape from daily life in the arms of another man. The story of Emma Bovary shows the situation of a nineteenth century woman from whom society expects obedience to her husband, and obedience to moral norms. The story ends tragically, in the suicide of both its hero and heroine.

It would appear that Flaubert intended to express himself that *Madame Bovary c'est moi* (Madame Bovary, its I), which would suggest that the author identified himself psychologically with the heroine of his own story. Many scenes, which are found in that story, including erotic ones, were based on the author's own experiences. The famous scene in a carriage is very similar to what happened during a ride in the company of Louise Colet. The agonizing hallucinations of Emma are based, in large part, on his own experiences during nervous breakdowns. The funeral account is reminiscent of an occurrence at the funeral of Alfred de Poittevin, and at the funeral of his own sister. Although the previously cited words, "Madame Bovary, it's me," are not of the author's origin, but were attributed to him by some biographers, does not change the fact that many threads of the story have a connection with his own experiences.

Multiple editions and much enthusiasm about *Madame Bovary* made of Flaubert a person generally known and respected. His following works were not as famous as that novel, yet everyone stressed the uncommon concern about style and precise expression of thoughts by the author. His creativity had an influence on other writers, such as Guy de Maupassant, the de Goncourt brothers, Alphonse Daudet and Emile Zola. Someone spiteful could notice that three of them, de Maupassant, Jules de Goncourt and Daudet were in solidarity with the master to such an extent that they became infected with syphilis, the disease that tormented Flaubert during his entire adult life.

To other, better known novels of Flaubert belong *L'Education sentimale,* published in 1969, and later, *Three Tales* (1877), consisting of three stories, "A Simple Heart," devoted to George Sand, "The Legend of Saint Julian the Hospitaller," and "Herodias." Flaubert began still another novel, *Bouvard et Pecuchet*, which he did not finish, and which was published only after his death. Flaubert also tested the extent of his skills in the drama, *Le Candidat*, which, however, did not attain success.

The social life of Flaubert, as a person of established reputation, a popular writer and celebrity, was conducted between Rouen and Paris. The writer was a frequent guest at dinners hosted by the Princess Matilde Bonaparte in the latter city. He invited guests to Croisset and liked to be seen in the company of influential people. He boasted of his friendship with Gambetta, the chairman of the Lower House of the French Parliament, later the Premier of France. (39) During one of Princess Matilde's dinners, at which George Sand was also present, the authoress spoke to Flaubert using the familiar *Tu* (you), which gave rise to gossip that something more than just friendship joined them. (40)

However, this was only gossip, as nothing points to Flaubert being interested in Madame Sand. During weekends in Croisset, Flaubert, at the request of friends, would read trials of texts on which he was actually working. During one such meeting, the writer read to his friends a fragment from notes from a journey to the Near East, prepared for printing, in which, in addition to descriptions of nature, were tales of obligatory marches, hours spent in the saddle, days without water and nights spend among insects, wanting to impress his friends with accounts of his health, his infection with syphilis, and descriptions of diarrheas that were reactions to mercury treatments. (41)

Flaubert went through at least several courses of mercury treatments, which, speaking gently, did not belong in the pleasant category. The author describes the "sialorrhea that occurred after taking mercury, swelling of the oral cavity and tongue that frequently exceeded that of an ox's protruding lips, which could not be closed . . . ." He mentioned sleepless nights, as well as numerous days during which he ate nothing. In addition to mercury, Flaubert used iodine preparations, took laxative agents, and applied leeches. He planned a visit to Dr. Philipe Ricord, then the authority on treating syphilis, but probably never actually did it. (42) Accounts of the ailments tormenting the author contain information about stomach pains, skin reactions that caused him to appear leprous, ulcers the size of hens' eggs, coughs and fevers. (42) It is not possible to confirm whether these changes were caused by the disease or were side effects of treatment with mercury, allergic reactions to iodine or bromide, or simply furunculosis caused by bacterial infections of the skin.

Flaubert was likewise tormented by problems of a psychological nature, although he was completely functional intellectually during the entire time. He often complained of weakness and depression. Once, he wrote that, as a result of sleeping a long time (10-12 hours at a time), he feared that his brain was undergoing softening. (43) During the Franco-Prussian War in 1870, his friends were concerned that at the moment of occupation of Rouen by the Prussians, Flaubert would explode! (44) Fortunately, nothing like that happened, and the writer lived through a short Prussian occupation without any further problems.

We do not know why his friends had such concerns, as Flaubert behaved during this time in a way that can be described as "patriotically pragmatical." He did not leave France, as did many people in his surroundings. He remained in Croisset, which, to some extent was dictated by the necessity of taking care of his seriously ill mother. At a certain point he presented himself to his doctor brother as a "nurse-volunteer." Next, he joined the National Guard, completed the appropriate training, and, with rank of Lieutenant, was commissioned as the commander of a detachment of volunteers composed of his neighbors. During training, he presented patriotic lectures, declaring "Anyone who shows cowardice will find my sword in his belly," and requested that he be treated the same way should that apply to him. When the Prussians took Rouen, and ten Prussian dragoons took up residence in Croisset with their horses, Lieutenant Flaubert had to lower his tone. "Weeping after the executioners," he had to carry hay for the Germans' horses, and complained that they "neigh right in my face," which, as he wrote in letters to his sister, he considered a personal offense. (45) This last sentence allows one to believe that, despite an undeniably difficult situation, the author of *Madame Bovary* retained his sense of humor.

Despite the fact that, over the course of years, Flaubert's disease progressed, his death was rather a surprise. On May 8, 1880, preparing to leave for Paris, he had a warm bath in the morning, then became weak and fainted. The doctor who was called found him still alive, while de Maupassant, who immediately came to Croisset, wrote that he "saw his huge body on the carpet, with a swollen neck, upon which [I] noted a black collar." The first accounts said that the cause of the writer's death was apoplexy (a stroke) or an attack of epilepsy, which he had not had for a very long time. (46). Others spoke of a heart attack, syphilis, and also the possibility of suicide, of which the black collar around the dead man's neck was supposed to be an indication. The supporters of this latter theory drew on the frequent self-identification of the author with the heroine of *Madame Bovary*, who committed suicide, but there is no convincing evidence for this.

Gustave Flaubert was buried in his family town, while after 10 years, thanks to the efforts of friends, among others, of de Goncourt, de Maupassant and Daudet, a monument to him was unveiled in Rouen.

JULES DE GONCOURT (1830-1870)

Jules de Goncourt was one of two Parisian brothers known for their art collections and as art critics, authors of novels and theatrical works. Jules and Edmond de Goncourt are the authors of the well-known *Journal des Goncourt* (The *des Goncourt* Diary), which made them famous (Fig.5b.5). For many years the brothers worked together and always presented themselves as coauthors of their creations. The men not only worked together, but also lived together, and they would never spend even a single day apart. Supposedly, they promised each other that they would never marry. Friends and acquaintances would always invite them together. They went to dinners, theaters and art exhibitions together, visited friends and took part in gatherings together, traveled together, and visited foreign countries together. Together, they picked up women, for whom they would buy dinner, and then went to bed with them – but together? – that, I don't know. Together, they visited bordellos, which "took up 5 hours weekly – from six to eleven." (47)

According to some, there was something more than just brotherly love between them, while others even suggest that Edmond was a homosexual. It is possible that such a small difference in sexual preferences protected Edmond from sharing the fate of his brother. Jules was eight years younger than Edmond, yet died 26 years earlier than he; the cause of Jules' death was syphilis. Even earlier, Jules became infected with gonorrhea, (48) which Edmond also avoided; this could serve as evidence that the brothers took advantage of the services of different persons, and did not sleep together. In the *Journal* there is not a word that could attest to the sexual preferences of either, but remember that the brothers lived at a time when homosexual activities were carefully concealed, although, in France, in contrast to other countries, they were not punished by imprisonment.

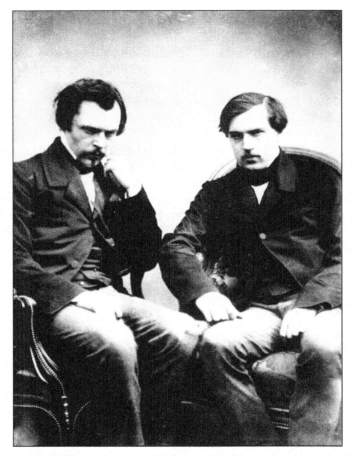

Figure 5b.5 Photograph of Edmond (left) and Jules (right) de Goncourt by Felix Nadar

Jules and Edmond came from French aristocracy, but lost their parents at an early age. The estate that they inherited allowed them to have a fully satisfactory life, leaving them plenty of time for entertainment and involvement in the arts, not necessarily concerned about income. Involving themselves with art criticism, mostly of painting and literature, they became part of the aristocratic-literary world of Paris of the second half of the nineteenth century. In their social circles were found princesses and poets, politicians, writers and journalists, as well as courtesans and high-class prostitutes. Among their close acquaintances were Flaubert, de Maupassant and Daudet, mentioned in this chapter, but also Emile Zola, George Sand, Victor Hugo, and a Russian writer who lived in Paris, Ivan Turgeniev. About half of these were known syphilitics, which allows one to suppose that the disease was very popular in these circles.

The creativity of the de Goncourt brothers was, according to their own opinion, undervalued. The brothers had an unusually high opinion about themselves, and what they did and published, and considered it bad of the whole world that their works were not met with the same enthusiastic acceptance as the tales of Flaubert, or the novels of de Maupassant. This situation changed, but only after the death of Jules, when, in 1887, there appeared the first volume of their *Diary*. This turned out to be a publishing hit, and during the first nine years nine volumes appeared. The publication of each of these produced a reaction reminiscent of putting a stick into an anthill, as the material contained, namely indiscretions, gossip, and private affairs, often intimate, compromised friends equally as enemies of the de Goncourts. Partly as the result of the reactions of the 'heroes and heroines' of *The Diary*, the final volumes – and there were 33 – appeared only many years after the death of Edmond (1896) and of the people about whom they wrote.

The *Journal* of the de Goncourts is a chronicle of happenings that took place in France, and particularly in Paris, during the course of a half-century. Information contained in it concerned mostly persons from the literary-artistic community, and their subjects were not happy with what they read about themselves. The majority of the heroes and heroines of *The Diary* felt belittled, ridiculed, and offended. Remember that these were people from the front pages of newspapers, belonging to the social and political elite.

As a sample of The Diary, and writing of the secrets of the bedroom of the Prussian monarch, here is an entry dated September 25, 1886:

This morning, we spoke about copulation. This is a subject that is never boring. A friend of a friend had a mistress, who asserted that she slept with the future Kaiser Wilhelm II. She was advised to wait for him completely undressed, except for overly long black gloves that reached above the elbows. He went to her equally undressed, and their arms tangled ... and after a brief look at her, he "hurled himself upon her" throwing her to the floor, and satisfying his sexual desire in a bestial frenzy.

To the extent that one can understand this attempt to ridicule the future monarch of a nation with whom France had been at war not so long before, completely *not* understandable is gossip insulting persons who were numbered among good acquaintances, including author friends, such as George Sand. In one of the earlier volumes of this Journal an entry from 1852, noted: A squabble between Mrs. Sand and Clesinger (the sculptor-husband of her daughter). Mrs. Sand: I will do my best that everyone gets to know about your actions ... Clesinger: 'And I will sculpt your ass. Everyone will recognize it,' (49) which had to mean that more than one man in Paris had seen her *au naturelle*.

About Emile Zola, a member of the same social circle, they wrote that "he has a second family," revealing to the public a fact maintained in complete secrecy by the renowned author. It is obvious that the subjects of this gossip had a right to be insulted or feel betrayed by the publication of these types of revelation.

Alongside reports of current events and information of a gossip nature, there were also entries testifying as to their keenness and their ability to arrive at correct conclusions. A good illustration of this is an entry from March 23, 1890, concerning the aforementioned Wilhelm II:

> The young German leader, this neurotic mystic, passionate admirer of the religiously war-like dramas of Wagner, who, during sleepless nights dreams of the white armour of Parsifal and shows signs of feverish mental activity, appears to me very disturbing, unless they lock him up. (50)

As later history reveals, Edmond de Goncourt (this was already after Jules' death) was right. Wilhelm II was one of the main culprits responsible for the outbreak of World War I in 1914, a senseless armed conflict that caused the deaths of millions of Europeans and slowed development on that continent for many years.

In addition to entries of a gossip or journalistic character, relating to artistic and political events (or impressions from the authors' travels), *The Diary* presented the personal opinions of the des Goncourts, which were often very controversial – if it cannot be said, disgraceful. Their opinions on the subject of women are, from today's point of view, frankly shocking, although I suspect that they were a reflection of those of a large portion of society at the time. Here are several of them:

> People such as ourselves do not need women to be well-mannered or educated, necessarily, [but], by nature, [to be] be cheerful and amusing; [they] will comfort and cheer us like a beautiful animal of which we can grow fond. (51)

Or,

Women can do something outstanding simply by sleeping with many men and, so to speak, draining them spiritually: Madame Sand, Madame de Stael. I think it impossible to find a virtuous woman whose intelligence would be worth a broken farthing. Virgins never created anything. (52)

The *Journal* is full of this type of golden thoughts, but these are not what is most important for me. From the point of view of a physician and venereologist, the des Gouncourt diary is a font of knowledge about well-known persons with syphilis. It contains rarely published information about the private lives of known syphilitics, speaks of their sexual habits, their life problems as related to the disease, which were previously unknown or were passed over by biographers, as well as about attempts to cure it. There are also descriptions of specific signs and symptoms appearing in the late stages of lues: descriptions of the changing outlook of the ill person and his/her behaviors, which varied in relation to the progress of the disease, as well as detailed accounts of the last months, days and hours of someone suffering from syphilis.

Of great value to me as a venereologist are the notes of Edmond de Goncourt speaking of the last months of life of his brother, Jules, while he was losing his battle with the disease. In the choice of texts available to me, I did not find any information describing the time or circumstances of his infection with syphilis. Similarly, there is nothing on the subject of treatment with mercury, the then current medication used in the treatment of lues. The first description of Jules' illness, a somewhat enigmatic one, comes from January, 1870 in which hydrotherapy is spoken of, without giving details of who received it or why. One cannot exclude that Jules did not obtain standard treatment for lues (similarly as his gonorrhea had not been treated earlier), while trying alternative methods such as hydrotherapy, which was used then for very varied illnesses, particularly those of a neurologic basis. (53)

The first notes pertaining to the final stage of Jules' illness are from January 1870.

> After many months, I am taking up the pen that fell from my brother's hand. At first, I wanted to end this journal with the last notes-entries of the dying one, who is returning to his youth and childhood. ... 'My literary career is finished, my literary ambition has died.' ... 'Today, I think as yesterday, yet there is a certain sweetness in relating to myself the months of despair and agony – but maybe also an unclear longing to strengthen that, which is tearing asunder, for the friends of his memory.' ... 'I am, therefore, undertaking the journal, returning to notes sketched during nights of tears, notes similar to shrieks, in which physical suffering seeks relief ....' (54)

End of February:

> Today, he feels well, unusually well, and he who was earlier our common will, but [now] allows himself to be convinced of something with such difficulty ... proposing a walk to the waterfall (in the Bologne forest) ... During the walk he asserts that "I do not want to go anywhere, I do not want to show myself to people: he said to me that he is ashamed of himself. (54)

March:

> Tactfulness was his share. No one was equally subtle in serving himself with tact in an instinctive and thoughtful manner. These so very aristocratic talents he is losing now, and lacks the gradation of politeness in relation to types of people whom he meets; already, a lack of gradation of intelligence

appropriate to that of the people with whom he comes into contact. ... For some time – and visibly worse every day, he mispronounces certain letters. (54)

<u>April 8</u>.

A mystery, an inconceivable and unfathomable mystery, is that, in this brain atrophy, certain strengths, certain abilities remain and make a gallant stand; a mystery that, out of the lethargy that is becoming generalized, words, thoughts, lively or deep descriptions escape ....

Later there appears a description of the intellectual degradation.

On this beloved face, where intelligence, irony, subtle and charmingly sarcastic expressions of humor lived, minute by minute is superimposed the wild mask of muddleheadedness. Gradually, sincerity is lost, dehumanization occurs; others stop existing for him and once again there is born in him the cruel egotism of a child. ... His own illness is not sufficient for him; he is constantly troubled by imagined illnesses, looking with alarm and a pained expression at [every] white or red mark squeezed onto his skin by a fold of his shirt. Awful in these repulsive illnesses of the mind is that they are not satisfied [just] with intelligence; with time, and mysteriously, they destroy in the individual whom they reduce to bestiality, sensitivity, tenderness, attachments; they kill the heart ... I no longer see and do not meet the friendship that we shared greatly, and [which] was my fortune. No, I no longer feel his love; for me it is my greatest grief, and no matter what I say to myself, nothing is able to assuage it. ... His face has become submissive, ashamed; he flees from looks – the spies of his fall and degradation. (54)

About April 30th:

Neither the weakening of his intellect, nor the loss of memory, nor anything of this type causes me to despair, but I am afraid of something undescribed, a different creature that he is becoming. His profession, which occupied him so much, even to giving up work, has stopped interesting him; his relationship to his books is as though he had never written them. Stupefaction, immobility lasting a half-hour, and only rapidly revolving eyes beneath blinking eyelids .... (54)

About May 30:

Like a little child only what he eats and wears concerns him; he rejoices *hors d'oevres*, is happy about new clothes."

June 5:

Long moments when, while sitting next to me in the bedroom, he is not with me. Where are you, my dear? – I asked him yesterday. He responded after a moment's pause, "In space ... in empty space.

June 18:

It's two o'clock in the morning. I arose and am relieving Pelagia (the maidservant) at the bedside of my poor, beloved brother, who has not regained consciousness and speech from two in the afternoon on Thursday (about three days)... "I listen intently to his rapid and labored breathing. In the shadow of the curtain, I see his motionless stare. Every few moments he touches me with his arm stretched out from the bed..... from his lips exit incoherent words that weep with one another ... Despite taking a threefold dose of potassium bromide in a quarter glass of water, he cannot sleep even a minute, his head in unceasing motion turns from left to right; something not apprehended clamors in his paralyzed brain, from his lips fall outlines of sentences, fragments of words, unarticulated syllables, repeated violently, at first, and ending as a sigh.

[During his last months, Jules experienced epilepsy-like seizures.] Suddenly, he threw his head backwards, and shouted so hoarsely, throatily and horribly, that I had to close the window. Immediately, contractions contorted his pleasant face, deforming all its shapes, changing all its features; terrible convulsions jerked his body and arms as though wanting to screw them on, from his distorted lips fell a bloody foam. Sitting behind him on his pillow, I held his arms and pressed his head to [my] heart; its deadly sweat wet my shirt, and ran down my thighs. After this attack, other, less violent ones occurred, his face became again the one which I knew. In turn, a calm arrived, one full of delirium. He would raise his arms above his head, experiencing a vision with kisses. He was transported like a wounded bird to flight and on his now calmed face with bloodshot eyes, pale forehead, lowered and bluish lips appeared an expression, which had nothing human – an inscrutable and mysterious look, as though from Leonardo da Vinci. (54)

The above and further reports constitute accounts of delusions and hallucinations that are typical features of general paresis:

Even more frequent were moments of fear, of frightened retreats, as though the body was seeking shelter under the bedclothes, as if hiding from a ghost, stubbornly hiding in the depths of the curtains; against it, he would direct his unformed words, and stretch out his finger in surprise, once even shouting clearly 'go away.' "Tatters of sentences uttered in an ironic tone flowed in a torrent. ... At times, under the action of an unremitting fever and hallucinations, he would repeat all of his daily activities, by gesture indicating that he was donning his spectacles, raising his weights, over which I tormented him during the last few months, fencing, writing, pretending to write.

The neurologist (dr. Beni-Barde), who examined the patient, told me that 'everything was finished, that a decomposition of the brain at its the base, at the rear of the skull had set in, that there was no longer any hope.' (54)

Monday, June 20 (5 o'clock in the morning):

In his eyes, [there is] an expression of unspoken suffering and misery. To create a being such as he, so talented, so intelligent, and to kill him in his thirty ninth year of life. Why? (54) [Jules died several hours later.] 'He is dying, he has died! Thanks be to God! He died after several soft sighs, [as though of a] sleeping child." (54)

This rather long citation is an account related by Edmond de Goncourt from the final month, days and hours of his brother, who was dying as the result of lues. It is simultaneously an account of the signs/symptoms of third-stage syphilis, and specifically, of general paresis seen through the eyes of a member of his family and the person taking care of the sufferer. It is very moving, but also very authentic, and, thanks to that, more understandable for the average person than a dry account of the disease, as can be found in a medical handbook intended for students and physicians.

ALPHONSE DAUDET (1840-1897)

Alphonse Daudet belonged to the same social-literary circle as Gustave Flaubert, Guy de Maupassant, the de Goncourt brothers, and several others. He came from a not very wealthy family, as his father did not do well in business (Fig.5b.6).

> At home, there was not a penny, while the father changed his profession and type of business every day, while Lyons, with its constant fog was loathsome for this tiny being who was in love with the sun. He read greedily – he was only 12 years old – he read poets, books of fantasy, which, together with sipping alcohol, stimulated his thoughts, he read all day on a boat, which he would push off from the shore. And in the flowing splashes of both rivers (Saon and Rodan), intoxicated with reading and alcohol, near-sighted by nature, lived as though in a dream or hallucination, outside reality, which had no access to him. (55)

This is how Alphonse Daudet reminisced about his childhood during one of the visits of Flaubert in February, 1875. From school, he brought the worst possible reminiscences. He was slighted by teachers, and bullied by his classmates. After finishing his education, Alphonse obtained work as a teacher, but after only a year, he'd had enough work in school and went off to his brother, who worked as a journalist in Paris. Soon, Alphonse also obtained work with the widely read, Parisian paper, *Le Figaro*. Simultaneously, he began to publish his own works: short stories, poems, and even theatrical works. This was not

Alphonse's literary debut, as he wrote his first story and first poem at age 14, and published them in a little tome titled *Les Amoreuses* (The Lovers), when he was eighteen years of age.

The next stage in Daudet's career was to take on work as a secretary to one of the more important ministers of Emperor Napoleon III. This job greatly improved Daudet's social status, and facilitated the publication of the author's subsequent creations. In the course of the next 30 years, Daudet published a series of works that were more or less popular. Some of them were: *Chose* (The Little Thing), in which he describes, in a rather embellished way, his recollections from school; *Lettres de Mon Moulin* (Letters from my Mill), the adventures of the comic hero, Tartarin, described in *Tartarin de Tarascon* (Tartarin of Tarascon), and *Tartarin sur les Alpes*, (Tartarin in the Alps). In one of his later works, written in the style of a memoir, *La Doulou* (Pain), Daudet gave an account of symptoms produced by *tabes dorsalis*, which the author experienced at the end of his life. Unfortunately, his family made a number of changes in it likely with the aim of protecting the author's good name. (56) This book appeared many years after Daudet's death, and was also translated into English in 2002 by James Barnes, under the title *In the Land of Pain*.

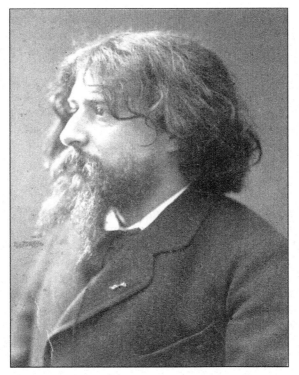

Figure 5b.6 Alphonse Dauded by Felix Nadar

To other, better known creations belong the patriotic stories, "Monday's Tales," as well as realistic works describing the times during which the author lived and worked, "Sapho" and "The Nabab." The last clearly reveals the author's racist outlook. It is worth adding that among in the circle of Daudet's friends, in addition to well-known French literary figures, there were also well known anti-Semites of the period. One of these was Edouard Drumont, the founder of the Antisemitic League of France, as well as the owner and editor of the anti-Semitic newspaper, *Le Libre Parole*. In his *Journal*, Edmond de Goncourt describes a series of dinners that took place in Daudet's home, in which Drumont and his friend, Jacques de Biez, another well-known anti-Semite of the period, took part. The last was the French delegate to the first Congress of Anti-Semites that took place in Bucharest in 1886, and also was the author of the cry, "France for the French!" During the dinner mentioned above, the gentlemen dreamed of organizing disturbances in France directed against the Jews, and greatly lamented that they could not gather the funds needed for this purpose. (57)

I do not know if excessive eroticism is one of the characteristics of racists, but if that were the case, then Daudet would be one of the best examples. He lost his virginity at age 12, and then is supposed to have undertaken the seductions of the wives of his friends. He got married when he was 27 years of age, his chosen one being Julia Allard, an authoress writing under the pseudonym "Karl Steen."

Alphonse was not a faithful husband. In the *Journal* of the de Goncourt brothers is found a description of a meeting, during which Daudet describes one so-called marital *faux pas:*

> Daudet related to Heredi (the poet Jose-Maria Heredia), how he was surprised by his wife. As he had no doubt that Madame Daudet had gone out, he like his 'love' disrobed, he was completely naked, his little beauty also. The door opened. A muffled shriek. The door closed. Silence from both sides; a half year passes without a word. But, his wife 'gets the vapors,' she is ill. Daudet risks an apology. Mrs. Daudet says: "I wanted to jump out of the window, but I thought about our child ... Nevertheless, I am warning you that if it happens again, I will kill myself.

Mrs. Daudet was sufficiently a Breton as to keep her word. And Daudet added, "And now, my dear fellow, take a look at what it means to be surprised in this way. All my rights were taken away; every morning, my wife looks through my mail, and throws any from women into the fire etc., etc." (58)

I do not have the date nor the circumstances related to Daudet's infection with syphilis. There was gossip to the effect that, supposedly, he became infected by a highly placed woman, a court stenographer, a woman from the 'upper crust.' I do not know whether, or when he might have had signs of early lues earlier. The first accounts of his illness come from 1884, a time when signs revealing damage to the nervous system (and, specifically, *tabes dorsalis*) had already appeared .The first signs of this condition usually present from several to 13-19 years after infection, while one can assume that Daudet most likely became infected before 1880. For a while, it was felt that Daudet had tuberculosis, and that his disturbances in movement were related to rheumatism. The first physician who made the diagnosis of syphilis in him was the well-known French neurologist, Dr. Jean-Martin Charcot. Charcot was the one, who, ten years earlier, had described "gastric crises," and associated them with late syphilis, and, specifically, as one of the signs of *tabes* dorsalis. Alphonse Daudet suffered, not only from gastric crises that caused severe stomach pains and vomiting, but also had problems with walking and urination. Additionally, he experienced so-called *lightning pains*; these are extremely severe pains radiating to the extremities, and are frequently so severe that patients cannot suppress shrieks when experiencing them. One of the manifestations of *tabes dorsalis* is ataxia, which includes, among other things, movement disturbances, and influences the patient's manner of walking. Daudet would fall often, and went up and down stairs with difficulty, which was observed by the then-still-little Misia Godebska-Sert, later a friend of many well-known French artists of the end of the nineteenth century. Although walking with difficulty, Daudet would visit her family, and Misia, together with the other children, watched how he came down the stairs with amusement, expecting that he would fall at any moment. (59) Another example of Daudet's ataxia comes from an account of a reception in London, in which he participated, together with George Meredith, the well-known English author-syphilitic, who also suffered with *tabes dorsalis*. It is said that both men, while wanting to 'clink' glasses filled with wine during a toast spilled it on the lady sitting between them, as a result of handicapped coordination. (56)

Dr. Charcot sent Daudet to spa, where he tried traction therapy, an experimental treatment method devised in Russia. In 1884, as the result of severe swelling of the scrotum, Daudet agreed to a consultation with the famous Parisian venereologist, Dr. Alfred Fournier. Some type of surgical procedure was then performed, and iodine preparations were recommended. Despite the treatment, the disease progressed, while the patient became aware of approaching severe problems. In entries from July 14, 1890, Edmond de Goncourt noted:

> Poor Daudet, one thought persecutes him: he is scared of degradation, that is, the physical appearance brought about by paralysis. And when one wants to raise his spirits, he relates that in Lamalou (a spa in southern France) he compared the advance of his disease with that of others, that this awaits him in a year, that in two .... (60).

Ten days later, there appears another entry concerning Daudet:

> After a longer moment of concentration, Daudet says, with head lowered toward his poor, dead legs in felt shoes: "Every night, I dream that I am walking ... on beaches, while people say to me, 'How well you walk over the stones!' And waking up ... Oh, waking up is terrible. (60)

Less than a year later (May 10, 1891), we have the next information concerning Daudet.

Oh, how that Daudet is suffering! Today, in my garret, he was unable to speak at times, he was writhing, and stretching out his painful legs, while his face was so anguished, so tired. During two hours, he thrice gave himself an injection of morphine. (61)

Despite the physical crippling caused by *tabes dorsalis*, Daudet remained intellectually functional. He took part in the social and cultural life of Paris, wrote and published. Edmond de Goncourt noted spitefully that the quality of his writing underwent a change for the worse, and that the author published mainly for the money necessary to support his family (62). Alphonse Daudet died December 16, 1897, at age 57.

GUY DE MAUPASSANT (1850-1893)

Guy de Maupasant, younger than Flaubert by close to 30 years, came from a wealthy family living in Normandy (Fig.5b.7). When he was 11 years old, his parents separated, and Guy, together with his younger brother, lived with his mother. Guy's mother, Laura de Maupassant, was an independent person of strong character, well read and a lover of classical literature, particularly that of Shakespeare. Laura was the sister of Alfred Le Poittevin, a friend of Flaubert, and very good friends with the writer, himself.

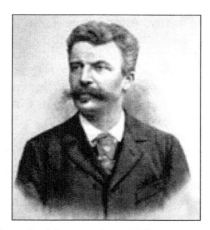

Figure 5b.7 Guy de Maupassant. Photograph form 1888 by Felix Nadar

We know that de Maupassant's uncle, Alfred Le Poittevin, was a childhood friend of Flaubert. Older than Flaubert, he was a model to emulate, an authority in artistic matters for the latter, an oracle in philosophical matters, and an adviser and confidant in erotic matters. It is said that it was he who was the first to be a bad example for the young Flaubert, showing him the road to bordellos and encouraging him to avail himself of the services of women of loose morals. Similarly to Flaubert, Alfred Le Poittevin later studied law in Paris, and took advantage of such entertainments as the capital of France offered at the time. He was interested in philosophy, poetry and literature, particularly of the romantic and ancient periods. Unfortunately, he was an alcoholic, and suffered from tuberculosis and syphilis. He died, destroyed by all these diseases, at age 32.

Similarly to his uncle, even in his school days Guy de Maupassant was interested in literature and poetry, although an equally strong passion of this young man throughout his life was water sports. After finishing his education in Rouen, de Maupassant began the study of law in Paris, but the Franco-Prussian war soon broke out, and the young student signed up with the army. After the war, he stayed in Paris, where he worked as a clerk, first in the Department of the Navy, then in the Ministry of Public Education. He was clearly bored at work, while he passionately took part in water sports, rowing on the Seine, frequently for many hours at a time. A second passion of de Maupassant, and later also a main source of his income, was writing. Even during his school days, he stayed in contact with Flaubert, who encouraged him to write, and as an experienced author, dispensed valuable advice. Guy was very grateful to Flaubert for everything that he did for his career as a writer. Near the end of his life, when Flaubert had financial problems, Maupassant took advantage of a position he held at the Ministry of Public Education and arranged a government pension for him. De Maupassant was not only a student and a friend, but also a guardian, frequently visiting Flaubert, both in Paris and in Croisset.

We do not know if the advice Flaubert provided to the young de Maupassant concerned only writing, as, observing his relationships with women, one can get the impression that the latter could have been mimicking his master equally in erotic matters. Claude Quetel wrote that "de Maupassant demonstrated the same sexual ardor and the same pride in wounds of victory as Flaubert, and makes mention of the sick psychology, which also finds its reflection in his deeds." (63) Frank Harris, who befriended de Maupassant from 1880, writes in his memoirs of the boasts and sexual deeds of his friend. He maintained that de Maupassant was more proud of his sexual achievements than of his stories. (64) Many biographers of the writer refer to accounts in "The Diary" of the de Goncourts that speak of the "wild nights of de Maupassant, who was said to bring himself to the highest state of sexual excitement." They write about relations with six prostitutes in the course of less than an hour, and about an episode when one day de Maupassant painted a primary chancre, there when it normally appears (on the penis), and showed it to his female partner, whom he then raped, asserting that he had gifted her with syphilis. (65) Jokes about topics related to syphilis were reborn in time with an unamusing reality. De Maupassant became infected with the disease, a fact that he did not initially realize. It is assumed that he became infected when he was 20 years old from a girl with whom he undertook a boat ride on the Seine, as he himself, expressed it, "from some Mimi or Nimi from Bezons, or another *marchandes de spasms*." (66) It also cannot be excluded that the infection took place at a time when de Maupassant enlisted in the army, and took advantage of the sexual services of some "patriotically inclined" female citizen.

Unfortunately, the author learned about his disease only after some time, and that, without any possibility of an exact determination of the time and source of infection. In a letter from 1877, addressed to a friend, he wrote:

> You would never guess what a wonderful discovery my doctor made ... As my utterly lost hair never grew back, and because my father shed tears over me while my mother's laments reached from Etretat even to here, I grabbed my doctor by the collar and told him, 'scoundrel, either you find out what is the matter with me, or I will beat you up.' He replied: 'lues.' I admit that I did not expect this – I felt ridiculed; finally, I asked: 'What medicine?' He replied, 'mercury and potassium iodide.' I went to another Aesculapian, who gave me the same diagnosis, narrowing it down to old syphilis, of about six or seven years. ... In brief, for five weeks, I have been taking four centigrams of mercury and thirty centigrams of potassium iodide daily, and feel fine. I am afraid that mercury will become a constant feature of my everyday diet, become my everyday food. My hair is starting to appear ... the growth is thickening on my butt ... I have lues! Finally! The real thing! Not gonorrhea,

worthy of contempt, not ecclesiastical *crystalline* {doubtless referring to genital herpes}, not the bourgeoisie *condyloma acuminata* or vegetative cauliflowers – no – no, the great lues, that from which Francis I died. Majestic and straightforward syphilis; elegant syphilis ... I have lues ... and I am proud of it, damn it, and I scorn in advance all bourgeoisie. Hallelujah – I have lues, as a consequence of which, I am no longer concerned that I will catch it, and [can] kiss street girls [and] disreputable women beneath the [city] gates, and then say to them, 'I have lues.' And they are scared, while I laugh. (67)

I don't think that this was funny for de Maupassant! A young, athletic and healthy person until then, he must have realized what the consequences of the infection were, and in the letter to his friend, he was "putting on a strong face." His words remind one of the boastings of Flaubert on the same topic.

Another question that presents itself during the reading of this text is the date of his infection. The physician who examined de Maupassant asserted that infection took place six-seven years earlier. Balding as a result of syphilis *(alopecia syphilitica)* usually appears several months after infection, and is a sign of secondary syphilis. In untreated lues, balding may remit spontaneously usually after six-twelve months. Is it then possible that de Maupassant was infected later than we judge thought? And another point: in the ending fragments of the above citation, de Maupassant boasts that he has lues, and not some *crystalline* - which, in today's terminology is described as genital herpes, caused by infection with a virus of the *Herpes* group, and not *bourgeoise condyloma*, which we now call venereal warts, caused by the human papilloma virus (HPV). The latter virus has a variety of manifestations in addition to common warts, which we find commonly in children, includes some strains that are also the cause of cervical cancer in women, and penile cancer in men. I want to bring attention to the fact that even from second half of the nineteenth century, genital herpes and genital warts (*condyloma acuminata)* were distinguished from lues, although both are transmitted sexually.

In literature, Guy de Maupassant is considered the world's best short story writer. Besides his shorter works, he also wrote narratives, travelogues, and poetry. His first great literary success was the narrative, *Boule de Suif* (Ball of Fat), whose action unfolds in 1970 during the Franco-Prussian War, although the best known are *Pierre et Jean* and *Bel Ami.* In the course of the following 10 years, he published close to 300 items. Some of his biographers cite unsubstantiated opinions that those ill with lues, generally during the period before symptoms involving the nervous system appear, are more intellectually fertile, of which de Maupassant is supposed to be a good example. (68) His stories and novels are devoid of any sentimentality or idealism, and, similarly to his mentor (Gustave Flaubert), de Maupassant tries to be a realist to the point of exaggeration. He was interested in the emotional problems of people coming from different social classes. Women and their problems are a frequent topic, as also are venereal diseases. In one of his stories,"*Le lit 29"* (Bed No. 29), the author brought up the topic of conscious (premeditated) infection with syphilis, a topic which had been the subject of the little squeamish practical joke by de Maupassant, recounted earlier. In the story's narrative, whose action takes place even before the outbreak of war, de Maupassant relates the story of Captain Epivent, an attractive man, famous for his innumerable romantic conquests. Captain Epivent, whose external attributes remind one of the appearance of the author himself, falls in love with a beautiful girl by the name of Irma. The war breaks out, and the captain, before heading for the front lines, spends the night in Irma's arms. After the war ends, when he returns to the town with the aura of a front-line hero, with medals for courage, she looks for her love, and learns that she can be found in the hospital. The doctor he meets treats him rather harshly, after which it turns out that his beloved Irma is in Bed No. 29, in the ward designated for those ill with syphilis. The woman is physically changed, and has a foul odor, similarly to other sick women on this ward. Irma explains that the Prussians physically forced her to sexual relations, and infected her with syphilis. "But why did you not get treatment?" the captain asks. Irma, with flashing eyes, replies that no, she "wanted revenge, inasmuch as [she was] going to die from this terrible disease!" "And so, I also infected all of them, just as many as I could. I did not get treatment as long as they remained in Rouen." (69) When Epivent reproached her that, after all, she should not have messed with the enemy, Irma replied that her war effort was even greater than his as a hero captain, and that she doubtless liquidated more enemy soldiers than he as a captain in the French army.

De Maupassant's books, even during the author's life, enjoyed enormous popularity, often having between thirteen and nineteen editions yearly. The author became a celebrity and moved around in the best social circles, although he was generally a loner and avoided contact with people. He travelled a bit. He was a wealthy man, had his own yacht, bearing the name of one of his stories, *Bel Ami*. Among his friends were Gustave Flaubert, Emile Zola, Edmond and Jules de Goncourt, and even the famous Alexandre Dumas.

The first accounts concerning de Maupassant's health problems come from 1880. It was then that he complained that he may lose his sight, as he had stopped seeing out of his right eye. After an examination by the ophthalmologist, Dr. Abadie, it turned out that the problem was a paralysis of accommodation in the right eye. Another ophthalmologist, Dr. Landolt, noted an enlargement of the pupils, and determined that the problem did not lie in the eye, itself, but was the result of a disease of the ophthalmic nerve. Despite not overly accurate accounts, one can assume that this was most likely *ophthalmoplegia interna*, which is an element of palsy of the optic nerve, without, generally speaking, paralysis of the external muscles of the eye. Besides an absence of response to light and accommodation, dilated pupils or derangement of the accommodation may be present. Changes pertain only to one eye, and in close to 75% of cases, was the result of syphilis. Dr. Landolt knew that these types of problems testified to advance of the disease, and had no illusions that things would end in any way other than tragically. (70)

Edmond de Goncourt described a joint trip with Zola and de Maupassant in November 1890, when they were going to Rouen for the unveiling of a monument to Flaubert:

> I am struck by de Maupassant's sorry appearance, his sunken face, clay-like complexion, his excessive expressiveness, and sickly immobility of glance. It does not look as though he can live long ... When we crossed the Seine, just before Rouen, [and] stretching out his hand to the river hidden by fog, he said, 'I am indebted to my morning rowing on this water for my condition today'. (71)

It would be interesting to know whether, by saying these words, he wanted to relate that, if not for his physical training associated with his passion for rowing (boats), his state of health would have been worse – or whether he wanted to confer the idea that he attributed the beginning of his health problems to his mutual rowing excursion with a woman ill with lues.

Not only his friends, but de Maupassant himself was increasingly worried about the state of his health. Psychiatric signs/symptoms that were difficult to conceal appeared. In the course of one of his visits to the editorial office of *La Nouvelle Revue* ("The New Revue"), he began to behave very suspiciously, and when the lady with whom he was speaking remarked that he was behaving like a madman, he said that he understood that he would land in an insane asylum one day, and that his brother, who also was ill, was already there. Several years earlier, de Maupassant had helped to admit his younger brother, Herve, to a hospital for the mentally ill, due to a general paresis produced, most likely, by luetic infection. (72) Guy had to have been aware of the seriousness of the situation, and that in several years he could follow in his brother's his footsteps.

One of the physicians taking care of de Maupassant at the time was the famous Parisian physician, Dr. David Gruby. He proposed a special diet to the patient, which was supposed to improve the state of his health. It consisted of boiled potatoes, a large quantity of eggs and milk, and saltwater fish for every meal, as well as meat and poultry in any quantity. The diet forbade eating fresh vegetables, wild game, and wine. It is difficult to understand what guided my famous medical colleague, as the dietary recommendation above had no influence on the basic illness from which de Maupassant suffered, unless the patient were emaciated, and required a high-protein diet.

Despite the increasingly frequent signs of insanity, de Maupassant continued to write and to publish. During this time, there appeared two narratives, *Le Horla* and *La Preur*, in which the psychologic experiences of the characters are narrated with great precision, as though he had experienced them himself. Psychiatric problems caused de Maupassant to travel frequently, as though wanting to free himself from thinking about his approaching death. Paris irritated him; he could not stand the smoky air and noise in the city, which gave him headaches. Guy compared himself to a howling dog, one that howls from suffering, but whose howling is addressed to no one, reaches no one, and says nothing to anyone. (73)

Edmond de Goncourt, in *Le Journal*, dated August 17, 1892, informed us that:

[T]he newspapers write about an improvement in health of de Maupassant," and cites a conversation with a Dr. Blanche: "Maupassant spoke almost the whole day with imaginary persons – exclusively bankers, stock-brokers and financiers – and cried out, suddenly, "Are you making fun of me? So where is the 12 million that you were to bring me today?

Dr. Blanche added:

He doesn't recognize me, and calls me doctor, but, for him, I am some other doctor, not Dr. Blanche," and speaks sadly of de Maupassant's appearance, which now has the physiognomy of a real maniac, a faulty gaze and inanimate lips. (74)

The ill author, fearful of his increasing insanity, spoke of suicide. In periods of remission, he was aware of his state of health, and recorded his experiences very precisely. In November 1892, he wrote:

There are whole days on which I feel I am done for, finished, blind, my brain used up and yet still alive ... I have not a single idea that is follows the one before it. I forget words, names of everything, and my hallucinations and my pains tear me to pieces.

It appeared to him that the saltwater irrigations he had been giving his nostrils had started a salty fermentation in his brain, and that his dissolving brain was flowing back through his nose. He maintained, also, that he had become a count, and insisted that this title be used when addressing him. (75)

In December, while on a boat trip in the company of two women, he had visual hallucinations – he asserted that he had actually seen a ghost. During the first day of the New Year, his servant found him lying in a pool of blood with a cut throat. It was reported that he tried to shoot himself, but that the wound was not particularly serious. After physicians dressed the wound, it was decided to confine him to a strait jacket. The author later imagined that war had broken out, and that he had to go to the front lines. On January 6, 1893, de Maupassant was taken to the psychiatric hospital in Passy, in Paris, run by the aforementioned psychiatrist, Dr. Blanche.

The following months were periods of return to his senses, interwoven with periods in which the writer suffered from hallucinations and aggressive episodes. From April onward, the state of his health steadily became worse. The patient asserted that he is the wealthy younger son of the Mother of God. He planted small branches in the garden, awaiting their growth as small de Maupassants. He licked the walls of his cell, and stored his own urine, which, he maintained, was made of diamonds and other jewels. He would ask people whether they saw the thoughts that had escaped from his head. He was delighted when he found them in the form of butterflies of various colors, depending on his mood: black were sad; pink, merry; and violet, adulterous.

During his last days, as a result of a heightened level of violence and the danger to himself and to his surroundings, Guy de Maupassant was mechanically restrained. He died on July 7, 1893.

OSCAR WILDE (1856-1900)

Oscar Wilde, poet, writer of prose and dramatist, was born in Ireland in a medical family (Fig.5b.8). His parents were among the intellectual elite of Dublin. Having a French *bonne* and a German governess, Oscar learned those languages even as a child. He studied, first at Trinity College, Dublin, where he is remembered as an exceptionally talented student, and later at Oxford, where he quickly became a celebrity.

Thanks to his above average intelligence, colorful personality and uncommon lifestyle, and, above all, to his writing talents, Wilde became the subject of many biographies. Most of these (R. Ellmann, F. Harris, H. Pearson, and H. M. Hyde) consider him to have had syphilis, and that he died as a result of it. Not all, however, agree with this opinion, the dispute turns on two points. In the first, the authors question whether Oscar Wilde ever became infected with syphilis, and in the second, whether syphilis – if he, in fact, suffered from it – was the cause of his death. Richard Ellmann writes: "It was at Oxford that an event occurred that was to alter his whole conception of himself. Wilde contracted syphilis, reportedly from a woman prostitute." This author further clarifies:

My belief that Wilde had syphilis stems from statements made by Reginald Turner and Robert Ross, Wilde's close friends present at his death, from the certificate of the doctor in charge at the time and from the fact that the 1912 edition of Ransome's book on Wilde and Harris's (1916) life (book of which Ross oversaw), give syphilis as the cause of death. Opinion on the subject is, however, divided and some authorities do not share my view of Wilde's medical history. Admittedly, the evidence is not decisive - it could scarcely be so, given the aura of disgrace, shame and secrecy surrounding the disease in Wilde's time and after and might not stand up in a court of law. Nevertheless I am convinced that Wilde had syphilis and that conviction is central to my conception of Wilde's character and my interpretation of many things in his later life. (76)

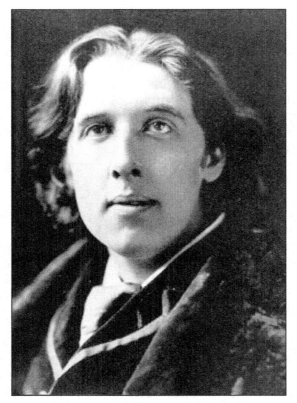

Figure 5b.8 Portrait of Oscar Wilde (New York 1882)

On the same page, Ellman writes further:

As a doctor's son, he had been inclined to minimize illness, so this came as an especially crushing blow. In 1870, medical authorities followed Sir Jeremy Hutchinson's advice [that] anyone contracting the disease should wait two years before marrying and [should] undergo a course of mercury treatment. The main physical effect of mercury in Wilde was to turn his slightly protrusive teeth black, so thereafter he usually covered his mouth with his hand while talking. (Mercury did not cure the disease, though it was reputed to do so, but the mental effect was profound). Like his father he had been subject to fits of melancholy; now there was a new warranty for them. (76)

The last sentences of the cited text are not very convincing, as the state called *melancholia* by Ellmann is very common, and does not need syphilis as its cause. Blackened teeth are also not evidence of lues, although we know that mercury treatment causes inflammation of the mucous membranes of the oral cavity, often ending in the loss of dentition. On the other hand, important and convincing arguments speaking for lues are the cited revelations of the author's close friends, who may have known details concerning Wilde's health that were hidden from a wider public opinion.

There is no lack of opposing opinions, whose authors maintain that Oscar Wilde never suffered from syphilis, or, more exactly, that there is no proof of it. (77) Indeed, until now, no medical documents corroborating the type of diagnosis in which *expressis verbis* is written have been found, i.e. that the writer's health problems were the consequence of syphilis. Even the death certificate drawn up by physicians in Paris says that the cause of Wilde's death was meningitis or meningoencephalitis, without giving details of the etiology of his illness – of which there is quite a variety, including lues.

Oscar Wilde, a handsome, young and intelligent man was the object of interest for many women. He also was interested in them, and was able to appreciate their charms. It appears, however, that even from his early youth, he was also interested in boys, and this interest was more than the average, of which young Oscar, at least initially, was unaware. As Neil McKenna wrote:

Oscar's path to erotic self-realization was twisted and stormy. In his published poems, he publicly celebrated the glories of Greek love {the word, "homosexuality," appeared in the English language only at the junction of the nineteenth and twentieth centuries}, and in private he rhapsodized poetically over the physical charm of boys. Yet it seems that Oscar was able to successfully separate his sexual yearnings from his sexual identity. He could have sex with young men, and yet still cast himself as a conventional lover of women. And he could convince himself – even lie to himself – that his sexual contacts with men were of a different order from his sexual contacts with women. (78)

Information about his first flirtations with young women comes from 1875, when a mother caught Oscar with her daughter, Fidelie, whom Oscar was secretly kissing, on his lap. She wrote a letter to Oscar, informing him of his inappropriate behavior toward Fidelie, as not worthy of a gentleman. From about the same time, there was a flirtation with a Miss Eva, whose aunt declared that the young woman was ready for marriage, if Oscar's intentions were honorable. The next young woman that interested Oscar, and with whom he probably fell in love, was Florence Balcombe. Oscar drew a pencil portrait of her (which has survived to the present), and gave her a small, gold cross for Christmas. The young people wrote to each other for a time, but what at first looked like love, transformed itself into just a friendship that lasted three years. It is worth noting that at the same time as Oscar was sighing about Florence, he was having sexual contact with Frank Miles, a man, whom he met in the spring of 1876. This mixing of Oscar's emotional-erotic behaviors repeated itself over many years – of course, in a variety of configurations and with various partners.

Frank Miles was a year older than Oscar, lived in London, and was a beginning portrait artist. After several months from his first meeting, Frank introduced Oscar to his friend and sculptor, Lord Ronald Gower, also a homosexual, whom Oscar presented theatrically in his later work (*Dorian Gray*), in a rather negative role, as Lord Henry Wotton.

Despite the fact that the friendship between Oscar and Frank Miles lasted quite a long time, it appears that no greater mutual feelings were created, and this was more a simple friendship, renewed, from time to time, with sex. This relationship was diminished over time, which may have been partly caused by the fact of Frank having a mustache that Oscar clearly did not like. Another element limiting the relationship between the two men was lues, which Frank acquired from one of his numerous sex partners. Frank Miles died at the age of 39, in a mental asylum where he spent his last years because of *general paresis*. (79)

Even during his friendship with Frank Miles, Oscar was maintaining contact with other artists, including Arthur May and Walter Pater, but these relationships did not interfere with his being interested in women. Among the latter whom he adored, was one, Lillie Langtry, a so-called "professional beauty," who posed for painters, among them Frank Miles.

Lillie, nicknamed "Jersey Lillie "(she was from the island of Jersey), was considered an unusually beautiful woman, and it is no wonder that she had many admirers. She chose her lovers very carefully – one of these was the Prince of Wales, the later King Edward VII. It was said that Oscar also fell in love with Lillie: "There were rumors that he was deeply in love with her, and that he presented her with a single pale lily every day." He also said, "I would have rather discovered Mrs. Langtry than have discovered America." Wilde wrote a poem, "The New Helen," praising her beauty, and sent her a copy inscribed "To Helen, formerly of Troy, now of London." (80) Beautiful Lillie was featured in a 13-part television serial, appropriately titled *Lillie,* in which, in almost every part, Oscar

Wilde appeared very frequently. In one scene, he professes his love to Lillie, but when she clearly encourages him to its consummation, Oscar is presented as visibly embarrassed, and asserts that it would be inconsistent with his nature.

Other women with whom Oscar liked to be seen included the actress, Ellen Terry, as well as the then-well-known star of the French theater, Sarah Bernard. Apparently, when Sarah arrived in England, Oscar placed a bouquet of lilies at her feet, which action was eagerly noted in the society chronicles of many newspapers. (81)

Oscar did everything he could to be talked about and written about. He dressed very colorfully, if not eccentrically, wore his hair long, and supposedly once took a walk in London, dressed in knee breeches, with a flowing velvet jacket, and holding a lily in his hand.

Encouraged by his mother, but also for other reasons, Oscar started to think about marriage. Mama dreamed of a "suitable match" for her famous son, but before he found this perfect person, Oscar proposed to at least two women. The first to whom he proposed marriage was the sister of his university friend, one Charlotte Montefiore, who did not want to marry Wilde. Charlotte clearly gave Oscar to understand that she did not love him, and it appears that he likewise was not certain of his feelings toward her. The next candidate for Mrs. Wilde was Violet Hunt, the beautiful daughter of a well-known landscape painter, Alfred Hunt, and his wife, the also well-known authoress, Margaret Hunt. The young people liked each other, almost from their first meeting and saw each other quite often, especially on weekends. Oscar would visit the Hunt home, or invited Violet, together with her mother, to his own, where he invited guests, including Frank Miles, with whom he then resided. Nothing came of a possible marriage, when it turned out that the Hunts were not as wealthy as it had appeared to Oscar. Additionally, the young lady's parents came to the conclusion that the sexual orientation of their daughter's intended future husband was at least ambiguous, an indication of which was said to be a caricature that appeared in the magazine, *Punch*, characterizing Oscar as effeminate. (82)

Shortly after this, Oscar met a woman who did become his wife. She was Constance Lloyd, the daughter of an already deceased, well-known attorney, and, at the same time, the sister of a friend of Wilde's from Oxford. Constance was a young, tall and slim woman, of a rather boyish appearance. She was an intelligent person, well-educated, and appeared to be an excellent match. Frank Harris had a different opinion, and maintained that Constance had no special attributes, nor was she beautiful, and suggested that Oscar could have married her for a steady income that she inherited from her father. (83) From the first day of their acquaintance, Constance was fascinated with Oscar, and full of admiration for his talents. It is in fact at this time that Oscar published his first collection of poetry, *Poems,* and was a person spoken of with acknowledgment.

Shortly after meeting Constance, Oscar received an invitation for a series of lectures in America, where he spent a whole year travelling from one end of the continent to the other, and also to Canada. He gave about 150 lectures before tens of thousands of listeners. It should be remembered that, despite his marital plans and feelings he professed toward Constance, he did not stop being interested in 'boys'. It is written that during his stay in New York, he engaged in an affair with what was most probably a male prostitute that he met on Fifth Avenue, during which he lost the enormous sum (at that time), of $1,200. This was doubtless contrived, and Oscar took the matter to the police. This unfortunate affair clearly indicates that Wilde's difficult to control sexual drive induced him to risky behaviors, which were to be repeated in the future, and which, as a consequence, led to the calamity of the poet's life.

After returning from America, Oscar was invited to Paris. There, the writer met many colleagues who had been corresponding with him, among others, Edmond de Goncourt, upon whom he did not make the best impression. This was May, 1883:

> Dinner at the Nitts' [residence] with the English poet, Oscar Wilde. This personality of dubious sex, a sailor's speech and tendency to humbuggery, comically describes a town in Texas: its inhabitants are criminals, the revolver shapes customs, while in places of amusement hang signs [saying] 'Don't shoot the pianist, he's doing what he can." He describes a theater hall, which, as the largest in the town serves as the place for holding court; after the play, an execution on the stage, and he happened to see the [gallows-bird] clinging to the scenery, and the audience shooting at him from their seats! (84)

During this stay in Paris, Oscar met Robert Sherard for the first time. The men became friends, and many years later, Sherard published several books on the subject of Oscar. It was Sherard who first wrote that, in the course of 17 years of acquaintance, he saw no signs of syphilis in Wilde, while later declaring that Oscar Wilde suffered from congenital syphilis, which, as a consequence, led to his death. This last assertion is clearly nonsense, as Oscar Wilde had no signs or symptoms that would provide evidence for a congenital origin for his illness, while, additionally, one can accept that Oscar's father, who was a physician, could not have infected Oscar's mother – who would also have had to have been infected in order to give birth to a child with congenital lues! Sherard appealed to Oscar very quickly, but was decidedly heterosexual, and tolerated Wilde's flirtations with great aversion. He was very embarrassed when Oscar kissed him on the lips in greeting, and was surprised that the poet rarely took advantage of the services of female prostitutes.

Sherard did record Wilde's single encounter with a female prostitute in Paris. Oscar announced one evening that "Priapus was calling," and left Sherard in order to visit the *Eden*, a notorious music hall where he met the famous *demimondaine* Marie Aquetant, whose lover later slit her throat as she bestrode him during sex. "What animals we all are, Robert," said Oscar when they met the next morning. (85)

In contrast to his friend, Robert Sherard took advantage of prostitute services very frequently. The French writer, Pierre Louys, described a night spent together that ended with breakfast at dawn in the company of two 16-year-old prostitutes, who had oozing lesions, the size of a walnut, caused by syphilis, on their bodies. (85) It is no wonder that Shepard very quickly became infected with that disease, let alone the serious problems of alcoholism.

Travelling around America, and visiting France, Oscar did not forget about Constance. He often wrote to her, which, in a young woman, only increased her feelings toward the poet, and confirmed her desire to be his wife. Their friendship had already lasted two and a half years, and was ripening toward a resolution. One cannot exclude that Oscar deluded himself with the hope, not uncommon among young homosexuals, that marriage to a woman that he liked and desired could be a cure for his homosexuality. This type of opinion was very popular in those days, and even now, over a hundred years later, many believe one "can be cured of homosexuality," if one greatly desires to be. It is known that, shortly before his marriage, Oscar went to see a doctor. Some explain this as a need to make sure that the lues, which he contracted from a prostitute at Oxford, was cured, and that he was no longer infectious for his wife-to-be. Others speculate that during this prenuptial visit, Oscar asked for advice as to whether, in the case of a candidate for marriage who had a clear interest in men, marriage to a woman made sense, and whether it would allow him to get rid of the former passion. One cannot exclude that the doctor gave him a green light, believing, consistent with medical opinions of the time that it could help. Andre Gide, a French writer about whom more will be said later, had a similar situation; his physician attempted to convince him that, despite his clear interest in boys, marriage to a woman whom he found attractive would be a good solution: "Get married! Marry without a fear. And you will soon see that the rest only exists in your imagination." The specialist told him he was, "like a hungry man trying to make a meal out of gherkins." (86)

Oscar became convinced that he was capable of marriage; he believed that it would allow him to quiet rumors on the subject of his homosexual tendencies, as well as to calm his mother's fears, and would give a new impulse to his literary career. What's more, he was convinced that he loved Constance, something about which he attempted to convince his friends many times, even many years after the breakup of his marriage.

For their honeymoon trip, the newlyweds travelled to Paris. There, Oscar met Sherard, who congratulated him on his wedding. Sherard remembered that when they went for a walk and passed near a florist shop, Oscar bought a great bouquet of flowers, and had it sent to the hotel where his wife had stayed. It did not hamper him from visiting bars and bordellos a few days later in questionable districts of the city, however. At the time when the Wildes were spending their honeymoon in Paris, there was a lot of talk there about Huysman's book, *A Rebours*, which can be translated as "Against Nature." Reading it, brought to Oscar's attention that the emotions and bond that joined him to his wife probably would not block his desire for contact with men.

Some consider this to have been the moment when Oscar started to realize that he had made a mistake. Many homosexuals acquire a distaste or even a disgust at the sight of a woman's body, particulalrly the genital area. Pregnant women are considered deformed and repellant, while the pregnancy itself possesses nothing noble. Feelings of this type were not foreign to Oscar, although, according to McKenna, at the time when Constance was pregnant, Oscar, most likely remained a faithful husband. (87)

Not long after the birth of their first child (Cyril), Oscar met a young man, a student at Cambridge, Harry Marillier, with whom he entered into a homosexual relationship, while soon thereafter, he began a new friendship with yet another young man, Douglas Ainslie from Oxford. This type of behavior was consistent with a motto uttered by the poet: "How much more poetic it is to marry one and love many." (88)

Oscar Wilde's sex life after he reached physical maturity coincided in time with a wave of anti-homosexual attitudes in England, where it was decided to deal with a reportedly increasing wave of that practice, whereas its penalization until that time was not very coherent. In 1885, committing sodomy was subject to a penalty of life imprisonment, but a definition of sodomy was very imprecise, as, for example, mutual masturbation between men or fellatio were not included in it. It was considered that sexual contact between men in which penetration was not attained (meaning anal sex), was not subject to penalty, even though it was considered deviant. Another factor making conviction of the guilty parties difficult was the need to prove that during the act of penetration, ejaculation occurred. The new law introduced an amendment, which said that:

> Any male person who, in public or private, commits, or is a party to the commission of, or procures the commission by any male person, of any act of gross indecency with another male person, shall be guilty of misdemeanor, and being convicted thereof shall be liable at the discretion of the Court to be imprisoned for any term not exceeding two years, with or without hard labor. (89)

I cited this fragment of change in British law, because one of its first and loudest objects was Oscar Wilde. Continuing the gallery of Oscar Wilde's male partners, I wanted to introduce 17-year-old Robert Ross, who first became his partner, then his lifelong friend. The exact circumstances of meeting by the two men are not well known, although Frank Harris maintained that Oscar told him that he met Robbie in a public lavatory. (90) Public lavatories for men were, and still are, a place for making acquaintance among homosexuals; however, there is no certainty that Robbie and Oscar did, in fact, meet under such circumstances, nonetheless, according to the account of a Scotland Yard inspector, Robbie often was seen in such places in the company of suspicious men. (90) Ross was a declared homosexual, preferring receptive contact with men, and it is considered that probably while in such contact with Robbie, Oscar for the first time committed an act of sodomy, as defined by an earlier version of British law. Despite the fact that Oscar and Robbie had many sex partners, their friendship lasted many years, and the latter was one of but a few of the poet's friends who later came to Paris to take care of the terminally ill Wilde.

Regardless of his contacts with men, Oscar still was married, and fulfilled his marital obligations. Oscar's second son, Vyvyan, was born in November 1886, but his father had already stopped living with his wife for several months. It is suggested that this could have been caused by a return of syphilis, but appears to be of low probability. (91) Signs and symptoms of relapsing syphilis appear not later than two-three years after becoming ill, and, if any skin changes had appeared in the meanwhile, they could have been early signs of third-stage disease, which are no longer infectious – or signs of some skin disease not related to lues. Wilde's terminating the relationship with his wife did not mean terminating contact with men. At this time there appear and disappear the names of various young men, whom I will not identify due to the limited space, which I can devote to writing about syphilis and Oscar's erotic life. I cannot, however, fail to mention several persons whose presence in Oscar Wilde's life weighed on his fate or had an influence on his literary creativity. One of these is Lord Alfred (Bosie) Douglas, whose acquaintance became the beginning of the end of the poet's career, or another, John Gray, who was the inspiration for the novel *The Picture of Dorian Gray*.

At some time in mid-1889, Oscar met the young poet and writer, John Gray. He was, as McKenna wrote, a "devastatingly handsome" young man, and compared the encounter to Shakespeare's meeting the probably fictional addressee of some of his sonnets, Willie Hughes: "There was the young man, the ideal boy incarnate, who could inspire Oscar's passionate adoration and his strange worship." Oscar fell in love with John Gray at once." (92) But Gray did not immediately respond to Oscar's advances, which only intensified the poet's feelings to the newly met ideal of male beauty. John came from societal lowlands, but thanks to his intelligence, industry and handsomeness— qualities particularly attractive to homosexuals—he obtained an education and a certain status. In Gray's biography, many who helped him are mentioned – the majority were rich, older men. Oscar's efforts to win John's affections lasted several months, but were finally successful. "Sex between them did take place but it was sex more as a rite of passage, a rite of possession. For Oscar, sex with John Gray was an act of worship. For John Gray, it was confirmation of his social and literary status." (92)

In August 1889, Oscar signed a contract with the American publisher, Lippincot, for a story, and thus arose *The Picture of Dorian Gray*. Friends and acquaintances of the poet were aware of the fact that it was actually John Gray, Oscar's new lover, the model for Dorian Gray. A letter written by John to Oscar has survived, in which John signed himself as Dorian, and Oscar sometimes spoke of John using the name, Dorian. As McKenna maintains, Wilde changed the name, John, to Dorian, calling to mind the memory of a certain tribe living in ancient Greece that promoted pederasty. "The Dorians were a tribe of ancient Greece, inhabiting the major cities of Sparta, Argos and Corinth. They were famous for their customs of institutionalized "*pederastia*" by which an older man became the lover and the teacher of a youth. The Dorians were generally held responsible for the spread of *pederastia* throughout ancient Greece. (93)

Similarly to Oscar, one of the characters of the tale, Basil Hallword, a painter, falls in love with Dorian at first sight. The entire account is permeated with discrete eroticism, including homoeroticism, while its telling allows one to surmise that its author is himself a homosexual. This type of exhibitionism, while somewhat veiled, was very risky, and even dangerous. English society at the end of the nineteenth century was far from tolerant in regard to "those who love differently," something about which the author was soon to learn about the hard way.

In the meantime, the renown with which publication of Dorian Gray was met increased the number of admirers of the writer's talents, particularly among homosexuals. One of Oscar's new admirers was poet Lionel Johnson, who lent a copy of the book to his young friend, Lord Alfred Douglas, who was enchanted by it. It is no wonder that it was the young Lord's dream to meet the author as quickly as possible, and that occurred three months later, when Johnson brought Alfred Douglas to the Wildes' house.

Lord Douglas was twenty years old. He was said to be an unusually handsome youth, and had the nickname, "Bosie," as a result of his very boyish appearance (Fig.5b.9). The writer became enamored of him, almost at first sight, as the young man had several attractive traits. He was not only handsome, but also intelligent; he was a poet, and came from an aristocratic family, which greatly impressed Wild.

Bosie's reaction at this first meeting with Oscar was rather cool. The young man was not immediately enchanted by the famous writer, perhaps because it was Bosie who, until that time, picked out his sexual partners, who with certain exceptions were younger than he. Bosie began his homosexual life even while at school in Winchester, and until the meeting with Oscar his partners were mainly young boys of his own age, from various social classes, and did not exclude male prostitutes coming from the working class.

Oscar was very busy at this time; he wrote articles for newspapers, prepared a theatrical play, and traveled to and from Paris. He maintained contact with his male partners, and met new men. He didn't forget about Bosie, however, and met and corresponded with him. Their contacts became less frequent in late autumn, 1892, when Bosie became the victim of blackmail, during which Oscar provided him with wide-ranging assistance. Blackmail of homosexuals, particularly rich ones and those coming from affluent families, was something very common, partly due to the restrictive British laws concerning homosexuality. Many people derived a livelihood from this practice, while homosexuals who took advantage of *rental boys* tolerated this state of affairs, considering it an unavoidable cost of satisfying their sexual inclinations. Oscar helped Bosie extricate himself from a certain affair in which he was being blackmailed, and by this means won his friendship. For Oscar, Bosie became, over time, "the personification of ideal love, the fulfillment of undying love with a beautiful boy. "

This type of emotional state did not by any means indicate avoiding other partners, however. Oscar and by Bosie were enormously promiscuous, seeking new sexual sensations, both together and separately; apparently, sexual activities conducted with other partners in each others' presence did not evoke feelings of jealousy or of betrayal. Swingers are not just a discovery of the tw^{entieth} or twe$^{nty\text{-}first}$

centuries; these types of sexual games have been played since time immemorial.

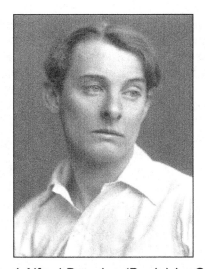

Figure 5b.9 Lord Alfred Douglas (Bosie) by George Charles Beresford (1903)

Oscar's publication of two new works dealing with the problems of homosexual activity (*The Portrait of Mr. W. H.* and *The Picture of Dorian Gray*) clearly contravened the then recently strengthened British law, and was of advantage to the adherents of de-penalization of homosexuality in England. It is worth remembering that at the same time in France, where the Napoleonic code was in force, sexual contact between males was not subject to any punishment. This fact resulted in the number of proponents of toleration for "loving differently" to increase steadily, and to encourage the veiled homosexual propaganda found in works of Wilde and the poems of Bosie. I think that both men may be described in today's terms as "gay rights activists," but the times were different, and their activity was subject to far greater risk than presently. This does not mean that contemporary homosexual activists have an easy life, despite not being threatened with incarceration, as happened to Oscar. Increasing sympathy for those who loved differently and the slogans they used somewhat emboldened our heroes and lulled their vigilance. The two men rented rooms next to each other in the Hotel Savoy, where they hosted orgies with newer paid male prostitute partners to their rooms, and even invited or lured underage thirteen and 14-year-old boys working in the hotel for kissing and fondling in return for very large tips.

According to depositions of witnesses in the proceedings against Oscar, they went as far as acts of sodomy, namely anal intercourse, which in England was carried a punishment of imprisonment from ten years to life. According to McKenna, Bosie acted exclusively in the role of the active partner (penetrator), while Oscar felt good in both roles, equally as penetrator as the person penetrated. (94) Evidence in the case included the dirtied bedclothes, which the hotel employees testified they had to change and clean, with great distaste. One cannot be surprised that after several months, the hotel management asked Oscar and Bosie to vacate their rooms. Other problems also appeared.

Robbie Ross, Bosie, and to a lesser degree, Oscar, were caught having contact with young boys; but, this time, not with "rental boys," but with the sons of wealthy parents. These were 16-year-old youths whose parents hired detectives and took the matter to court. However, as because the court's judgment in the "Bruges Affair," as it was called, could have resulted in the imprisonment of not only Robbie, Bosie, and possibly Oscar, but also of the boy victims, the parents abandoned the complaint, having in mind the good names of their sons. Nonetheless, the danger of the court case and the prospect of imprisonment hung by a thread. Robbie Ross hid in Davos, Switzerland, while Bosie, at the entreaties of his mother and the urging of Oscar, left for Egypt. Then, Bosie's family got the idea that maybe a diplomatic career would be appropriate for their son, and that a stay in Egypt could be an introduction to it. They deluded themselves with the hope that the change in environment and the separation from Oscar would have a curative effect on their son, but nothing more mistaken could have been the case! The Near East and Northern Africa were then a sex-tourism destination, and not only for homosexual men (to recall the travels of Gustave Flaubert in this region). After several days' stay in Egypt, Bosie set out to search for lanky young boys of olive complexion, and after a short while it turned out that their supply exceeded the sexual possibilities of a tourist /diplomat. Oscar, uncertain to the end how his cards would fall in connection with the Bruges affair, left for Paris.

In February 1894, Bosie left Cairo, for Istanbul, where he was supposed to become the honorary *attaché* to the British ambassador in Turkey. Along the way, he decided to stop in Athens and visit a friend who worked there for the British Society of Archaeology. During his stay in the Greek capital, he learned that the ambassador, who had promised him the position in Istanbul, had changed his mind, doubtless as the result of signals from colleagues in Cairo shocked by Bosie's behavior in that city. This news did not have any special effect on the would-be *attaché*, who had already started to long for Oscar's company, and determined to meet with him. Oscar, who had planned a longer holiday from Bosie, did not exactly yearn to meet him, but after countless urgings by Bosie, which included threats of suicide, agreed to meet him. After a short, stay in Paris, both partners returned to London, and it was there that that they met the experience, which had a significant influence on the career and future of Oscar Wilde.

One March day in 1894, Bosie's father, the Marquis of Queensberry, looking out of the window in his hotel, noticed a cab, and in it, his son caressing Oscar. Agitated by what he saw, he wrote a letter to Bosie and Oscar, demanding the immediate breaking up of their friendship. The Marquis was a person of high impetuosity, stubborn, and vindictive, while his own private life left much to be desired. Having been divorced for a long time, he decided to marry a young woman, whom he met on vacation. The wedding took place in November 1893, and the only person taking part in the celebration other than the newlyweds was the Marquis' valet, who was one of the witnesses. The marriage lasted barely several days, after which the wife of the Marquis applied for an annulment, giving as a reason, "malformation of the parts of generation and frigidity and impotency." (95) There can be no doubt that the newly wed husband felt ridiculed and humiliated, and was furious. His feelings of humiliation deepened, as a result of gossip about his two sons: the older, Francis, Viscount Drumlanrig, and the younger, Lord Douglas, known to us as Bosie, who were both accused of homosexuality.

Half a year before the affair with Bosie and Oscar, the Marquis was disgraced as a result of a scandal, accusing the ruling premier, Lord Rosebery, of a romance with his older son, Viscount Drumlanrig. Due to the intervention of the Prince of Wales, the scandal was hushed up, while the Marquis had to reconcile himself with defeat. No wonder that Queensberry, catching Oscar with his son in a situation confirming the gossip, decided to act decidedly; he demanded that the lovers break up immediately. It is not difficult to understand him. Accused by his last wife of impotence, and defamed by gossip concerning his sons, he felt the need to defend the family's honor. The Marquis, like most of society then, considered homosexuality to be a deviation. I must remind the reader that it was not until the seventies of the tw[entieth] century that the American Psychiatric Association removed homosexuality from the list of diseases, regarding it a natural phenomenon.

After the quarrel with his father, Bosie left for Florence, where Oscar soon joined him. It is possible that they deluded themselves with the idea that getting themselves out of the sight of the Marquis of Queensberry would quiet the latter's nervous state, but they were mistaken. Shortly after Bosie's return from Italy, the Marquis paid a visit to the Wilde's home, where he created a disturbance, and threatened to take Oscar to court if he did not break up with his son. In revenge, Bosie threatened to take the Marquis to court for baseless accusations against him and his friends. It happened that the Marquis knew many more details of the lives of the two men. For some time, he had been investigating the actions of his son, and had Oscar followed, trying to gather as much evidence as possible to prove their criminal behavior.

At the time when Queensberry was making a row with Oscar and his own son, anti-homosexual sentiments in England increased. In September 1894, there appeared in the London press news about the arrest of eighteen men who would meet on Fitzroy Street. Several of them, evidently transvestites, were dressed in women's clothing, and in such surroundings were quite open about their lifestyle. Many of those arrested were later released, due to of a lack of evidence of having committed a crime; nonetheless, the police became interested in homosexual groups, which included many persons who belonged to Oscar's social circle, or were at one time his partners. In October of the same year, Bosie's brother, Viscount Drumlanrig committed what was most likely suicide, which was attributed to his participation in a homosexual affair with Lord Rosebery.

The beginning of 1895 was very promising for Oscar Wilde. His stage play, *An Ideal Husband*, presented in London, was successful, and his next play, *The Importance of Being Earnest*, was in its final phase of rehearsals, with a premiere planned for February. Wilde hoped that two stage plays performed at the same time would markedly improve his financial situation, which was not the best at that time. Wilde earned a great deal, but spent even more. Feeling confident in future theatrical and financial successes, he left for a short vacation, together with Bosie, to Algeria, at the time one of the main sex-tourism destinations, preferred especially by homosexuals. He wrote, "There were beautiful boys wherever they turned, seemingly all of them smiling sexual invitations . . . Several shepherds fluted on reeds for us," wrote Oscar – which, to him, apparently signified a readiness for oral sex. (96) Oscar and Bosie had no difficulty taking advantage of the paid services of underage boys without hesitation, whether the sexual services offered by underage Arabs, or English teenage boys in London.

After a week's stay in Algiers, Oscar and Bosie set out on a trip to Blidah, a historical town about 50 kilometers (30 miles) from the county's capital. They stopped in a hotel where resided Andre Gide, their mutual friend from Paris. Gide, a well-known writer, who would be a Nobel laureate in 1948, entered the annals of syphilology with the famous statement, "It is unthinkable for a Frenchman to arrive at middle age without having syphilis and the Cross of the Legion of Honor." I believe that this famous author was unfair toward his countrymen, as not everyone managed to attain the Legion of Honor at such a young age, while, in regards to syphilis, and speaking seriously, France was no exception among European countries when it came to a high rate of lues in the general population.

When Andre saw that Oscar and Bosie had stopped in the same hotel, he wanted to leave unnoticed, but was late for the last train leaving for Algiers that day. The three men met at supper, after which they went for an evening walk together about the city. In the course of this brief trip, Bosie took Andre by the hand, and confessed to him that he couldn't stand women, and had sex with young boys exclusively. Gide, who until this time did not consider himself to be a declared homosexual, and did have sexual relations with women, knew that there was something awry with himself, as he was also attracted to young men. He was in a state in which he desired and simultaneously rejected the possibility of sex with a man.

After an exhausting vacation in Algeria, Oscar and Bosie returned to London. One of two important reasons for the return to England was the pending premiere of Oscar's new play, *The Importance of Being Earnest*. The other, a more private one, was the venereal disease that Oscar contracted during this time, most likely, gonorrhea. Wilde sought help, not from his own family physician (as we would say nowadays), but from a Dr. Vernon Jones, who specialized in venereal diseases. He stayed under his care for 3 months – as confirmed by the unpaid bills for his treatment! (97) Treatment of gonorrhea in those days was long and painful, and, even if the patient conformed to the recommendations of the physician, was often of little efficacy. Wilde took a variety of medications used for the treatment of gonorrhea at that time, including, probably, strong analgesics containing opium. (97).

Just before the premiere of his new play, Oscar learned that the furious Marquis of Queensberry planned to announce the scandal during opening night. Bosie's father intended to plaster the author (who was to appear on stage after the final curtain), not only with accusations of sodomy, but also with rotten vegetables. After consultation with Oscar, the theater's management wrote to the Marquis, who was getting ready for the premiere, that the ticket that had been sold him was invalid, attaching a refund of its price. The Marquis looked for Oscar in various places, and finally left his business card – on which he wrote the insulting phrase, "For Oscar Wilde, ponce and sodomite" – at the club to which the poet belonged. This was a publicly measured slap on the face, to which Oscar did not know how to react. His friends in this matter were not of one mind in their advice. Some counseled against, others encouraged, referring the matter to the courts. Bosie was of the latter opinion, encouraged Wilde to summon his father to court, and Oscar came to the conclusion that he had to react. The attorney to whom he turned for legal help asked him for a declaration that the insulting words had no basis, and that Oscar denied being a sodomite and procurer.

Even the first hearing that was held turned out to be a disaster for Wilde. Several days before its start, Queensberry directed a so-called "Plea of Justification" to the court. In it were presented the contents of many of Wilde's works, including *The Picture of Dorian Gray*, which, in the opinion of the defense was an apotheosis of homosexuality, describing "the relations, intimacies and passions of certain persons of sodomitical and unnatural tastes, habits and practices." (98) At the time of the trial, there was talk of other publications of similar tone, which were against the moral principles of the time. Next, were presented several cases of matters related to Oscar's being blackmailed on the basis of his letters and intimate contacts with male prostitutes. The case acquired such a disadvantageous turn for Wilde that his attorney advised him to withdraw the complaint against the Marquis of Queensberry, who, in his specifications in legal procedure had even more than enough evidence to call Oscar what he had called him. Wilde admitted that he "'posed as a sodomite' at least as far as the literary part of the case was concerned. (99) The judgment of the court in Wilde's suit against the Marquis was in favor of Queensberry, who was found not guilty, and it became clear to Oscar that this was just the beginning of his real troubles. After the end of this trial, the Marquis' defending counselor is said to have told his wife in private conversation, "I have ruined the most brilliant man in London." (100)

The testimony of the witnesses left no illusions that the next stage of the court procedure would be the arrest of Wilde, and accusation of sodomy. Queensberry triumphed as a defender of morality, while the majority of public opinion was on his side. After numerous legal deliberations, Wilde was accused of "various counts of indecency," what was far milder than accusations of sodomy, for which very large punishments threatened. Two court hearings were conducted, in the course of which persons, who were direct participants in the sexual orgies of Oscar and his friend, testified these included male prostitutes, underage boys working at the Hotel Savoy, maids, and others who corroborated the charges placed in the act of accusation. The judgment was "two years at hard labor." Wilde still had time to avoid the punishment by leaving immediately for France, but did not take advantage of this possibility, and went to jail for two years.

After completing his prison sentence, Wilde very quickly left London for France. Despite numerous expressions of sympathy on the part of certain communities, mostly literary ones, he was not very successful at finding a place for himself. In London a collection of his prison poems, *The Ballad of Reading Gaol,* was published, receiving good, but not enthusiastic acceptance. Many former friends did not want to maintain contact with him, although his old friends, particularly his earlier sex partners, remained faithful to him, among them including Bosie. Constance, his wife, who had applied for a separation and change of surname, died shortly after unsuccessful surgery of the spine, leaving Oscar a small financial grant. Wilde took advantage of "non-returnable loans" from friends, as well as private invitations for short stays in their homes. He began to drink and returned to the dangerous habit of taking advantage of the services of an increasingly lower category of male prostitutes.

In the summer of 1889, Wilde developed a skin rash, which he described as mussel poisoning. The changes were pruritic (itchy), and were localized on the arms, chest and back. One of the doctors described this as indicating neurasthenia, and excluded food poisoning. In September, a problem with his ear appeared. Supposedly he had had this earlier, during his stay in prison, but it was disregarded by a prison physician. At this point the problem appeared sufficiently serious that the physician summoned from the

British Embassy in Paris, a Dr. Tucker, acknowledged a need for surgical measures. The operation was performed in Wilde's hotel room by the Parisian surgeon, Dr. Paul Cleis. There is no exact account of what the operation consisted, while Richard Elleman, on the basis of the opinions of modern physicians, suggests that it could have been a paracentesis of the eardrum, or removal of polyps. (101)

The post-operative period passed without significant complications, although Oscar felt weak and, in letters to his friends, informed them of his approaching death, often in a dramatic tone. Nineteen days after the operation, Wilde got up from bed, and, although still weak, went for a walk in the company of Robbie Ross. During the walk, they stopped in the coffee house where Oscar ordered absinthe, the drinking of which his physicians had forbidden. (102) The following day, Wilde developed a fever, while pain from the affected ear increased. Pus appeared in the ear, together with symptoms indicating infection of the middle ear (*otitis media*). According to Reggie Turner, who was taking care of his friend during the last weeks of these symptoms, they were, in the opinion of the physician, signs of third stage syphilis, a disease that Wilde had acquired in his twenties. (103) The pains increased, and, in addition to frequent changes of dressings, Oscar required strong anti-pain medications (analgesics), i.e. morphine, opium and chloral hydrate. Despite a proscription against drinking alcohol, Wilde drank champagne, while the male nurse changing his dressings used hot compresses over the affected ear, despite a clear prohibition by the physician; this probably provided some relief of the pain, but was clearly contraindicated in this situation. At the end of November, Wilde's state worsened, and his temperature rose, while on November 25th, signs of brain involvement appeared, diagnosed as inflammation of the brain membranes and brain (meningo-encephalitis). Oscar Wilde died on November 30th, 1900.

For many years, authors studying the life and works associated with the person of Oscar Wilde have considered the question of whether the poet had syphilis, and whether it could have been the cause of the illness that led to his premature death. The crowning argument of those who believe that Wilde never had syphilis is the fact that, until now, no written evidence confirming syphilis has been found, information about his putative lues coming from accounts of acquaintances and friends. (76,103) This argument is not convincing, however. In those times the word syphilis was assiduously avoided even in medical documents, due to its stigmatizing effect, which disgraced the patient in the eyes of his family and friends, not to mention the wider public. Using Wilde's style, one could say that this talented person was not only a believer in "love that does not dare to speak its name," but also suffered from the disease whose name one did not dare to mention!

Avoiding the word *syphilis* in accounts of the medical problems of those who acquired the disease was not a characteristic exclusively of England; it was a rather common and widely accepted social custom. I must remind the reader about syphilitics discussed earlier, who, in private discussions or private correspondence did allow the disease to be called by its name, sometimes even in a somewhat defiant manner, whereas, when in official situations, they almost never bragged about it. I would also recall the *Journal* of the de Goncourt brothers, in which there is an abundance of information about persons ill with syphilis, yet this word is not mentioned, not even once. Analyzing these accounts, we can easily diagnose them as signs of lues, mainly third-stage syphilis, but can one proceed in this manner in the case of Oscar Wilde? I will begin with the skin ailment that first manifested in the summer of 1899, and which was described as mussel poisoning and even neurasthenia. (104) According to today's knowledge, such signs as were observed then in Wilde do not fit either of the two. Accepting Ellman's statement that Wilde became infected with syphilis in his 20s, one can consider whether or not the signs described above, are signs of skin changes of nodular or noduloulcerative tertiary syphilis (105). Available accounts of the skin changes (104) are very unprofessional, and do not permit one to take just one side. One can say with a great deal of certainty that they were not, as Wilde judged, caused by food poisoning, but rather an allergic reaction or something entirely different. The timing of their appearance, their recurrent character, their appearance bringing to mind leopard skin, or the location of "red splotches on his arms, chest and back,"(104) could indicate tertiary noduloulcerative syphilis. However, in none of the accounts are the lesions described as nodular or noduloulcerative today, nor as changes with central healing and a tendency to circular expansion, which are typical of this form of syphilis. (105). Bear in mind that the accounts come from people who were not specialists in dermatology, and who might not have noted certain details important from the point of view of a skin doctor.

The skin changes of late lues often co-existed with gummas, which were common changes of tertiary syphilis developing from bones or subcutaneous tissues. The problems that Wilde had with his right ear could also suggest a gumma of the inner ear – which could have penetrated to the middle ear to cause a purulent drainage from the ear canal, with pain and fever. However, they could also have partly been a consequence of errors committed by the patient and his caregivers, and do suggest inflammation of the brain membranes (meningitis) and brain (encephalitis). This conclusion takes into consideration the reaction and actions of the physicians, who, during conversations with friends of the patient were to have said that Wilde's ear problems had their origin in the disease that he had acquired in his youth, i.e. syphilis. (103)

Oscar Wilde would not have been himself if in a confrontation with a serious disease he had not retained a sense of humor and his talent for making brilliant associations of ideas. It is from just this time that his famous saying, "My wallpaper and I are fighting a duel to the death. One or the other of us has to go," came. But, he did not know that he was taking part in an uneven duel, as the silent ally of the wallpaper could well have been syphilis!

JAMES JOYCE (1882-1941)

James Joyce is considered one of the most significant writers of the early twentieth century (Fig.5b.10). Among his best known works are: *Ulysses*, with a title borrowed from Homer's Odyssey, but whose action takes place in Dublin; a collection of stories entitled *The Dubliners*; autobiographical tales under the title, *Portrait of the Artist as a Young Man*, based on events from the author's childhood and youth; and one of his last novels, published in 1939, *Finnegan's Wake*. Joyce is considered the representative of *avante garde* modernism in the literature from the beginnings of the twentieth century, although his works are not easy to accept for the unprepared reader.

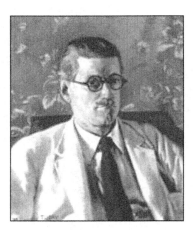

Figure 5b.10 Portrait of James Joyce by Patrick Tuohy (Paris 1924)

James Joyce appears on the pages of this book because according to specialists studying his works the problem of syphilis is woven into many of his novels; some maintain that the author himself was ill with it, and even that he died from it. In the biography, *James Joyce, a Portrait of the Artist*, authored by Stan Gebler Davies, is found an appendix in which we read, "James Joyce undoubtedly contracted venereal disease on several occasions but there is no positive proof that he ever had syphilis. His father, however, most certainly had it, and Joyce could have inherited it. (106)

Dr. F.R. Walsh of Kilkenny contributed an illuminating article on the subject to the *Irish Medical Times* of May 9, 1975:

> John Joyce, (father of James) in his old age, was in the habit of consorting with medical students. In 1919/20, he confessed to Dr. Walsh, then a student, that while himself a student at Queens College, in Cork, in 1867, he had discovered a syphilitic chancre and treated it himself by the then usual method – cauterizing with carbolic – which might remove the symptoms but by no means guaranteed a cure. Eye failure can be a consequence of syphilis. [Dr. Walsh quotes W.A. Boyd, "The Book of Pathology (1961)," to the effect that there is no symptom which it cannot cause, no syndrome for which it may not be responsible]. John Joyce was himself treated for iritis and conjunctivitis in 1909. His first child lived only a few days, two were stillborn, two did not survive adolescence, and the last, like the first, died after a few days. Mary Joyce (mother of James) died at the age of forty-four of a disease was variously diagnosed as cancer of the liver and cirrhosis. Syphilis, too, can attack the interior organs. James Joyce died of a perforated duodenal ulcer and

peritonitis which followed an unsuccessful operation. Gastric syphilis, says Dr. Walsh, is rare but not unknown. Bailey and Love [, in] "Practice of Surgery," say [that] the differential diagnosis is difficult. Erosion of a mucosal gumma could presumably lead to ulceration, hemorrhage and perforation - an unlikely, but possible event." It is possible therefore, if impossible to prove, that John Joyce, that amiable ruffian, carried in his blood an agency which, untreated, blinded - perhaps even helped to kill - James Joyce and could conceivably also have killed his own wife and several of his children. Dr. Walsh has made a considerable study of James Joyce's medical history and finds it surprising that he was not, when his eyes were being treated in middle age, ever tested for syphilis. He advances the theory that it simply never occurred to Dr. Vogt of Zurich to suggest such a thing to so eminent a man of letters. (106)

Even in the first sentence of this rather long citation, it is said that James Joyce suffered from a venereal disease (diseases), and that, several times, although there is no certainty that among them was syphilis. It is emphasized that it is almost certain that James' father, John Joyce, had become infected with syphilis, and that in two instances his wife gave birth to a stillborn child, which may be evidence that these children had succumbed to congenital syphilis. It is also suggested that James' health problems could be the result of congenital lues, and even the cause of his early death, as a perforated duodenal ulcer could be a sequel to a gumma of this organ. Deliberations on the subject of syphilis in Mary Joyce (James' mother), who died of liver cancer, as well as the premature deaths of some of the Joyce children requires a commentary.

As we know, syphilis, known as "the great imitator," could produce signs and symptoms similar to those of illnesses of a different etiology. One must, nevertheless, remember that physicians practicing at the end of the nineteenth and the beginning of the tw^{entieth} centuries, had to deal with a greater number of cases of syphilis, and were more sensitive even to its lesser manifestations. It is thus very unlikely that they would not consider lues in the differential diagnosis of the unsuccessful births of Mrs. Joyce; or that, after confirming a first case of congenital syphilis in the Joyce family, would not have either treated the mother, or forbidden her to become pregnant during a certain (normally two-year) period following completion of therapy. Additionally, shortly after the discovery of *Treponema pallidum* in 1905, a blood test, known as the Wasserman test, was introduced to the diagnosis of syphilis. This rendered the diagnosis of lues far easier, and with a higher probability of accuracy. James Joyce, who suffered from inflammation of the iris of the eye (iritis), would have had this test done. The text cited also suggests that the writer's eye problems may have been manifestations of late congenital syphilis, although the view that James Joyce became infected with syphilis on his own, and that his eye diseases were the result of acquired third-stage syphilis is more popular. The cited fragment speaks of a primary chancre that Joyce James' father treated with carbolic acid, and says nothing of any other longer treatment of the disease whatsoever, such as with mercury, iodine-containing preparations or Salvarsan. It seems quite unlikely that John Joyce, an intelligent and educated man, who came into contact not only with medical students, but also with experienced physicians, would not know how one should proceed after infection with syphilis! John's wife, Mary Joyce, died from cancer of the liver, which, as we know today, is a frequent complication of hepatitis B or C. These diseases in a large proportion can also be transmitted by the sexual route, and here, the infidelity of her husband could have had some significance, as nobody accuses James' mother, a religious person, of any transgression whatsoever against the 6th Commandment.

In its last sentence, the citation speaks of the efforts of Dr. Walsh, who was unable to find any confirmatory evidence of the performance of any laboratory tests for syphilis; this seems of low probability considering the fact that some of the writer's eye ailments could really have been a sign of late congenital syphilis or acquired tertiary syphilis. One can assume that test results were hidden or destroyed, with the aim of preserving the writer's good name, or, similarly to the example of other famous people – for instance Oscar Wilde and others – family, friends, or close acquaintances would know something on the subject and such news would, sooner or later, come to the public's attention. It seems to me that James Joyce, as a result of his lifestyle and tendency to alcohol abuse, was exposed to, and suffered from some venereal diseases, but whether or not syphilis was among them, one cannot unequivocally confirm without more convincing evidence than that "syphilis can mimic every other disease."

James Joyce was born in Dublin. His father, John Stanislaus Joyce was from a reasonably well-off family from Cork that gradually yielded to poverty, partly as the result of John's lack of ability in running a business, and partly as a result of his tendency to abuse alcohol. His mother, Mary Joyce, also came from a wealthy family, while her father made a fortune from the wine trade, and had business contacts with James' future father. The family had ten children who survived infancy. James was the second-born, but the first who survived, as the first child (a boy) died shortly after birth and before being christened. (107,108)

James began his education in a school run by the Catholic Jesuit order, who, with short interruption, were his teachers up to the moment when he entered the university in Dublin in 1898. Young James studied modern languages, mainly English, French and Italian. He was active in student educational circles involving literature and the theater. Quite early on, he began to be interested in the opposite sex. When he was fourteen, he was interested in a servant girl, who was many years older than he; according to reports by his brother, Stanislaus, she was over twenty years old. James generally felt quite comfortable in the company of young women, and this had a calming effect on his parents, who may have suspected him of hidden tendencies toward homosexuality. (109) James lost his virginity at the age of fourteen; having at his disposal a certain sum of money that he had received as a prize in a literary school competition, and while returning one evening from the theater, he allowed himself to be caught by a street prostitute with whom he spent some time. This fact was noted in one of his novels, *Portrait of an Artist*, in which the author, utilizing the name, Steven Dedalus, relates his own memories from school, his early religious experiences and his first sexual encounter in the arms of a prostitute. (110, 111)

After finishing his studies in Dublin, James left for Paris in 1903, with the idea of studying medicine. Nothing came of his medical studies; instead the young Joyce spent his money on visits to the theaters and local bordellos, about which he informed his friends in letters. (112 113) The remaining time in Paris, he spent in libraries, studying the works of the ancient philosophers. In April, James received news from home that his mother was dying and was waiting for the return of her son. Mrs. Joyce was ill with liver cancer, suffered greatly, and died at 44 years of age. As already mentioned, some biographers are of the opinion that James' mother died of syphilis, specifically of luetic gummas that, situated in the liver, could produce signs and symptoms resembling cirrhosis or cancer of this organ. These are mere suppositions, and are not founded on any convincing evidence. The death of his wife deepened the tendency to abuse of alcohol by James' father, who began to spend money earned by his now-maturing children for the purpose. (114)

After returning to Dublin, James Joyce became a frequent guest in so-called "Nighttown," where he partook of such amusements as were available there, not excluding paid sexual services. In his best-known novel, *Ulysses*, are scenes remembered by the author from his own experiences. He described the place as a "regular death-trap for young fellows of his age." (115) After one of these visits, in March, 1904, James wrote a letter to his friend, the later-to-be otolaryngologist and poet, Oliver Gogarty, asking for "the name of a doctor willing to treat ailments of a sexual nature," (116) or, as stated by R. Ellmann, "the name of a physician who would cure a minor ailment contracted during a visit to Nighttown." (117) According to Ulick O'Connor, Gogarty's biographer, the disease was supposed to have been syphilis. (116)

> This could have contributed to Joyce's later eye trouble. There is also the possibility that he may have inherited the disease. Arthur Power tells me that he remembers speaking to a Dr. Sullivan, a Dublin physician, who told me that he had treated John Joyce for syphilis.

Dr. J.B. Lyons, in his "James Joyce in Medicine" (Dublin 1973), disagrees saying that there is no evidence that Joyce had syphilis. (116)

Correspondence between James and his friend, Gogarty, contains many allusions and double meanings. In one part, Gogarty writes of "Ellwood Poxed," attaching a verse from his poem in which he speaks of "Hunterian swelling," that "the canker had attacked Art," and "Poxes the part that they love, "and now he prays to Mercury." This type of verse could suggest that the disease that afflicted Joyce was syphilis, although in another place he writes about so-called *gleet*, a term that describes a prolonged state of inflammation of the urethra, a characteristic of chronic gonorrhea or non-gonococcal urethritis, (118) or something else.

In July, 1904, some four months after infection, Joyce informed his friend that "Elwood" nearly cured," and that he plans a meeting with a certain young lady – which could have indicated that he considered himself a cured person and no longer contagious.(119) Such a short period of therapy and sexual abstinence would speak in favor of gonorrhea, whose treatment was shorter and more efficacious than that for syphilis. Not long thereafter, in October of the same year, James started to sleep with a woman with whom he spent the greater part of his life, whom he married, and who was the mother of his two children. (120) In those times (*cf*. Oscar Wilde), physicians recommended, observation and at least two years of sexual abstinence for patients treated for syphilis, the latter supposed to protect wives or regular sex partners from infection.

Without a doubt, Joyce, taking advantage of the services of prostitutes and consorting with women of suspicious reputation, "rubbed against syphilis," but there is no credible evidence for his ever having been infected himself. Even during his stay in Dublin, he resided, together with Gogarty, in the so-called "Tower," for a short time, where there also lived a beautiful girl about whom it was said that she had lues. Apparently, Gogarty kept a long distance away from her, which cannot be said about Joyce. (121)

James spent most of his adult life abroad. In the Fall of 1904, together with a newly-met woman, Nora Barnacle, he went to Switzerland, where he had a supposedly promised job as a teacher of English at the Berlitz Language School. After arriving in Zurich, it turned out that there was no work for him there, but that the same school in Trieste on the Adriatic needed English teachers. In Trieste, it similarly turned out that there was no position, and Joyce started to teach English in Palo, a town situated not far from Trieste, where there was a base of the naval fleet belonging to the

Austro-Hungarian Empire (currently Croatia). After some time, he got a job in Trieste, where James and Nora lived for many years. It was in this city that their first child, a son, Giorgio, came into the world, without any complications – which could have occurred even had Joyce and his wife suffered from syphilis. There are also no indications that Nora had, or was treated for lues.

During James' stay in Trieste, the Joyces were needy, and were not delighted with life on the Adriatic. James abused alcohol, and often visited the area in Trieste that we would today call the "red light district." The writer went to Rome for a short time, where he got a job as a bank clerk responsible for English language correspondence, which, after a short while, he hated, and returned to Trieste. Also during his stay in Rome, Joyce would get drunk, and visit places of suspect reputation. In July, 1907, Mrs. Joyce gave birth to a daughter; the birth took place on a ward designated for impoverished women. During this time, Joyce also stayed in a hospital, where he was treated for arthritis, which he asserted was, "the aftermath of [my] carefree nights in Rome and Triestine gutters." (122)

Adherents to the theory of Joyce's infection with venereal disease seek a venereal etiology for his joint symptoms (arthritis), citing handbooks of medicine containing accounts of complications of gonorrhea, and infection with *Chlamydia trachomatis*. The fact is that untreated gonorrhea can, indeed, be the cause of arthritic inflammation of the large joints – knee or ankle – and *Chlamydia trachomatis* infection, even today (though rarely), can also be the cause of the arthritis of Reiter's syndrome. In addition to the arthritis, other manifestations of Reiter's are urethritis (inflammation of the urethra), conjunctivitis (inflammation of the conjunctivae of the eyes), and, sometimes, iritis (inflammation of the iris of the eye). Remember that the last of these was one of Joyce's afflictions for many years, and plagued him practically until his death. In Reiter's Syndrome, one frequently encounters a particular type of skin changes, although patients in whom this occurs may also often be suffering from psoriasis. (123) None of James Joyce's biographies speak of Reiter's Syndrome; they refer exclusively to inflammation of the joints, and these may have a very varied etiology, the most frequent being streptococcal infections, such as the so called "strep throat." During James' illness and the birth of his daughter, the Joyces were in such a bad financial state that Nora, leaving the obstetrical ward, received financial assistance, as a service to impoverished patients, in the amount of twenty crowns. After leaving the hospital, James again began "looking into the wine glass;" his younger brother, Stanislaus, who also lived and worked in Trieste, wrote in his journal, on December 9, 1908, that he had saved his brother and the latter's family from starvation six times. (124) To James' credit it must be said that though lying in a hospital bed with swollen and painful joints, he wrote a couple of chapters to one of his first novels, *Portrait of the Artist as a Young Man*.

In June 1909, James set out for Dublin, together with Giorgio; other than boasting about his son, he was to take care of publication of his new work, *Dubliners*. There, he also met his old friends, Gogarty and Cosgrave, the latter of whom had once tried to get the attention of Nora, but was rebuffed, as the lady preferred Joyce. During the meeting in Dublin, Cosgrave declared that his pursuit of Nora had been successful, which completely unbalanced Joyce. Despite assurances from his wife that Cosgrave had not been her lover, and assurances from Stanislaus side, to whom Cosgrave had said that he had never slept with Nora, Joyce could not be calmed down. He despaired over his imagined ill fortune, and even wondered whether Cosgrave might not have been Giorgio's father. (125)

Soon after returning to Trieste, Joyce again left for Dublin, this time with business aims, as a representative of a firm that was to open a first cinema, "The Volta Theatre," in

Dublin. After an initial success, the cinema business went bankrupt shortly after Joyce's return from Dublin.

During James' travels, the married couple corresponded with each other, and the contents of their letters, particularly James', are saturated with eroticism. One can see clearly that the couple derived sexual satisfaction from reading each other's letters, about which we can easily be convinced by reading fragments of their correspondence, of which the majority, unfortunately, were destroyed. One of James' telegrams to Nora read: "Be careful." He meant her not only to be careful to keep the letters out of anyone else's sight but to be careful not to get aroused after reading them, so that she would seek satisfaction otherwise. He got hot too. "I got your hot letter last night" says one (censored) letter, and "did as you told me." "But the only thing I hope is that I haven't brought on that cursed thing again by what I did." "Pray for me dearest. Lest Nora feared a recurrence of the cause of his malady, he assures her that he will stay clear of whores." (126) While in Dublin, Joyce went to a hotel where Nora once worked, and looked at the room she had occupied. Joyce was clearly excited by the sight of the rooms once occupied by his wife: "Waitress let him see the room where Nora had slept. He did, and was excited at the thought of her undressing her fair young body there." (127) In one of his letters to Nora, he writes:

> I am your child as I told you and you must be severe with me, my little mother. Punish me as much as you like. I would be delighted to feel my flesh tingling under your hand. Do you know what I mean, Nora dear? I wish you would smash me or flog me even. Not in play, dear, in earnest and on my naked flesh. I wish you were strong, strong, dear, and had a big full proud bosom and big fat thighs. I would love to be whipped by you, Nora, Love! (127)

This last citation reeks of masochism, but probably only in the imaginary sphere, as I found no other evidence confirming this type of inclination in Joyce.In 1913, the Joyce's financial situation improved somewhat, when James obtained work in a school, which provided the opportunity of giving private English lessons. One of his private students was a Miss Amalia Popper, the daughter of a Jewish businessman by the name of Leopold. James Joyce came to like his new student greatly, while her new teacher of English pleased her, also. Their probably innocent romance had fruit in the appearance of the person of Amalia as Emmy in *Portrait* and, in part, as Molly Bloom in *Ulysses*.

After the outbreak of World War I, the Joyce's financial situation, being subject to the British, became troublesome once again, as England found itself in the camp of nations hostile to Austro-Hungary. Although, at the time, internment was not a threat – Joyce's brother, Stanislaus, was interned, however – the Joyces decided to leave for Switzerland. More or less at this time there appeared in Joyce's life a Miss Harriet Show Weaver, an English feminist and publicist, who, in contrast to other women in James' life, was not a mistress, nor even tried to romance him. Miss Weaver knew literature, and was delighted with Joyce's published works to that time, and, what was important for the writer – who struggled with financial difficulties – became the person who helped him materially and strove to publish and market his new creations. One could be tempted to say that, from the time of Harriet Weaver's appearance on the scene, the financial troubles that had been a constant vexation for the author ceased to exist, or, maybe more accurately, knowing the thriftlessness of the family, were greatly reduced. Shortly thereafter, there appeared a new admirer of Joyce's talent, a Mrs. McCormack, who funded a stipend of 1,200 franks annually. Being assured of a base for material existence, Joyce could devote himself completely to writing, and so began the first chapters of *Ulysses*.

The idyllic life of the Joyce family in Switzerland, surrounded by nations engaged in a ruinous war was disturbed by the writer's health problems, however. Although some of these had appeared even during his time in Trieste, serious ocular pain and problems with vision clearly increased during his time in Zurich. These troubles were diagnosed as an iritis (inflammation of the iris) with glaucoma (increased ocular pressure).

> An attack of glaucoma was so severe that he could not move for twenty minutes from pain. His ophthalmologist insisted on iridectomy on his right eye. It was necessary, but it permanently reduced his vision. ... Miss Weaver's money enabled him to take his doctor's advice and leave the unhappy climate of Zurich for Locarno for the duration of the winter. ... The condition of Joyce's eyes had prevented him doing much work on "Ulysses," but he was understandably reluctant to undergo the operation prescribed. ... "I dislike the idea of cutting out pieces of the iris at intervals. (128)

It is worth noting that James' father, John Joyce, was treated several years earlier for a similar problem with his eyes, described as conjunctivitis and iritis (129), which were supposed to be signs of late syphilis, from which he allegedly suffered. Adherents to the theory of James Joyce having syphilis are of a similar mind, suggesting that the ocular problems of the writer were the signs of congenital syphilis, while, if that doesn't appeal to someone, then of syphilis acquired during the course of the writer's adult life. Here, I will allow myself to cite from the handbook of Syphilology, from 1970, in which it is said that ocular changes in congenital syphilis are most frequently those of luetic chorioiditis and chorioretinitis:

Ocular changes are the result of spirochetal bacteremia, which develops in the last months of fetal life or the first months after birth. After resolution of active inflammatory changes, which normally resolve spontaneously, there arise characteristic changes on the retina, described as "salt and pepper." These changes do not involve the iris, nor cause glaucoma!" (130) As for late congenital syphilis (*lues congenital tarda*), most often the changes are those of *keratitis parenchymatosa* (interstitial keratitis), which frequently coexists with chorioiditis. These signs usually appear between 6 and 20 years of age, and very rarely beyond 30 years of age. Changes in the cornea may accompany a strong inflammatory reaction in the iris (iritis). Ocular changes in congenital late syphilis are rarely singular and frequently occur together with other signs, for example, characteristic changes in dentition and hearing, forming, with those of vision, the so-called Hutchinson's triad. Serologic tests (the Wasserman test or others) are, as a rule, but not always, strongly positive. (130) Inflammation of the iris (iritis), from which both male Joyces suffered, usually accompanies inflammation of the cornea, a dominant sign, which was diagnosed in neither of them. It is worth adding that, in adults, these changes are, in general, no longer active, and do not produce such stormy symptoms as appeared in James Joyce. Iritis can have a variety of etiologies: viral, fungal, and bacterial (not excluding syphilis). It can also be the result of an allergic reaction, and accompanying inflammation of the joints. This illness, in the pre-antibiotic era, when antibiotics were not known, frequently appeared in persons in whom a chronic, pus-forming inflammatory reaction had been present are found in several places, e.g. on the tonsils, in decayed teeth, or in the gall bladder. Iritis caused by syphilis was commonly of the chronic type, in which the symptoms were less evident, while in the iris itself, there appeared yellowish or grey, tuberous infiltrates, occasionally visible to the naked eye. Other than syphilis, the causes of such changes were also sarcoidosis and tuberculosis. (130)

During his stay in Zurich, Joyce met Frank Budgen, a painter, who, during the war, added to his income as a clerk in the British Consulate in Zurich. Budgen really liked Joyce's writing, and the latter reached out to his friend, a while later, for advice during the writing of *Ulysses*, then later for *Finnegan's Wake*. Even at the start of the friendship, Budgen became entangled in one of Joyce's romances, namely in Joyce's romance with Miss Martha Fleischman. Miss Fleischman was a young woman with her own, modest income, which allowed her to rent an apartment in Zurich. She occupied herself mostly with herself, which means that she liked to dress up, smoked cigarettes, read modish romances, and bestowed her favors on a gentleman named Rudolf Hiltpold, an engineer, who added to her finances so that she would be at a loss for nothing. Martha lived in a building next to Joyce's apartment, and the writer noticed her for the first time through an unshaded window. Joyce turned his attention to her, as she reminded him of a woman wading in the sea, whom he remembered from Dublin - and whose *persona* appears in his books. James started to write love letters to her, and delivered them personally to her home. He also sent her a copy of "Chamber Music," with an appropriate dedication, not knowing that the lady did not know English, while her knowledge of French did not allow her to read his correspondence accurately. In the beginning, Miss Martha appeared not to be interested in a new admirer, yet after a while, when she recognized that he was more than the average immigrant, began to look upon him with a somewhat more favorable eye. Joyce noticed that the lady was becoming more approachable, and determined to take advantage of the fact that Budgen had access to the artist's studio of a friend, and invited the lady for a meeting. He also asked Budgen to sketch a picture representing a naked woman, as what could be found in the studio was erotically neutral. When Joyce brought along Martha and introduced her to Budgen, the latter was somewhat disappointed, as he had expected that this new object of his friends sighs would be more attractive. After looking at the nudities drawn by Budgen, and a short conversation, Joyce took the lady home. When, that same evening, the men met again, Joyce gave his opinion, which everyone can freely interpret for himself: "I have explored this evening the–coldest and hottest parts of woman's body." (131) Joyce's romance with Martha came to an end the moment engineer Hiltpold realized what was going on, and demanded that Joyce return to her the letters she had written to him. One of the characters in *Ulysses*, Gerty MacDowell, the Nausicaa, inherited a limping leg, a characteristic of Martha Fleischman.

In the middle of 1920, Joyce left for Paris, together with his family. It was intended that they stay three months there, so that James could finish *Ulysses*, but the writer liked the city so much that he lived there almost to the end of his life. Paris at that time was the cultural capital of the world, and swarmed with well-known names of every kind of artist, not excluding writers. It was in Paris that the work of his life, Ulysses, appeared in print for the first time, in large part thanks to the efforts of a Miss Sylvia Beach, an American, and the owner of a bookshop and book-lending establishment in Paris. It was here that Joyce's international fame began, and in a short time, he became a celebrity, a man for whose acquaintance other writers and intellectuals would contend. Along with acknowledgment of Joyce's writing talents, there appeared a greater income, coming mainly from sales of *Ulysses*, but also, of other works by the author, which sold better and better. It must be added that in the beginning phase of *Ulysses'* success, the book was included among erotic literature.

Ulysses attracted many other, sometimes quite strange, visitors to "Shakespeare and Company" (the name of Miss Beach's bookshop). The work appeared in catalogues of erotica alongside *Fanny Hill* and *The Perfumed Garden*. A review that appeared in *The Observer* acknowledged the author's genius, but criticized the obscenities of some fragments of the book. (132)

It has been said that in every barrel of honey, there is always a tablespoon of tar. Literary successes and international recognition improved the family's financial situation; perhaps for the first time, they did not have to worry about money, yet the fullness of their good fortune was disturbed by Joyce's health problems, as well as by those of some of his family members. For a long time, James had been suffering with recurring iritis and associated glaucoma, to which cataracts were later added. The author received treatment from the well-known Parisian ophthalmologist, Dr. Louis Borch, recommended by Miss Beach. In the course of almost 10 years, he underwent at least nine operations. During painful recurrences of his illness, Joyce could not work; Nora took care of him, bringing him immediate relief with compresses over the eyes. (133) Another physician recommended removing all his teeth, probably judging that purulent infections of the teeth might contribute to recurring acute iritis. Adherents to a putative syphilitic infection could acknowledge this as evidence of earlier treatment with mercury, which, as it did to Oscar Wilde, might have damaged Joyce's teeth and gums.

Another of the author's serious problem became drunkenness. Joyce got drunk often, both alone and in the company of friends. One drinking companions was the American author Ernest Hemingway, a later Nobel Prize laureate in literature. It appears that the American had a stronger head than Joyce, as Hemingway would often bring a drunken Joyce home. The following fragment of text, authored by Hemingway, describes Joyce's situation: "He really enjoyed drinking, and these nights when I'd bring him home after a protracted drinking bout, his wife, Nora, would open the door and say, "Well, here comes James Joyce the author, drunk again with Ernest Hemingway." (134)

In the 1930s, Joyce frequently traveled to Switzerland, where he would be treated by the famous ophthalmology professor, Alfred Vogt. A rather detailed description of Joyce's ocular ailments that I found in his biography does not show that the renowned ophthalmologist linked those ailments with any previously acquired venereal disease. (135) Similarly, there are no data dealing with serologic tests (already popular in those times), which could help establish the etiology of his illness. It seems to me very unlikely that they would not have been done, as the poor effectiveness of syphilis treatment then would have caused it to be considered in the differential diagnosis by Joyce's physicians. Some followers of the syphilis theory of Joyce's illness would say positive results confirming syphilis were removed, in order not to disgrace the famous man; others, that these tests would not have brought in anything new, as the classical serologic tests in late syphilis may be negative.

Another cause of the family's frustration of was the illness of the Joyce's daughter, Lucia, in whom schizophrenia was confirmed, and who, after many years of trying home and hospital treatments, was placed into a closed psychiatric ward. Nora also became ill. She was diagnosed with uterine cancer, and, at the end of 1928, underwent surgery and a series of radium treatments. At the beginning of 1929, Nora again found herself in the hospital, where she had a hysterectomy. Adherents to the syphilis theory, who say that all of Joyce's and his family's misfortunes had a venereal origin, may suggest that cervical cancer can be considered a disease transmitted by the sexual route. In fact, in the majority of cases, the malignant process affecting the cervix is initiated by infection with the human papilloma virus (HPV), some serologic types of which (particularly HPV-16, 18, 31, 33 and 35) are considered to be carcinogenic. HPV viruses may be transmitted by the sexual route and, in addition to cervical cancer, may produce vaginal cancer in women and penile cancer in men. As Nora was faithful to her husband, one logical explanation of the cause of her illness (if it indeed was cervical cancer) would be her unfaithful husband, who, as I have demonstrated sufficiently, was hardly a celibate angel!After the outbreak of World War II and the entry of German forces into Paris, the Joyce family moved to Zurich. For a long time before they left for Zurich, James had complained of pains in his digestive tract that came and went. In January, 1941, after a dinner with friends, he had severe stomach pains, which were not relieved until he was given morphine. The following morning, the pains appeared again, and Joyce was taken to the hospital, where an X-ray was done. The result showed the presence of a perforated duodenal ulcer, from which, as was supposed, Joyce had suffered for many years. (Some believe that the ulcer that perforated was caused by a syphilitic gumma on the duodenum, for which, in my opinion, there is no convincing evidence). The patient underwent surgery, which went successfully, and, after waking up from anesthesia, was in good spirits. Unfortunately, on the following day, his condition worsened, and James fell into a coma. When he regained consciousness for a short time, he asked for his family, but when they arrived, James Joyce was no longer alive.

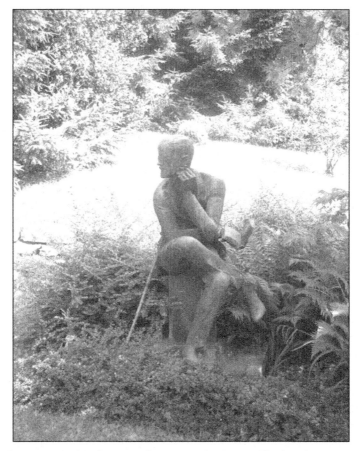

Figure 5b.11 Grave of James Joyce in Zurich Fluntern Cemetery. Photo: E. Mroczkowska

James Augustine Joyce died on January 13, 1941. He was buried in the Fluntern Cemetery in Zurich two days later (Fig.5b.11).

KAREN BLIXEN (1885-1962)

Karen von Blixen-Finecke is one of but a few women merited for her contribution to the arts who suffered from syphilis (Fig.5.12). Considered to be

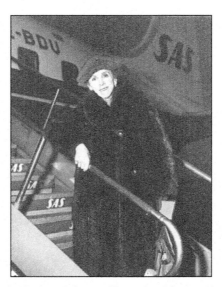

Figure 5b.12 Karen Blixen-Finecke (Copenhagen 1957)

a Danish writer, she also wrote in English and French. Twice nominated for the Nobel Prize in literature, she never received it. The majority of her creations were published under the pseudonym Isak Dinesen, with several others as Osceola and Pierre Andrezel.

Karen Blixen was born in Rungsted in Denmark on April 17, 1885; the parents of the future writer were Wilhelm Dinesen, a retired officer with some literary achievements, and Ingeborg Westenholz, a person involved in politics and social action. Karen spent her childhood on the family estate, where she received a careful and proper upbringing, as her family had an aristocratic background, though they did not possess a title. When Karen was 10 years old, her father committed suicide. It is felt that the cause was infection with syphilis and a conviction that the disease would drive him to madness. (136)

At age twenty-eight, Karen became engaged, and married the Swedish Baron Bror von Blixen-Finecke, receiving the title of Baroness. As will become apparent later, this was not the only "wedding present" that Karen received by marrying the Baron. Here, it should be noted that the nobleman was only second on the list of candidates for a husband, as number one was his twin brother, Hans von Blixen-Finecke, in whom Karen was in love, and probably romantically involved; Hans, however, did not want to marry. Shortly after the wedding, the new von Blixens left for Kenya (then British East Africa), where, near Nairobi, they established, using family money, a coffee plantation.

The marriage was not a good match, either in interests or in temperament. Bror, shortly after the wedding, began to be unfaithful to his wife, and by the end of the first year of marriage, signs of syphilis were seen in Karen. The source of the infection was her faithless husband, of whom it was said that he contracted the disease from Masai tribeswomen, among whom the disease was supposed to be endemic. Another version held that Bror had become infected from a white woman belonging to their circle of friends.

Karen's illness was not diagnosed immediately, but only several months later, when she came under the care of a British physician in Nairobi as a result of excessive use of sleep medications. The physician recommended mercury treatment, although Karen must have still felt quite well, as, during the same month, she went on a two-month safari to the mountains – from which she returned with a fever. This time, the physician recommended a return to Europe, where she had a better chance of taking good care of her health.

An account of the early period of the writer's disease and her treatment comes from her friend, Aage Henriksen:

The decisive turning point in our relationship occurred one Sunday afternoon in July, when we were sitting alone on her veranda. She said she wanted to tell me something in complete confidentiality. She then told me the story of her illness, and I repeat it here from memory, without consulting the information that has been published about it in recent years. In 1915, she said, she traveled from Kenya to Paris to be treated for the syphilis infection she had incurred in her marriage. The doctor who examined her asked her in astonishment how long she had been sick. When she told him it was about two years, he said, shaking his head: "My dear child, you must have lived the life of a cavalry officer. The disease is already in its third stage". He advised her to go to Copenhagen, where she could receive treatment that at the time was the best in Europe." (137)

According to the above account, in which the author cautions that he is writing from memory, Karen Blixen learned from her physician in Paris that her lues was already in its third stage, which would indicate that the doctor noticed signs of third-stage syphilis in his patient. Old handbooks of syphilology describe cases of syphilis with a particularly virulent course, in which the signs of third-stage lues appeared even after just several to over a dozen months after infection. These cases are called *lues maligna, tertiarismus praecox*, or secondary-tertiary syphilis, and it is considered that they are either caused by treponemes of greater virulence or are associated with a markedly lowered immunity of the patient.

Cases of this type are almost unknown today, due to the availability of more effective methods of treatment, as well as much better methods for the diagnosis of syphilis. In Copenhagen, the writer came under the care of the well-known Danish venereologist, Professor Carl Rasch, at the

Rigshospital; he recommended the use of a new medication from the arsenobenzene group, Salvarsan, then already in use in Europe. This agent, though of greater efficacy than mercury, like the latter was not health-neutral, and had unpleasant side effects. These appeared even after the first course of treatment, and Karen did not want to agree to a second series of injections. Professor Rasch, who took care of her for close to ten years, also backed away from oral treatment with mercury, which caused loss of hair and skin darkening, and instead, used mercury cream rubs, which also were not innocuous for health. Despite frequent visits to the doctor and numerous hospital stays, it was possible to maintain secrecy about the patients' illness. Even her closest family did not know exactly why the writer was hospitalized, as she was not on a ward designated for syphilitics, but on the general ward. It was maintained that Karen was being treated there as a result of some tropical disease. (137)

Karen also tried more innovative forms of treatment of her disease, as initiated by Dr. Julius Wagner-Jauregg, about whom I have already written that he tried to treat syphilis by injecting malaria parasites to cause a rise the body's temperature. She also took advantage of the then more modern arrangements, for instance using steam boxes, into which patients were placed with the aim of raising the body temperature by several degrees. This did not last long, as it turned out that she suffered from claustrophobia, which did not allow a continuation of this treatment method.

Despite her serious health problems, the authoress retained her intellectual functions to the end of her life, thanks to which readers of good literature were provided a series of interesting publications. The best known of Karen Blixen's works is the novel, *Out of Africa*, which appeared for the first time in 1937. This narrative, which describes her stay in Africa, gained greatly in popularity after its being made into a film in 1985 by the well-known director, Sydney Pollack. The film had an excellent cast of actors, with Meryl Streep in the role of Karen, Klaus Maria Brandauer in the role of Bror, her husband, and Robert Redford as Dennis Finch Hatton, the heroine's friend and paramour. The merit of this film is not just the select cast, but also the beautiful cinematography of the African landscape and the exquisite music including works by Mozart, with fragments of his beautiful clarinet concerto. *Out of Africa* begins with the words, "I had a farm in Africa, at the foot of Ngong Hills," is a nostalgic story of the life of a white woman in still-colonial Africa, who, after separation from her husband, runs a coffee plantation. The story is not completely autobiographical, as some of its threads are not consistent with the real biography. The authoress does not reveal all the details concerning her private life, representing her contacts with Dennis Finch-Hatton as platonic and more friendly than romantic, while we know that they lived together, the result of which were two abortions. Supposedly, Finch-Hatton did not want to have a child, and encouraged her, in his letters, to get rid of their unborn children. The personal life of Karen Blixen had a sad conclusion, as did her interests in Africa. Dennis Finch-Hatton died in an airplane accident, while the coffee plantation went practically bankrupt.

Out of Africa was not the Danish writer's first publication. In 1930, there appeared a collection of stories under the title, *Seven Gothic Tales*, described by critics in England and the U.S.A. as a masterpiece. Despite her origins, Karen, although a Dane, preferred to write in English, which, according to those who know literature, was unusually beautiful. I will not list all of the writer's works, of which many did not appear until her death. I will mention one more, namely a collection of tales entitled *Anecdotes of Destiny*, which appeared in 1958. One of the anecdotes, "Babette's Feast," was filmed, similarly to *Out of Africa*, and that film also like the latter, received several awards. One more of the authoress' films attained a film adaptation, namely *An*

Immortal Story, which was adapted by none other than Orson Welles!

In the medical world, there has long been a discussion on the subject of what constituted the main cause of the writer's health problems in her latter years. If syphilis and the secondary effects of its treatment were been involved, could there have been something entirely different? In 1995, Dr. Kaare Weismann published an article in "Sexually Transmitted Diseases," entitled, "Neurosyphilis or chronic heavy metal poisoning: Karen Blixen's lifelong disease." (138) The author seeks to convince us that Karen's health problems after her return to Europe were the result of mercury poisoning, which she began to take in 1915, while she was still in Africa. At the time when she returned to Denmark, and Dr. Rasch's care began, both anemia and inflammatory changes of the oral cavity were found, and were diagnosed as mercury poisoning. As already mentioned, Dr. Rasch recommended Salvarsan and mercury cream rubs, neither of which medicines were without effect on the general state of her health.

There is no doubt that medications used in the treatment of syphilis at that time could be more dangerous than the disease itself and determining in which cases their use made sense, and in which they missed the target, was practically impossible. To this day, we do not know, and can only speculate why in some people lues appears to stop its development, while in others, despite treatment, it progresses to the appearance of psychiatric, neurologic, or cardiovascular changes that lead to the death of the patient.

A solution to that dilemma, or to that of whether Karen Blixen's health problems were caused by syphilis, and specifically *tabes dorsalis*, or by poisoning by heavy metals (mercury and/or arsenic), I consider impossible to determine; discussions on the subject are very academic, even more so, given that one has also to consider a third element to the puzzle, i.e. that there could be other diseases involved, including psychosomatic illness. In her later years, Karen overused prescription drugs, and had symptoms suggestive of anorexia. Among other illnesses experienced by the authoress must be named malaria, amoebic dysentery, unidentified tropical fevers, severe ("Spanish") influenza, sunstrokes, stomach ulcer and gallstones.

The history of Karen's gastric troubles was a very long one, the first reports of stomach pains coming even from the time when she lived in Africa. Some want to see *tabes dorsalis* in these, as so-called "gastric crises" can appear in that condition. However, such pains could equally be caused by prolonged use of mercury (we don't know how long she used it), or the beginnings of gastric ulcer disease *per se*. Because her pains often appeared in stressful situations (divorce, her sister's and mother's deaths, non-receipt of the Nobel Prize), some judge that these complaints could have had a psychogenic character, (139) or that they were an intensification of gastric ulcer disease, in which the emotional state can produce exacerbation of symptoms! In the 1930s, Karen's stomach pains were very intense and associated with vomiting, which, in turn, could indicate a syphilitic basis. We know that in addition to gastric symptoms the patient complained of pains in the extremities, a symptom suggesting lumbago – which could equally suggest *tabes dorsalis*. During neurologic testing from this period, a decrease in the patellar reflex was noted, as well as some derangement of sensibility, possibly pointing to *tabes dorsalis*. (139) Negative results in serologic testing of the cerebrospinal fluid performed at that time show nothing significant, as they neither confirm nor exclude *tabes dorsalis*. Close to half of patients suffering from this manifestation of syphilis have negative test results. (140)

We do not know exactly what Karen judged about the causes of her complaints. One cannot exclude that she did believe she had syphilis, which was then commonly considered incurable. One can also suppose that the family history and specifically the illness of her father and his having committed suicide could support her in such a conviction. It is considered, however, that at some period in her career Karen Blixen could have deliberately spread news about having lues in order to increase her attractiveness as a writer, and possibly to show that despite her suffering due to the disease, she could write interesting books. One cannot exclude that she believed (and not she, alone) that infection with syphilis helps in the development of talent, evidence of which can be the long list of talented people ill with lues, who created splendid works before the disease took them to the grave.

Beginning with the second half of the 1940s, due to her stomach pains, Karen began to use strong pain, anti-cramping, and sleeping medications, and also amphetamine and tranquilizing agents. Many of these could produce addiction, a fact not well known at the time. With the passage of years, the authoress' state of health worsened, and in the mid-'50s, as the result of a perforated stomach ulcer, Karen underwent a resection of her stomach, during which one-third of that organ was removed. After the operation, she ate even less, weighed but 80 lbs., and smoked cigarettes. She had problems with writing, but was able to have several radio broadcasts that were well received by her listeners. Despite her weak health, Karen Blixen managed to take care of her affairs. Taking advantage of the popularity of her books in the U.S.A., she undertook a trip to America in 1959, where she was received with great honors. Renowned American writers, among them Ernest Hemingway, Truman Capote and Carson McCullers, expressed themselves about her with great appreciation, while known dramatist, Arthur Miller, together with his wife, Marilyn Monroe, paid her a visit. The authoress, when going out, would call attention to herself by her appearance: shockingly thin, barely able to stand, and dressed in a black dress, which contrasted with her parchment-pale complexion and great, flashing eyes.

Karen Blixen died in 1962 in her family town of Rungsted, as a result of malnutrition, at the age of 77 years.

CHAPTER 5c

PAINTERS

EDOUARD MANET (1832-1883)

Edouard Manet, the mid-nineteenth century French painter, is well known to the public for his many splendid works, among which, attaining first place is the painting titled *Le dejeuner sur l'herbe* or Luncheon on the grass, painted in 1863 (Fig.5c.1). This painting is currently on display in the d'Orsey Museum in Paris, where it is one of the main attractions, and in front of which a large crowd of visitors always gathers. *Luncheon on the Grass* was presented to the annual painting exhibition (Parisian Salon) in 1864, but was rejected by the qualifications committee. Next exhibited at the so-called Salon of Independents, it was met with a great deal of interest by visitors, and, equally, with sharp criticism. One of the critics was Emperor Napoleon III, who is said to have remarked that this painting was an insult to morality, while the Empress ostentatiously pretended not to see it. (1) At a time when women wore dresses down to the ground, while the sight of a woman's foot adorned to the ankles produced excitement in men, showing a nude woman at a picnic with fully dressed men could be provocative, which was doubtless the painter's intent.

In the d'Orsey Museum, one can see many of Manet's canvases, besides *Luncheon on the grass,* many other of his paintings hang there: *Olympia, The Balcony, and The Piper,* to name the best known (Fig.5c.2). There is also among them a smaller canvas representing an older couple, titled *Portrait of Mr. and Mrs. Auguste Manet* (Fig.5c.3). In the center of the picture appears an older gentleman seated at table resting his right hand on a cane. At his side, and a bit behind him, is a woman holding a basket. This painting, in front of which fewer people usually stop than in front of other canvases of Manet, attracted my attention due to the face of the man, who appeared familiar to me. I couldn't understand from where I could have known this man, as the picture was painted in 1860! Nevertheless, it seemed certain to me that I had seen that face somewhere, yet simply didn't remember where. The riddle, to which I did not give very much time, was solved not very long ago, while, preparing this manuscript for a book about the history of syphilis, I began to study the biographies of famous painters who suffered from lues. Only then did I learn that the older gentleman in the painting – the father of Manet – also was ill with syphilis, while at the time of his posing for the painting, he already was in the terminal stage of the disease; more specifically, he was in the advanced stage of general paresis, with certain elements of *tabes dorsalis.* I remembered then that it was not the person who appeared so familiar to me, but the expression on his face, most particularly his eyes. His eyes, though open, seem to see nothing and this creates the impression that this man, while physically present, lives in another world; that his thoughts are wandering somewhere very far away from the place where he actually exists. I have seen such people; they were my patients. Yielding to cure by penicillin, and cured *de facto* of syphilis, they were hospitalized due to the necessity of psychiatric care and neurologic rehabilitation to which they were subjected as the result of symptoms of general paresis and *tabes dorsalis.* Some were fit enough to return to an almost normal life, but many of them vegetated in a variety of protective institutions to the ends of their lives. Edouard's father, Auguste Manet, remained at home while ill, being taken care of by his wife and closest family. The once-honored citizen, judge, and recipient of the Legion of

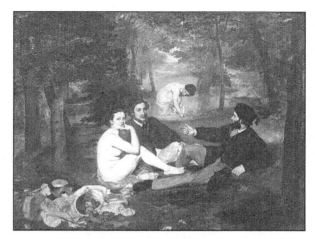

*Figure 5c.1 The Luncheon on the Grass by E. Manet (1863).
Musée d'Orsay*

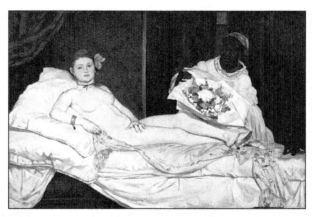

Figure 5c.2 Olympia by E. Manet (1863). Musée d'Orsay

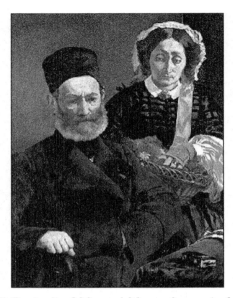

Figure 5c.3 Portrait of M. and Mme. Auguste Manet by E. Manet 1860. Musée d'Orsay

Honor was an invalid from about 1857 on, partly paralyzed, deprived of the ability to speak, and moving with difficulty with the help of a cane. (2) Of course, the fact of his illness was a closely held secret, while officially it was said that his crippling disability was the result of a stroke.

Edouard Manet was the firstborn son of judge Auguste Manet, and, what was a natural thing in such families, it was expected that he would not fail to reach higher honors in the French justice administration (Fig.5c 4). In school, Edouard did not stand out in anything in particular. He learned rather slowly, repeating the fifth year. More than the customary subjects, adjunctive lessons in drawing offered by the school interested him a great deal. It was in these drawing courses that he met a colleague, who remained his friend for life. This colleague was Antonin Proust, the later minister of Fine Arts, and author of memoirs about Manet, to whom we are indebted for many details about the painter's life. It is felt that the person who contributed to Manet's deepening interest in painting during his early years was his Uncle Edmond (his Mother's brother), who himself drew beautifully, and often took Edouard and his friend to the Louvre or to other Parisian museums, where he would show the young boys the works of outstanding painters. It must be added that it was Uncle Edmond who financed the drawing courses offered by the school – which Manet's father opposed, and for which he did not want to pay.

Pressured by his father to become an attorney, Edouard declined emphatically, and threatened that in the event of further insistence, he would move out of the house. He determined to enter the Naval Academy, to which his father, though unwillingly, agreed. In 1848, Edouard embarked on a schooling voyage to Rio de Janeiro, but after his return, did not pass the entrance examinations, possibly deliberately, as a naval career also did not suit him. In the course of the race trip, more than in the study of sailing, he was interested in the landscapes provided by the localities at which the vessel made port. He wondered from afar at the peaks of the mountains of Tenerife, one of the Canary Islands, and at the beaches of Porto Santo, a tiny island belonging to the archipelago of Madeira, where Columbus ones lived. The sailing ship did not reach Madeira itself, due to bad weather, and Manet had to admire this charming island from a great distance. During the stop in Rio, Manet was amazed at the manner in which the blacks were treated. In a letter to his mother, he wrote: "The Negroes have only a pair of trousers for clothing, sometimes a linen jacket, but as slaves they are not allowed to wear shoes. The Negressess are naked to the waist, some wear a scarf that falls over the chest. They take great pains in their appearance. (3) The future portraitist immediately perceived the beauty of those women, writing about the"magnificent black eyes of Brazilian women," although he must have met some faults on their part, as he also wrote, "Brazilian women are generally attractive but do not deserve the reputation for flirtatiousness attributed to them in France; no one is more prudish or stupid than a Brazilian women." (4) Regardless of any doubts one may have based on the previous sentence, one can clearly see that women and the natural attractions of the countries he visited interested Manet more than the mysteries of the art of sailing. During the entire period of travel, Manet did not stop sketching, and many things that he saw along the way he committed onto paper. After returning to France, it was already clear that nothing besides painting interested him and Father August agreed to finance appropriate studies for his son. Edouard signed up at the painting school conducted by Thomas Couture, where he spent the next six years.

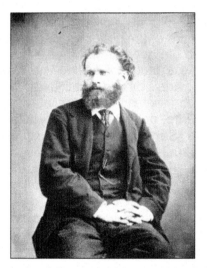

Figure 5c.4 Portrait of Edouard Manet (1874) by Felix Nadar

Even before beginning studies at Couture's school, there appeared at the house of the Manets a young Dutch woman, who had not been in France long. Her name was Suzanne Leenhoff, and she was hired by Manet's mother as a music teacher; she was to teach Edouard and his younger brother how to play the piano. Suzanne was nineteen years of age and, it was said, had come to Paris in order to improve her musical talents, which her father, the organist at the Groote Kerk church in Holland couldn't provide. Suzanne was warmly welcomed in the Manet home, equally by the parents as by the young students, particularly Edouard. She was nineteen and he, seventeen; she was lonely, and he was fresh from a long transoceanic voyage during which he had admired the beauty of South American women. Suzanne did not resemble the beautiful Brazilians in any way, having a type of beauty more to Rubens' taste. She was placid, plump, and looked older than her birth certificate would indicate. She was, nevertheless, not a bad pianist, preferring a romantic repertoire, with a particular affinity for the works of Robert Schumann. Suzanne rented an apartment not far from the painting school that Edouard frequented. One must admit that young Manet treated his studies very seriously, as, besides those at the Couture school, in the evenings he would attend the Swiss Academy, where, for a modest fee, students were allowed to paint live models. Because live models, and particularly female models, also posed naked at the Swiss Academy, and similarly to the Couture school the former was situated close to Suzanne's apartment, one might assume that Edouard did not devote every evening to art, unless one can so describe what he practiced with Suzanne.

At the end of January 1862, Suzanne gave birth to a child of male sex, who was named Leon-Edouard. On the birth certificate of Leon, there is a notation that the child's mother was Suzanne Leenhoff, while the father was someone with the surname Koella; no first name was listed. After giving birth to the child, Suzanne stopped teaching music at the Manets', since an esteemed family could not allow itself to provide a job to someone of "doubtful morals" in its home. Another cause was gossip that the father of the child could be Manet, but it was not known which one, as the paternity was equally suspected to be Edourd's as his father's. Further

307

behavior of the participants in this farce, and the later fate of Leon, indicate that Edouard was the more likely father of the boy, something to which, however, he never admitted officially. Suzanne's son was christened at age four, while his godmother was her grandmother, who had come to Paris in order to take care of her during the pregnancy, then, later, of Suzanne's child. The godfather [sic!] was Edouard Manet, most likely the biologic father of Leon. At christening, the child was given the name Leon-Edouard, which points even more at the principal of this chapter as the father of the child.

The camouflaging of the probable paternity of Manet for many years, even after his subsequent marriage to Suzanne, and while they all lived together, appears a bit strange. Manet continued to present himself as the godfather of Leon, while Suzanne began to relate that she was the older sister of the boy and his godmother. Helping to maintain this version was the fact that the true godmother of Leon, Suzanne's grandmother, had exactly the same name as she – namely Suzanne Leenhoff – which had corroboration in the birth documents. The whole story shows how prudish was the environment from which the painter came, and how hard they strove to maintain the pretense of propriety of the well-to-do.

In September 1862, after a long and difficult illness, Auguste Manet died. For the preceding five years, Edouard and his family had the opportunity to observe the gradual deterioration of the state of health of his father, and the progressive physical and mental deterioration. Edouard soon had the opportunity to observe the same process a second time, when his friend, about whom I wrote earlier, the writer and poet, Charles Beaudelaire, was dying as a result of late syphilis of the nervous system.

The death of Manet's father produced a new situation. After receiving his share of the inheritance, Edouard, became financially independent, and no longer felt obligated to observe the limits placed on him by Auguste. First of all, he married Suzanne, with whom he had been living anyway since the death of her grandmother, and now could devote more time to painting and social life. It was during this period that paintings, which would make Manet famous were appearing from his paintbrush, specifically *Luncheon on the Grass, Music in the Tulieries,* and *Olympia.* In the last two Victorine Meurent appeared as a model, with whom the painter collaborated for thirteen years. In both paintings, Mademoiselle Meurent appeared without clothes: in *Luncheon on the Grass,* in the company of two elegantly-dressed men, while in *Olympia,* half-lying on a settee, a completely unclothed beauty reminiscent of the figures in Goya's painting, *Naked Maya* or Titian's *Venus from Urbino.* When Manet met her, Victorine was eighteen years old, with a certain degree of experience as a model. She had posed earlier for painters belonging to Manet's circle, including Thomas Couture and Alfred Stevens, the latter of whom became her lover. She came from a family in the working class, where young women had little chance for a happy and ample life. Women of her sphere could marry men of an equal status, bear them children, and attempt to make ends meet with the goal of maintaining a family from the low earnings of their husbands. Capitalism was then in its plundering form, and workers' wages often were insufficient for supporting a family. Another solution was to become a model or mistress of a rich man, which was tied to certain obligations and limitations, but provided a greater chance of a more interesting and varied life. Some women worked in the just-born industries of the time, mostly in textiles. Young, often 15-year-old girls were hired for four-year contracts in Lyons' silk factories, where they worked seventeen-hour shifts under very unhealthy conditions. (5) Prostitution, often the only accessible occupation for many women, flourished.

Victorine was one of the first of Manet's steady models, and posed for very many of his paintings. Whether something else besides a model-painter relationship linked them, I leave to the conjecture of the readers. The long partnership may suggest a certain intimacy in their relationship, but one must admit that Mademoiselle Meurent was not deprived of talents, which Manet perceived and of which he managed to take advantage. Posing for a variety of paintings, she knew how to play a certain role as a painted figure that conferred a greater authenticity to Manet's paintings. One such example is Olympia that when exhibited in the Parisian Salon in 1863, provoked scandal and indignation on the part of the public. According to the account of Antonin Proust, only the vigilance of the Salon's organizers shielded the painting from destruction by the more prudish viewers. *Olympia* depicts a naked woman lying on a settee, facing the viewer, and in the company of a black servant. The naked woman is without a doubt a prostitute or, to say it better, a courtesan (the differences I will describe presently), testifying to which are certain accessories visible in the painting. Standing behind her, the black servant is holding a bouquet, doubtless sent by some admirer who desires to avail himself of her services. Victorine played this role excellently, looking provocatively, if not shamelessly, directly into the eyes of the viewer. Just as did to the earlier *Luncheon on the Grass*, so also, *Olympia* occasioned the press' discussion about obligations and the role of a woman in society, and, first of all, on the topic of prostitution. And there was much to write about!

In the 1830s, there were about 30,000 prostitutes in Paris, while in 1870, there were already three times as many. The letters of newly arrived Polish composer Frederick Chopin can testify as to how huge a problem prostitution and venereal diseases were in Paris. Chopin arrived in Paris in September of 1837, and described the impressions that the capital of France made on a visitor: "The city seemed huge and very modern. Splendid buildings, elegant new streets and boulevards appearing here and there, gas lighting, made Vienna, from where he had come, alongside Paris, a provincial townlet. The city struck him with its variety and bustle." (6) In this letter to a friend, young Chopin wrote, "Here, there is the greatest splendour, the greatest villainy, the greatest virtue, the greatest transgression, at every step posters about venereal disease – shrieks, clamour, rattle, more mud than one can imagine – one perishes in this paradise and it is convenient in that respect, that no-one asks how one lives here." (Letter to Kumelski) (6).

What struck the young composer most, aside from the bright lighting of the streets, was the number of prostitutes - "ladies of mercy" - accosting him at every step; *cantatrices,* tremendously willing to perform "duets," as he roguishly described it. He also said, "There was also a certain neighbor who proposed to him that they should warm themselves by a fire together on wintry days." (6) A major problem of the young man at this time was the "trouble" that he had contracted on the way to Paris, which would not allow him, as he wrote, to taste the forbidden fruit. (6) The word "trouble" means no less and no more than the venereal disease with which the young composer became infected during his trip from Vienna to Paris. This was most probably gonorrhea, with which young Chopin had become infected while on his travels through Bavaria. The infection took place at the cusp of July and August, and arriving in Paris in September, poor Chopin was either undergoing treatment, or was experiencing painful effects, which resulted in his inability to answer affirmatively to the unambiguous proposals made to him by the young Parisian women.

In Paris, each year, close to 3,800 new prostitutes were registered, and were employed in licensed categories divided according to the "quality" of the women providing services there, as well as the level of payments collected. Women working on their own without a license were subject to raids and arrest, and were placed into special prisons for women pursuing prostitution. In one of his stories, Emile Zola, who was a friend of Manet's, describes the scene of such a raid, in which police stop women suspected of the practice of prostitution, and demand to see their palms. Those, who had signs of the pricks of a tailor's needle (meaning that they worked at sewing or repair of clothing) were allowed to go free, but without such marks, they were considered unemployed and prostitutes. (7)

In the sixties of the nineteenth century, in the St. Lazare prison in Paris, there were 4,800 women arrested for pursuing prostitution. The inmates were separated into groups according to their ages and state of health. Those who had not completed their 13th year were kept separately from the older ones. Women who were diagnosed with venereal diseases were also kept separately. (8) Supposedly, during the (French) Second Empire, namely between 1852 and 1870, physicians employed by the police to examine prostitutes boasted that they were able to examine a patient (and determine her state of health) in 30 seconds. (9) Although this sounds improbable, such examinations certainly took place, to which attests the painting by Toulouse Lautrec (himself a syphilitic) showing women – prostitutes – standing in a row with dresses thrown up, waiting for an examination, doubtless only a look, by a physician. Just how low a value such examinations had is evidenced by the numbers of those venereally infected, not only prostitutes, but, generally, in the entire population. It is estimated that near the end of the nineteenth century, 20% of Parisians suffered from syphilis alone. (10) The low rate of diagnosis of these diseases, together with ineffective treatment, caused them to be daily companions of people; they were present in every environment, and almost every family. Since, for prostitutes, venereal disease was an occupational disease, using their services was equivalent to playing with fire, and Gustave Flaubert, also himself ill with syphilis, is supposed to have said that contemporary women were "hell under a skirt." (11)

But, let us return to Manet and his *Olympia*. First, I owe my readers an explanation of the difference between a prostitute and a courtesan. According to a certain writer from the eighteenth[h] century, "A courtesan was less than a mistress, and more than a prostitute. Less than a mistress because she sold her love for material gain, but more than a prostitute, as it was she who picked out her lovers." (12) The name Olympia was reserved for courtesans – somehow the upper class of women cultivating sex for money. "This upper class of the profession bore high-flown names taken from epic poems or the ancient world: Armide, Arthemise, Asparie, Ismene, Lucrece, Octavie, Olympe. As *noms de querre*, they went back to the courtesans of Rome and Venice." (13) In Manet's case, one can surmise that he chose the name Olympia, taking as an example the painting by Velasquez from 1649, who, while in Rome to paint the portrait of Pope Innocent X, also painted that of Olympia Maldachini Pamphilia, his widowed sister-in-law, who was reputedly also the pope's mistress. This story, which very few remember today, was generally known in Manet's time. (14) Another example of a courtesan by the name of Olympia and living in Paris in the 30s of the nineteenth century was Olympia Pelissier, a mistress of the Italian composer, Rossini, and whom he married after the death of his wife. (15)

The next woman associated with Manet, to whom the painter devoted much time and attention and who found herself in many of his paintings, was Berthe Morisot, the daughter of a family well-acquainted with Manet's own (Fig.5c.5). Monsieur & Madame Morisot belonged to the same social circle, and members of the family were often at each other's homes. Edouard began to visit the Morisots as early as in 1868, and did not hide his interest in one of their daughters. Berthe Morisot was not only an intelligent and beautiful woman, but was also interested in art. She, herself, painted beautifully, and was an admirer of Manet's paintings. Valued in artistic circles, she maintained contact with many famous painters of that time. Among her friends were Pierre-Auguste Renoir, Paul Cezanne, Camille Pissaro, Claude Monet, and many others. When Berthe met Manet, she did not yet feel secure as a paintress and often took advantage of his advice. Opportunities for this were very numerous, as, in addition to painting, Berthe often posed for Manet for his paintings, and what was easy to notice, was often their central figure. Berthe was enchanted with Manet's works – and with Manet as a man. Attesting to this is her letter written to her sister, as well as the paintings in which she is the central figure, where the expression on her face and her look suggests her bewitchment by the painter. As Beth Archer Bromebert writes:

> The years 1864-1872 were difficult ones for Berthe Morisot. The letters exchanged between mother and daughters, examined in the light of Manet's portraits of her, suggest that the relationship between Berthe and Manet went beyond that of model, younger colleague, or social acquaintance. (16)

As cited by Berthe Morisot's biographer, Anne Higonnet, these portraits were described as "elegant, sensual, beautiful, engaging, passionate and delicate." (17)

When Edouard met Berthe, he was already a married man, and took great care to maintain the appearances of fidelity toward his wife. The majority of his biographers, however, hold the opinion that something more than friendship and a mutual interest in art joined Berthe and Edouard. They stress the lack of attractiveness, equally physical as intellectual, of his wife, considering as an obvious thing in this situation, that the above-average artist could have had a romance with a beautiful and talented woman. As evidence that Berthe was bewitched by Manet is offered the fact that, not being able to join Edouard, she married his younger brother, who was very similar to the painter. In this way, she became a member of his closest family, reconciling herself to the fact that, not being able to have the original, she would be happy with his copy. Many art historians, among them Beatrice Farwell, wonder "what emotional undertones reverberated beneath the ostensibly proper relationship between this married man and the disturbingly attractive, still-young and unmarried colleague, who sat for him so often and who ended up married to his brother." (18) For those readers who would want to evaluate for themselves the emotional relationship between Manet and his model, Berthe, I recommend looking at several of Manet's paintings with Berthe as principal subject, and particularly, *Repose* from 1870; *Balcony*, Berthe Morisot with black hat, *Violets*, (1872) and *Berthe Morisot Reclining* (1873).

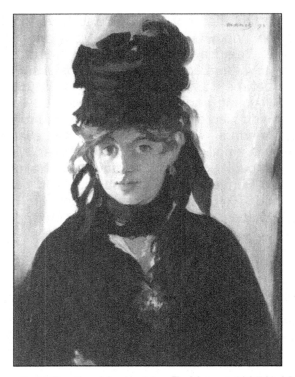

Figure 5c.5 Berthe Morisot by E. Manet (1872) Musée d'Orsay

The Berthe Morisot period in the life and creativity of Edouard Manet lasted over eight years, and it would appear that she was the only one of but a few women with whom the painter was authentically emotionally engaged. His later relationships with women – and there were many, particularly the flirt with Isabelle Lemmonier, or the long-term acquaintance with Mary Laurent – did not have the same character and meaning as the relationship with Berhe Morisot.

During the summer of 1870, the Prusso-French War broke out, and in mid-September, the Prussian armies began to encircle Paris. Edouard, together with his brothers, enlisted in the National Guard, while their family, that is their mother and Edouard's wife and son, left the city and took up residence in Oloron-Sainte-Marie in the Pyrenees. During the battles and the encirclement of Paris, Manet did not distinguish himself in any particular way. Together with his compatriots, he suffered the inconveniences associated with a lack of provisions as well as a dramatic deterioration of sanitary conditions in the city. During this time there appear for the first time changes in the artist's state of health. In a letter from March 1871, his brother Gustave asked, "Has Edouard finally recovered from the ailments he contracted during the siege, and does he understand at last how much he would have saved himself had he bought the essentials from time to time? He would not have fallen sick." Edouard, in turn, in letters to his wife, did mention his health problems, but, minimized their significance, not wanting to unnecessarily worry his family, or – and this is only my speculation – not wanting to inform his dear ones exactly as to the nature of his illness, in order not to arouse suspicions. Edouard wrote, very generally, that he had boils caused by long rides on horseback (one can speculate as their location), that he had a cold, and unspecified problems with his feet. (19) Because some biographers refer to the 1870s as the likely time at which Manet could have become infected with syphilis, one can wonder whether some of this niggardly and unprofessional description of his symptoms might not have been signs of early syphilis. Inasmuch as the boils, described as though caused by a long ride on horseback, were localized in the area of the groin or buttocks, one can speculate whether or not they were a primary chancre, the sign that commonly appears three weeks after infection, and which, if re-infected, can be very painful and bring to mind a common boil. Another manifestation of syphilis appearing as "boils" could have been flat *condyloma lata*, or pustular lumps, which are manifestations of secondary lues, and appear several months after infection. Very suspicious are Manet's unspecified troubles with his feet that he mentioned; if one can assume these to be of luetic origin, could have simply been the typical maculo-papular rash that appears on the palms and feet in the second stage of syphilis. I want to stress that these are purely my conjectures, though the conjectures of a venereologist aware that such imprecisely described signs in the letters could have been caused by other diseases and not necessarily syphilis.

Immediately after the war, Manet's health worsened to such an extent that, for a certain time, he stopped painting, and this happened to him very rarely! "Manet was wandering aimlessly from the Cafe Guerbois to the Mulhause to the Tortoni," which, as Tabarrant wrote was due to a nervous depression caused by his wartime experiences. (20) Based on a supposition that Manet could have been infected with syphilis during the wartime period, his "nervous depression" could have been a reaction to infection with the disease from which his father had died, and/or subsequent mercury treatment that did not belong to the most pleasant of these. Under the suspicion that Manet had become infected with syphilis during the war, a logical suggestion would be that he could have been treated in May/June 1871. Caring for Manet's health at this time was his friend and physician, Dr. Siredey, who did treat him (although we don't know with what), obtaining some improvement. Manet's psychiatric state of health nonetheless improved only very slowly, as the artist returned to painting only in the spring of 1872. Unfortunately, all the information concerning the painter's health from this period is very sparse, without detailed reports of illnesses or the types of medications taken, not to mention diagnoses or an identification of the disease by name. All of this may be without significance; nevertheless, avoiding definition of the causes of his illnesses could suggest that Manet suffered from, and was treated for a disease, of which, paraphrasing Oscar Wilde, one "didn't speak its name."

When Manet returned to health and began to paint once again in his studio, a young woman appeared. She arrived in the company of Alphonse Hirsch, a painter and neighbor of Manet. Manet, who was in an adjacent room, heard the voice of the woman, who expressed delight about the painting on which he had just been working, as well as about other paintings hanging in the studio. Intrigued by the enthusiastic appraisal of his works by an unknown woman, he asked, "Who are you Madame, and why are you appraising well that which many consider as very bad?" (21) According to the report of Proust, Manet frankly wept with happiness seeing in a woman, yet unknown to him, a person of uncommon intelligence, who was able to perceive in his painting something that others did not see. That woman was Mery Laurent, who later found herself in many of Manet's paintings, and who became his friend and, probably his mistress, for many years

Mery Laurent actual name was Anne-Rose, Suzanne Louviot, and she came from Nancy. She appeared in Paris when she was still very young, and beginning her career as a cabaret dancer to whom a role in an operetta was proposed. Her renown and the interest of, particularly, the male portion of the public, brought her the role of Venus in the opera of Jacques Offenabach, *La Belle Helene* (Beautiful Helen). Mery, in the role of Venus, appeared in a transparent costume, which, despite being a tight body suit allowed the unusually sexual build of her body to be seen. There, in fact, she met Thomas Evans, an American dentist living in Paris. Dr. Evans was the personal dentist of the Emperor Napoleon III, and was a popular and influential person who moved in the highest society circles. It was he who chose the very English-sounding artistic pseudonym of Mery for Anne-Rose Louviot, bought the then 17-year-old a beautiful flat, financed all her whims, and appeared publicly with her at the most important celebrations that took place in Paris. Mery Laurent was a most charming young lady, who turned the heads of not only the doctor, but of many other famous men of that time. To the circle of her admirers and friends belonged, among others, Guy de Maupassant, the poet Paul Verlaine, writer Emile Zola, and the composer and pianist, Emmanuel Chabrier. The last deserves a wider introduction, as he was not only a friend of Mery Laurent, but also a friend and neighbor of Manet's, an admirer of painting, and with whom he shared a certain misfortune, about which, more in a moment.

Emmanuel Chabrier, similarly to Manet, came from a juridical family (Fig.5c.6). In contrast to latter, young Chabrier continued in his father's footsteps, and finished the study of law in Paris, after which he took up work in one of the governmental ministries. He took his administrative work seriously, but quickly came to the conclusion that a legal career was not the field to which he wanted to dedicate himself, and that his passion and calling were music and composition. To the best-known and presently most often played compositions of Chabrier belong the musical poem "Espagna," the unusually charming "Habanera" and "Marche Joyeuse," as well as several piano compositions. Chabrier composed a number of operas, among which were *Gwendoline*, *L'Etoile* and *Le Roi Malgre Lui* (The King Despite Himself). The last, in my opinion, deserves a special comment for harmonic originality and unusual rhythms. Many fragments from this opera are widely known to the public, mainly from the orchestral version, which in my opinion is not enough; only a full execution, together with chorus, permits one to appreciate the unusual beauty and originality of these works. Here, I have in mind *La Fete Polonaise* and *Dance Slave*, as well as several other fragments of the opera, which, heard together with the chorus, are greatly benefited.

Emmanuel Chabrier had tremendous bad luck in his life; the fact that the creations of this talented artist are not sufficiently appreciated, and are rarely performed is just one bit of evidence. But, there are others. His opera, *Gwendoline*, rejected by the established Opera in Paris, was presented in Bruxelles. Unfortunately, after two performances, it was removed from the billing as a result of the bankruptcy of the producer. Also, *Le Roi Malgre Lui* was presented in Paris but saw only three performances, as the opera building was destroyed by fire. When Chabrier was already somewhat older, and sick, he lost the bulk of his money, due to the failure and insolvency of the bank where he kept it. Yet, his greatest bad luck touched upon his health. Not only did the composer become infected with lues, but he found himself among the one third of those with syphilis in whom the disease did not pause in its development, and led quickly to his death. Chabrier developed general paresis to such an extent that, in 1893, after the Parisian premiere of *Gwendoline*, when the audience was ready to give the composer a standing ovation, he was not in a state to understand that the bravos that he heard were intended for him. Bad luck did not leave Chabrier even after his death, as, although the composer's wish to be buried next to the grave of Manet, for some unknown reason, he was buried in a different cemetery, in Montparnasse.

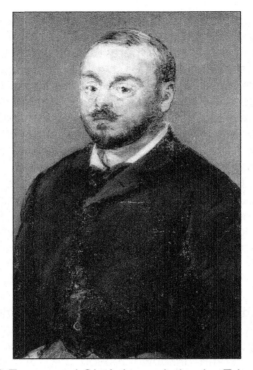

Figure 5c.6 Emmanuel Chabrier, painting by Edouard Manet. (Ordrupgaard Museum, Denmark)

Mery Laurent, the companion of Chabrier and Manet mentioned earlier, had much better luck in life—artistically, financially and socially. She was Manet's model as well as the muse of other artists namely, of Emile Zola, Marcel Proust, and the poet, Steven Mallarme. Mery was the model for the first part of Zola's novel, *Nana*, a fragment of which I cited earlier in writing about the raid on prostitutes in Paris. (7) She was one of the heroines (Odette Swann) in Marcel Proust's novel, *In Search of Lost Time*. She also was the muse and multi-year mistress of Manet's friend, the poet Steven Mallarme, with whom she became associated after the painter's death.

Mery Laurent was an emancipated woman, and it didn't bother her that, in public opinion, she passed for something between an actress and a courtesan, with emphasis on the second designation. The same cannot be said about Manet, who was a married man, universally known, concerned about his reputation, and desiring at all cost to pass for a Parisian bourgeois full of virtue. Manet took great care that details concerning his private life did not reach public opinion, and that any indiscretions of this type were unusually rare.

One of these rare indiscretions came from an account by George Moore, the Irish painter living in Paris. Moore describes an occasion when Manet and Mery Laurent were caught in a meeting about which no one was to know. One evening, as was customary, Mery was hosting Dr. Evans, who, as we remember, contributed to her upkeep and who, if one can call him so, was her official lover. On the pretext of a bad migraine Mery asked the dentist to leave her by herself, as she wanted to go to sleep early. Not long after exiting, Dr. Evans noticed that he had left his appointment book at Mery's and returned to retrieve it. To his astonishment, and certainly his indignation, he found his mistress on the stairs in the company of Manet; both were dressed as though they were going to some ball. Evans was insulted, but only for a short time, as after a few days, his relationship with Mery returned to normal; similarly his relationship with Manet did not undergo a change, as the gentlemen subsequently remained friends.

It was not only with Manet that Mery had secret meetings, although she spent many hours in his painter's studio in the role of a model. She posed for many of his famous paintings, and had no objection to doing so naked. In one of the paintings, entitled *In the Bath* (1878), Mery appeared as a woman washing herself in a bathtub standing, showing her charms from behind, a contrast to *Olympia,* which showed her from the front. In addition to these, Mery posed for many portraits for Manet, with a hat or without, as well as in many carefully chosen attires, such as *Autumn* and *Woman in Furs.*

In the summer of 1876, during a visit with friends at Montegeron, Manet began to feel unwell. The joint pains in his lower extremities, from which the painter had suffered for some time, clearly became worse. Until that time, he had considered the pain to be rheumatism – a frequent ailment in people over 50. The pain grew more serious, and I do not know whether it was in this period that Manet realized that this could be a sign of late syphilis. Indeed, during that year, he noticed numbness in his left leg, and pain and tingling sensations, for the first time. With no possibility of performing special tests – which were not available then – it would be very difficult to determine whether these were, in fact, signs of *tabes dorsalis*, or of something else.

We know that Manet considered the possibility that his rheumatic problems could have had a venerealogic basis, as in one of his later letters to Berthe Morisot, he wrote that one of his doctors "seems to believe in an origin that might allow for some hope." (22) Most likely, one of the doctors, when it was already evident that Manet could have syphilis, had suggested that his joint pains could be of gonorrheal origin, which provided a chance for cure. It was, unfortunately, otherwise, and two years later, problems with bending of the right leg appeared, as well as in coordination of movement of both lower extremities; these were acknowledged to be ataxia, a component of *tabes dorsalis.* Manet developed problems with movement, and began to step in a manner characteristic of tabetics, and described as a "stamping gait."

Whether or not Edouard was aware of the state of his health, is difficult to say. His biographer (Beth Archer Brombert) writes that, probably yes, as in this period he painted two self-portraits, as though he wanted to show his posterity a picture of himself at this period of his life. On one of them, Manet painted himself with a stiff right leg thrust forward, as though he wanted to say, see how I look in 1878.

Simultaneously we know that at this time, the artist was very attentive to his appearance, showing himself in public dressed blamelessly, as though trying to hide any worrisome physical ailments. We know also, that, in 1878, his physicians recommended hydrotherapy for him with the aim, as was said, of stimulating damaged nerves. Manet also tried unconventional methods, including homeopathy, recommended to him by his brother, Eugene, who had treated migraines in this way. (23) None of these treatments helped much, as in the following year, there appeared new manifestations of *tabes dorsalis*, so-called "lightning pains." On one occasion, while walking along the street, he fell to the ground, howling from the pain radiating along one leg. Dr. Siredey urged Manet to try the hydrotherapy offered in Bellevue outside Paris, where they specialized in the treatment of rheumatism and diseases of the circulatory system. Manet availed himself of the doctor's advice, and very reliably complied with the therapists' recommendations, submitting to massages, water baths and showers for four to five hours daily, believing assurances that these measures would ensure circulation of blood in the legs, would awaken nerves, and would restore proper function to the lower extremities. Then living on the institute's grounds, Manet still went for short walks about the area and painted a bit.

Tired of the advancing disease, and repetition of treatments at Bellevue, Manet found pleasure in painting scenes with the participation of beautiful women and the painting of their portraits. One of the ladies, whom Manet clearly found attractive, and with whom he was infatuated, was Isabelle Lemonnier. She is the main figure in several of his paintings from this period, including a series of portraits. It is believed that one of Manet's better-known paintings, *Chez le Pere Lathuille* (1879), in which a pair of young people are seen sitting at a cafe table and flirting, represents the painter imagining himself in the company of Mlle. Lemonnier.

Isabelle Lemonnier was a young, unmarried, yet independent woman. She was the daughter of a wealthy Parisian jeweler, whose older sister was the wife of the well-known and influential publisher, George Charpentier; he was the owner of a newly opened gallery that exhibited paintings, and whose firm also published the works of the modernists among then-renowned writers. (24) Isabelle had a lot of money and much free time. During 1879 she sat for Manet for six portraits, so we can imagine how much time they spent together, alone in the studio – of course without my making judgments about any inappropriate behavior by one or the other. For Mlle. Lemonnier, attention paid to her by the famous artist was certainly imposing, while Manet's humor improved in the company of a young woman, whose presence allowed him to forget the worsening state of his health.

Isabelle was not the only woman whom Manet painted during this time. During one of his treatment sessions at Bellevue, Manet rented a villa, which belonged to the opera singer, Emilie Ambre, the former mistress of the Dutch king. Manet painted her in the costume of Carmen from the opera of the same name by Bizet, for which the singer returned the favor by taking his painting, The Execution of Maximilian with her to the U.S.A. for exhibitions in New York and Boston.

From among the other women for whom Manet painted portraits, one must name the wife of the writer, Emile Zola, as well as the ballerina, Rosite Mauri, the mistress of his friend, Anthony Proust. It is at this time that Proust was named Minister of Fine Arts in the newly formed government, of which Gambetta became Premier. This opened up new perspectives for the painter, who for some time had dreamed of nomination to the Legion of Honor, which he certainly deserved, as he had already fulfilled all the criteria, which Andre Gide had mentioned. In December 1881, in the governmental bulletin, it was officially announced that Mr. Edouard Manet had become a Cavalier of the Legion of

Honor. This happened almost at the last minute. In less than a month, Gambetta's government tendered its resignation, and that included the Minister of Fine Arts, Anthony Proust. Regardless of the fact that acceptance of Manet to the Legion of Honor suggests personal favor, it is obvious to me that Manet deserved this honor, and not just because he was forty and suffering from syphilis!

The end of 1881 brought the painter not only important honors, but also increasing health problems. In a letter to Berthe Morisot (at this time, she was already Berthe Manet), he excused himself for not buying her a New Year's present on time, but was unable to go shopping, as he did not feel well. (25) At the same time, someone by the name of Potain prescribed for Manet ergot, an alkaloid obtained from the toxic parasitic fungus on rye. This medication, used appropriately for other illnesses, constricts the blood vessels and used for a long time could cause gangrene. Mr. Potain – we do not know if he was a physician – believed that Manet's problems did not have to be caused by syphilis, and that this medication could facilitate walking. Dr. Siredey warned his patient of the consequences of this type of therapy, and even wrote to Manet's friends to persuade him to stop taking it. Unfortunately, Manet, who was ready to do anything to improve the function of his lower limbs, did take ergot for a time, which, as we now know, ended tragically for him. In addition to ergot, Manet also tried vegetarian diets for a time, but these only worsened his general state of health. (26)

The beginning of 1882 brought a degree of improvement in the painter's health, about which his brother wrote in a letter to his wife. (26) In the first half of the year, Manet painted the seven portraits of Mery Laurent, about which I wrote earlier, and also prepared paintings for the annual artistic exhibition at the Parisian Salon. In summer, he rented a small house near Paris, in order to avoid the heat in the city. Unfortunately, problems with walking remained, and even increased, as there were days when taking a single step caused him severe pain. He painted intensively in order not to think of his illness, but did so mostly while sitting. He painted things that were mostly within the limits of his field of vision. The subjects in his painting from this period are fruits, flowers on a table, a view of the garden through the window, and the house in Rueil itself.

Disturbances in coordination of movement of Manet's upper extremities began to manifest themselves; we have evidence for this from a remark he made in a letter to Mery Laurent, in which Manet apologizes for his unclear writing, excusing himself for a bad pen. It would seem that the cause of the scrawls was a change in the character of his writing, related partly to ataxia, which had already been noticed two years earlier. (27) It is interesting that only the character of his *writing* underwent a change, while his ability to perform other movements with his hands remained as though unhandicapped, for the paintings that appeared during this time do not bear witness that Manet had any manual problems whatsoever. It is possible that any errors he eventually made were immediately corrected, but, not knowing the techniques of painting, I will say no more on this subject.

At the end of September 1882, the Manets returned to Paris rather unexpectedly, and Edouard went to a notary (lawyer), where his will was written. The heir of his estate was his wife, Suzanne, with the addendum that after her death, the entire estate was to go to her son, Leon. Despite preparations for the event of his death, Manet did not give up, and tried to work whenever the state of his health allowed. Much moral support for him came from the visits of his friends, particularly Mery Laurent, who would bring him flowers, which he would paint afterwards. To his favorites belonged lilac, but there were also others: roses, peonies and clematis. At the beginning of 1883, Manet stopped going to his studio, because attempts at walking threatened falls and hurting himself. In March, his mother wrote in a letter to a cousin:

> Edouard continues to suffer very much; his leg is now seized by attacks of fulginating pain that happily do not rob him of his appetite. He is beginning to accept his meals with some degree of pleasure, which makes me hope for a return to health! But I fear it will take a very long time!

In another letter written three days later, she observed, "The outcome of the consultation that just took place between the two doctors does little to quiet my fears. The foot is swollen and fever, chills have begun. I am very alarmed." (28)

Despite the worsening of the state of his health, Manet, just before Easter, appeared in his studio, to which also came Mery Laurent's servant, Eliza, bringing large Easter eggs and other presents from her lady. Edouard proposed to Eliza that she sit for a portrait for him, but this was one that he never finished. When Eliza returned the next day, her unfinished portrait hung on an easel, but Manet was no longer there. He lay at home, brought down by a fever and attacks of chills, as well as severe pains in his affected leg. The leg turned black, which irrefutably indicated gangrene, and it was clear that amputation awaited the patient. The operation was performed in Manet's house with the participation of a group of doctors, among whom Dr. Siredey was also. The operation was done with chloroform anesthesia, amputating the foot and the calf below the knee. The patient lived through the operation, but his general state did not improve. During the next ten days, Manet had a high fever, but was conscious to the extent that he could converse with visiting friends and his family. He died on April 30, at the age of 51. His admirer and later sister-in-law, Berthe Manet wrote, "it was a death in its most horrible form." (29)

One can ask whether Edouard Manet died of syphilis or as the result of inappropriate treatment. We do not know what the opinion of the doctors was in this case, but a painter friend had written to one of his own friends that he had no hope that Manet would recover, and that "that doctor Hureau from Villeneuve surely poisoned him with ergot." (30) This citation confirms other information that says that Manet used this preparation (ergot) for a long time, which most likely led to ischaemia of the foot and gangrene. Opinions that the cause of the gangrene could have been an ulcer of the foot (*mal perforans*), which can accompany *tabes dorsalis* also have to be treated seriously. This type of lesion, repeatedly infected on an ischaemic extremity, and caused by taking ergot, could have caused gangrene, to be followed by sepsis. The question of which of these versions is the true one will probably remain unanswered, as we have too little data to allow a definitive resolution of matter.

Manet was buried in the cemetery at Passy, and each year, in spring, when the first lilacs bloomed, Mery Laurent brought a wreath woven from them, and placed it on his grave.

PAUL GAUGIN (1848-1903)

Paul Gaugin, one of the better-known French painters of the nineteenth century, a post-impressionist and co-creator of a new style called synthetism, died on one of the islands of French Polynesia, not having exceeded the age of 55 (Fig.5c.7) The direct cause of the painter's death was probably a heart attack or an overdose of pain medicine, although some maintain that the basic disease, which ruined his health and led to his death was syphilis. Gaugin traveled a great deal, including in countries with tropical climates. He suffered from malaria, dysentery, and possibly yellow fever, each of which could have left its mark on the painter's later health. He was a habitual smoker and used alcohol to excess. He suffered from chronic heart disease and stasis dermatitis with ulcerations, which became a real nightmare for him in the declining years of his life. Widely talented, he was not only a painter, but equally a sculptor, did artistic ceramic work, and was a journalist and writer. Not appreciated during his life for a long time, he suffered from poverty, while his paintings, which found buyers with difficulty while he was alive, currently decorate the walls of the greatest museums in the world

Gauigin was not easy to get along with, while his personal life, except for a short period of a happy marriage, abounded with numerous short-lived relationships, most often with women much younger than he. Like many of his friends, he engaged the services of prostitutes, and it was one of these – but not until he was 47 years old – that infected him with syphilis. Despite treatment of the disease for some time, it poisoned his life, but it was not lues, in my opinion, that was the cause of his death. During most of his adult life, the painter suffered from heart disease, which had no connection with syphilis. It is a shame that he died so young, yet one must acknowledge that during his not very long life, he created many splendid things.

Paul Gaugin was born in Paris in 1848, his parents being Clovis Gaugin, a journalist employed by the pro-republican newspaper, *Le National*, and Alina Maria Chazal, the daughter of a known socialist activist, and a precursor of feminists, Flory Tristan. When Paul was a year and a half old, the family decided to leave for Peru, mostly for political reasons, where his mother's uncle, an influential and wealthy person, and former minister in the Peruvian government, lived. This uncle was not only an influential politician, but a capable businessman, who had made a great deal of money from growing sugar cane and the production of sugar. Gauguin's mother's family had Spanish roots going back to the Renaissance period, supposedly derived from the Borgia family. Another of its branches reached back to the times of the Conquistadors, and she was said to have descended from an Indian leader. (31)

The Gaugins' journey to Peru began with bad luck. During a stop in Port Famine in Patagonia, Clovis Gaugin suddenly became weak, and died on the deck of the ship, most likely as the result of an aortic aneurysm. (32) After a quick funeral, the ship sailed on, delivering to Lima the new widow and her two children, Paul and his older sister, Marie.

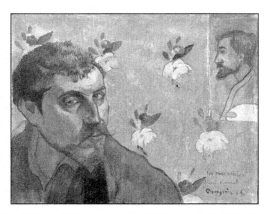

Figure 5c.7 Paul Gauguin Self Portrait 1888 (Van Gogh Museum, Amsterdam)

Despite the tragedy that happened during the trip, Paul Gaugin remembered his stay in Lima very positively. From the material standpoint, nothing was lacking him, while, thanks to his mother (who was interested in ancient Indian pottery), Paul came into contact with the art of the Incas for the first time.

At age 7½, Paul Gaugin and his family found themselves once again in France, residing in Orleans with grandparents from his father's side. Paul was enrolled in a Catholic boarding school, which, as it appears, did not appeal to him very much. When seventeen, he was asked what he wanted to do with himself, and he responded that he wanted to be an officer of the Merchant Marines, which, doubtless occurred to him from the earlier sea voyages to tropical countries that he still remembered from his childhood.

Consistently with the demands of his stated vocation, the future Merchant Marine officer had to begin his career as a cadet. Before sailing on his first assignment, Paul met an older colleague in Le Havre, who was a cadet on the ship, *Luzitano*; the cadet gave him a letter and a small package, and requested that he deliver it to a particular lady living in Rio de Janeiro, where his ship was headed. As it turned out upon arrival there, the addressee of the letter and package was a Mademoiselle Aimee, a 30-year-old French lady from Bordeaux, living in a cheerful district of Rio, on Rue d'Ouvidor. Miss Aimee was a well-known person in the town; she sang well, specializing in the repertoire of Jacques Offenbach, and also organized amusements, mainly for young sailors stopping at the port. Even a young cadet from the Russian schooling ship, who was the son of the Russian Tsar, did not resist her charms. Miss Aimee did not hide this relationship, and even boasted about it, emphasizing that, being the official mistress, even for a short time, of the son of the Russian Emperor, she made some good money.

Upon delivering the package and letter from his friend from Le Havre, Paul was greeted by Miss Aimee with the words, "let me look at you darling. How handsome you are!" – and was invited into her home. (33) Paul spent close to a month in Rio, and undoubtedly not just in the arms of the beautiful Frenchwoman. The same author writes that in Rio Gaugin "sinned for the first time in some sailor's brothel." (33) It is worth remembering that, seventeen years earlier, in December 1848, another would be sailor, sailed on a schooling ship for Rio de Janeiro, also from Le Havre, and also became a painter. He was Edouard Manet, who was very much attracted to Brazilian women, but to whom he attributed a lack of talent for flirting. Paul Gaugin had more luck, as, thanks to the recommendations of a colleague, he happened upon a countrywoman who was as beautiful as young Brazilian women, and could also be as charming as all French women. The experience Gaugin obtained from his acquaintance with Miss Aimee became useful during the return journey, as, now being experienced in his masculinity, he occupied himself with a fellow passenger, as he described in one of his letters:

> And Aimee certainly made my virtue cascade. The ground was no doubt propitious, for I became very licentious. On the voyage home, we had several female passengers, among others a plump Prussian woman. It was the captain's turn to be attracted, and he did his best, but it was quite useless. The Prussian woman and I found a delightful little corner in the sail-store, whose door gave on to the saloon by the companionway. Liar that I was, I told her a whole heap of nonsense, and the Prussian, who was very attracted, wanted to see me again in Paris .... (33)

Gaugin took part in two assignments of the *Luzitano* to Brazil, and, after promotion to second mate, left on a thirteen-month assignment around the world on a three-master, the *Chili*. During this latter trip, he had the opportunity to visit his father's grave in Patagonia, the shore and ports of Chile, the then-still-narrow Panama Canal, as well as Taboga island, which he again visited many years later. After his return from the voyage, Gauguin, now a seasoned mariner, enlisted in the French Navy as a stoker on the corvette *Jerome-Napoleon*, on the deck of which the Franco-Prussian War met him. Gaugin's corvette took part in battles on the sea, and seized four ships of the Prussian fleet, including the ship *Franziska*, on which he was a member of the prize crew for a time. We do not know how the young sailor remembered his games with the plump Prussian woman on the *Luzitano* during this time, although in the new situation, a romance of this sort would be considered very unpatriotic.

After five years at sea, Paul Gauguin concluded that he had had enough of being a sailor, and decided to try life on land. With the help of a friend of his deceased mother, Gustave Arosa, Gauguin obtained employment as a stockbroker in the Paris Bourse. For a person who had never had contact with business, young Gaugin did quite well, quickly advancing and earning considerable savings for a man of his means. He became friends then with some of the members of the Arosa family, who occupied themselves with amateur painting during free moments. One of these was the daughter of Gustave Arosa, Margarette, who gave him several lessons. It was probably at this moment that young Paul Gauguin became enamored with painting. Nevertheless, until Gauguin began to earn something from his paintings, he supported himself and his family for a long time with income obtained from his work at the stock exchange.

At the end of 1872, in a restaurant in a small hotel, where Gaugin used to eat lunch, he met two Danish tourists—Marie Heegaard, the daughter of a Copenhagen industrialist, and her lady companion, Mette Sophie Gad. The young people became friends, and after a short time, Paul fell in love with Mette. The young Danish woman, who earned her living independently, impressed Paul, and quickly filled the emptiness in his family life that had arisen after the death of his mother. Similarly for Mette, the young and energetic Paul, having steady work at the stock exchange, appeared to be a good match, boding quite well for the future. The young people married, and soon children appeared, of which there were five. Paul worked conscientiously at the exchange, but began to devote more and more time to his hobby, namely painting. Soon, he found friends who shared his passion, among them a colleague from the exchange, Claude Emile Schuffenecker, with whom he began to attend classes at the

Academie Colarossi, where they studied painting. Seeing her husband's painting trials, Mette recognized his talent, yet became concerned that Paul was becoming overly engaged with art, which started to reflect on his professional work and domestic obligations. Among Gaugin's acquaintances, there began to appear painters, and among them, Camille Pissaro, the later famous impressionist, who was born on the island of St. Thomas, which belonged to Denmark at the time (currently one of U.S. Virgin Islands). Pissaro was often invited to the Gaugin home, where he became friends with Mette, with whom he could speak in Danish. It was Pissaro who explained to Mette – who was disturbed by the excessive spending of her husband on paintings and other works of art – that the latter were a good place for locating capital, and represented a sure investment. Gaugin and Pissaro often painted together, mainly in the districts of Pontoise near Paris, where Pissaro lived with his family. Pissaro not only taught and perfected Gaugin's painting technique, but introduced him to the art community, which was composed mostly of impressionists. In 1881, Paul was invited to take part in an Impressionist Exhibition, where, for the first time, he met with approving opinions of art critics, among whom was J.K. Huysmans. (34)

Stocks on the Parisian Exchange were rising. Investors were earning money, as, also were the Exchange's employees. Increasing turnover on the Exchange demanded a greater engagement on the part of the people working there, which did not greatly please Gaugin. The beginning painter was ever more frequently coming to the conclusion that time spent at the Exchange was time lost, and felt that he truly lived only when he was standing in front of his easels and taking his brushes into his hands. (35)

January 1882 was a turning-point period in Gaugin's life. It was then that a crash took place on the stock exchange, and both big and small investors lost fortunes. A similar fate met the exchange's staff, for whom it was not enough that they lost their personally invested funds, but they also lost their jobs. This also affected Gaugin, who not only lost a lot of his own money, but had to say goodbye to his job, as well. The family was forced to move out of a large and comfortable home in Paris, and to move to Rouen, where the cost of living was lower. Gauguin had hopes that it would be easier to sell his paintings in his new surroundings, as well as to obtain orders for portraits. Unfortunately, that is not what happened. The local clientele was not interested in the works of an unknown painter, and there likewise were no orders for portraits; this resulted in the family finding itself without a livelihood, in a short while. After a half-year vegetating in Rouen, Mette was able to convince her husband it would be easier for him to find work in Copenhagen, doubtless counting on the help of her family who lived there. Unfortunately, here also, they met disillusionment. Gaugin, as a result of linguistic difficulties, was not able to find work, while his paintings did not find any buyers. Additionally, Mette's family did not demonstrate sufficient desire to help, considering him a freeloader, who wasted his time painting pictures for which there were no buyers. One source of income was French lessons given by Mette, as well as translation of French texts into Danish. Gaugin was in a depression, and thought of suicide. In a letter to Pissaro he said, "Every day I ask myself whether it wouldn't be better to go to the attic and put a rope around my neck." (36)

In June 1885, in the company of Clovis, his 6-year-old son, Gaugin returned to Paris. He had not a cent to his name, and availed himself of the hospitality of friends, living on small loans offered by them. He tried to find work, even at the stock exchange, where he had many friends, but there was no room for him. In December, Clovis became ill with smallpox, and thanks only to the generosity and protection of Gaugin's friends, did he manage to get well. In a short while, Gaugin's marriage came into question, as Mette set the condition that they could again be together, but Paul had to forget about painting, and had to find work that would allow him to support the family.

In July of the following year, thanks to a larger loan obtained from a friend, Gaugin sent Clovis to a boarding school, while he, himself left for Pont-Aven in Brittany, a small town situated on the Atlantic shore. This town had been popular for some time among painters, who gathered there from various countries, not just from France. A huge advantage of Pont-Aven, other than beautiful landscapes, was low cost of living and lodging. Gaugin, similarly to many other painters without a cent to his name, rented a room in a *pension* of Marie-Joanne Gloanec, perhaps the cheapest *pension* in the area, while its greatest advantage was that its owner allowed her tenants to pay their bills irregularly. It was here that, for the first time, Paul Gaugin felt like a painter, a free person, who could devote as much time to his talent as he considered appropriate. In addition to all this, he found himself among people who understood his passion, were able to discuss subjects in which he was interested, and respected his views on art. Gaugin wrote to Mette," I am respected as the best painter in Pont-Aven ... Everyone discusses my advice." (36) It was here that Gaugin befriended Emile Bernard, considered as one of the most important creators of the then new style of painting, called *Synthetism,* whose concepts he strongly supported. (38)

With the arrival of autumn, it was necessary for Gaugin to return to Paris, which was meant facing the sad reality that there was neither work nor buyers for his paintings. He tried to join the business of a friend occupied with the production of ceramic articles, unfortunately with the awareness that he could not count on significant income, if any. Engaging himself with ceramics gave him a lot of pleasure, even though the painter still needed a means for living. Gaugin's sister, whose husband, Juan Uribe, tried to start a business in Panama and needed an assistant, provided some help. Paul became enthusiastic about the idea, remembering his stay in that region during his schooling trip round the world. He was full of hope for a change of fortune, and saw himself painting in the tropics, free of material concerns, thanks to employment in his brother-in-law's firm. His imagination moved itself so far that in letters to his wife, he wrote that, after establishing himself in Panama, he would want to move his whole family there.

The trip to Panama, Gaugin planned for spring, while, in the meantime, winter and poverty were taking their toll. Malnutrition and low temperatures caused him to catch cold, and he landed in the hospital with a diagnosis of tonsillitis. The disease must have had a difficult course, as Gaugin spent close to four weeks there, which, for such a usually mild illness, appears suspiciously long, even though this was before the antibiotic era. We do not know how he was treated, but can assume that, at least, he was warm and not hungry.

As he had resolved, so he did, and in April 1887, Gaugin left for Panama in the company of another painter he had met in Pont-Aven. This was Charles Laval, ill with tuberculosis, whom Gaugin convinced that the change of climate would be beneficial for his lungs. After arriving there, it turned out that their hopes for a comfortable life in Panama had no chance of realization. Gaugin's sister's husband was not interested in collaborating with him, so he had to undertake work with the company involved with the building of the Panama Canal. This did not last long, because the firm went bankrupt, and Gaugin was again left without a job. After a short reflection, Gaugin and Laval determined to relocate to the island of Taboga, with the hope that it would be easier to find work, and that living costs would be lower there. Unfortunately, land prices and living costs had increased considerably from the time when Gaugin had been there earlier, and the men returned to Panama, stopping in Colon, a town situated on the western side of the isthmus. Gaugin tried physical work, but the high temperatures and humidity, as well as swarms of mosquitoes, did not allow them rest, even at night. The region in which they found themselves was known for its high rates of malaria, yellow fever and dysentery, and it was said that every kilometer of the railroad built there earlier had cost one human life. Gaugin comforted himself that these diseases supposedly concerned mainly the Blacks employed in the building of the Canal, but was wrong, as, in a short while, Laval became ill with yellow fever, and thanks only to the care of Gaugin, did not leave this world. Tired of Panama, the travelling painters determined to move to Martinique, a not-too-distant island belonging to France, and here, it seemed that their luck changed. A mild climate and a low cost of living permitted a reasonably comfortable life from a not-very-large fund that they had saved during their work in Panama. The inhabitants were friendly, and the women frankly incited to sin. In a letter to Mette, Gaugin wrote:

> A sixteen-year old Negress, and pretty too, had given [me] half a guava which she pressed against her breast. A mulatto had told [me] that this was a declaration of love and that the fruit had 'magic'. I can assure you the white man here has difficulty in keeping his clothes intact, for the ladies Putiphar are not lacking ..." But, he added, "You can sleep calmly as far as my virtue is concerned. (39)

I think, however, that after receiving this letter, Mette had serious doubts as to her husband's truthfulness.

The idyll on Martinique didn't last too long; after just a month from their arrival on the island, Gaugin fell ill with dysentery. For close to four months, he lay on his pallet, howling from the pain in his abdomen, often unconscious. "His illness had exhausted him. His head was cracked, he suffered from giddiness, reeled on his feet, shivered and sweated. He became terribly thin, [and] was no more, he said, than a mere skeleton. However little he ate, his liver tortured him." (40) The local doctors recommended a return to France, warning that if he didn't, he "would be ill with his liver and fever for ever." (40) Rather frightened, Gaugin turned to Schuffenecker with a plea for a loan or the sale, for whatever price of the paintings he had left in France. He wrote that he had to get the money as quickly as possible, otherwise, "I shall die like a dog!" I am in such a nervous state that all these anxieties prevent my recovering. I cannot stand on my legs. Come on, Shuff ... do your best." (40) Because the money was not forthcoming, the desperate Gaugin signed on as a deckhand to the *Master*, one of the ships sailing to Europe, and appeared in Paris at the end of November 1887, where he stayed temporarily at the Schuffneckers.

With nothing in view by way of an occupation that would bring in even a small income, as well as fading hopes for a sale of one or another of his paintings, Gaugin decided to leave for Brittany again. Wintertime in Pont-Aven in no way resembled spring and summer, when it was full of painters with whom one could drink absinthe and discuss art. The doleful atmosphere worsened his intestinal problems, which were causing Gaugin to spend three out of six days in bed as a result of dysentery. (41) I am not certain if the words "in bed" properly describes the place where the artist stayed during this time, although dysentery is characterized by abdominal pain, fever, and unrelenting diarrhea, which caused him to frequently outside the house, due to the complete lack of sanitary arrangements in the *pension* in which he lived.

During his stay in Pont-Aven, Gauguin established correspondence contacts with Theo van Gogh (Vincent van Gogh's brother), whom he had come to know earlier, and who succeeded in selling a couple of Gaugin's paintings. Theo tried to persuade Gaugin to join a so-called colony of artists of which Vincent van Gogh, then living in Arles, dreamed, and proposed giving him a small pension in exchange for one painting a month, under the condition that he would reside with his brother in Arles. Vincent van Gogh lived under similar conditions, as he could paint, thanks only to a regular pension paid by his brother in exchange for paintings. Gaugin accepted the offer, but did not hurry to leave. In Brittany, spring came, and with it painters whom Gaugin had befriended during earlier painting seasons began to appear. Among them were Gustave de Maupassant, the father of the writer, Guy de Maupassant, as well as Emile Bernard, who, together with Gaugin had formed an organization of critics of impressionism. Gaugin and Bernard were considered as followers of the then-new style called symbolism or synthetism, and believed that the aim of artists should be "to express their inner feelings and visions through their paintings rather than to depict reality or portray nature like the Impressionist. Gauguin wrote to Schuff, "Don't copy nature too literally. Art is observation; draw out from nature as you dream in nature's presence." (42)

Gaugin and Bernard spent time not only on mutual painting and discussions about art, but also visited the local bordello together; its atmosphere was particularly to Bernard's liking. Attesting to this could be the cycle of drawings by him, entitled *Au Bordel*, on one of which is found a footnote by one of the prostitutes, "No one can give a man as good a time as I can." (43) Despite Gaugin and Bernard were in agreement in regard to the general principles of the new style in painting, they disagreed very sharply about various particulars and even competed with each other for leadership in the group of the followers of synthetism. Their fights underwent a considerable assuagement after the arrival in Pont-Aven of Bernard's mother and sister, 17-year-old Madelaine, with whom Gaugin immediately fell in love. (44) Gaugin painted Madelaine's portrait, in which she appears rather more serious than her seventeen years, while Mlle. Bernard appeared much prettier in a painting done by her brother, bearing the title, *Madelaine dans le Bois d'Amour.* This painting is a good example of symbolism, and it was also asserted by Gaugin that this was one of the best paintings done by Emile Bernard. (45) Gaugin's feelings for Madelaine had a purely platonic character, and the painter behaved toward her more as an older colleague and teacher (Madelaine was a talented painter), than as an admirer or potential lover.

In autumn, as happened every year, Pont-Aven began to empty, and Gaugin began to pack his belongings. Encouraged by the advance of funds that he had received from Theo van Gogh, who had been able to sell some pottery, Gaugin was readying himself to leave for Arles. Shortly before leaving, however, symptoms of dysentery appeared, which fortunately did not last long, and at the end of October, Gaugin appeared in Arles, to be enthusiastically greeted by Vincent van Gogh. The reader can find a more detailed account of Gaugin's stay in Arles in the chapter devoted to van Gogh; here, however, I will only add that neither the town nor its inhabitants, equally, particularly appealed to his taste. During the day, both painters spent their time painting intensively, while in the evenings they quarreled mostly due to differences concerning artistic matters, though soothed by the consumption of large quantities of absinthe or visits to the local bordello. This did not cost them too much, and expenses for the purpose were planned for in their joint budget ahead of time, under the entry, "nocturnal and hygienic outings." (46)

Gaugin treated his stay in Arles as temporary from its very start, which greatly disturbed van Gogh, who was counting on his friend to stay with him longer. In December, just before the Christmas, during an attack of delirium, van Gogh tried to attack Gaugin with a razor, but the incident ended upon his cutting off a piece of his own ear, and landing in the hospital – which only hastened Gaugin's return to Paris. He did not stay there too long, as, after only a month, he again left for Brittany, where he remained for close to two years with interruptions practically until his leaving for Tahiti.

As always, Gaugin worked hard, yet was always without funds. He perceived some hope of selling his paintings at an exhibition that the French government organized in connection with the World's Fair held in Paris in 1889 on the occasion of the 100th anniversary of the French Revolution. Unfortunately, like other *avant-garde* painters, he did not find himself on the list of the Qualifying Committee. On the advice of Schuffenecker, rejected artists such as Gaugin, van Gogh, Schuffenecker, Bernard and others, organized a competing exhibition – which turned out to be a failure, as none of the paintings shown there were sold. (47)

After his return to Brittany, Gaugin changed his residence from Pont-Aven to La Pouldu, where it was less crowded and had better conditions for work. Many amateur artists had been arriving in Pont-Aven, which caused the little town to become crowded by tourists. In Le Pouldu, he availed himself of a studio rented by the Dutch painter, Jacob Meyer de Haan, who – importantly – covered the rental costs for the place. During this time, Gaugin painted a series of paintings considered as among his best, such as *The Seaweed Gatherers*, depicting the occupation of the local inhabitants, as well as *The Yellow Christ*, a work inspired by the wooden figure of Christ from the seventeeth century. (48)

In November 1890 Gaugin returned to Paris yet again, and as usual stayed with Schuffenecker. He felt at home there, to the extent that he began to invite guests there without any prior consultation with the owner of the house. Schuffenecker was always very much under Gaugin's influence, and allowed his friend a great deal, although at a certain point, acknowledged that he had exceeded the mark. Almost every Gaugin biographer writes about Schuffenecker's wife as a woman full of coquetry and disrespectful of her husband. All underscore that she flirted with Gaugin, and some even are of the opinion that their flirting may have resulted in adultery. (49)

Forced to leave his host's house, Gaugin rented a room on Rue Delambre, not far from the restaurant, *Chez Charlotte*, in which he took his meals. The restaurant was located opposite the *Academie Colarossi*, and often visited by its students. The owner of the restaurant was Charlotte Caron, who valued art, and who allowed impoverished artists eating there to pay past due bills by accepting their paintings. For this reason, her place was decorated with paintings by then little known artists – and whose current estimated value would be many millions of dollars. In the place of honor, there was a portrait of the owner by a poorly known then, Polish artist, Stanislaw Wyspianski. (50, 51)

Parenthetically, I cannot fail to add at this point that Stanislaw Wyspianski was not only a talented painter, but also an accomplished poet and dramatist; his historical drama, *Wesele* (The Wedding) has been in teaching programs of high school students in Poland until the present. Often presented on stage, his work also attained several film adaptations. Wyspianski was popular in his homeland even while living, though his life was greatly shortened as a result of serious illness. The poet died in Krakow (Cracow) in 1907, the result of syphilis, with which he became infected during a stay in Paris, though this is not completely certain. The last years of his life Wyspianski spent at home, practically tied to his bed, writhing with pain, as a result of the cutaneous (skin) form of third-stage syphilis. (52)

Louise Schuffenecker was not the only woman in whom Gaugin was interested during this time. Shortly after arriving in Paris, he funded for himself a young, 24-year-old mistress by the name of Juliette Huet. (53) She was a friend of the mistress of George Daniel de Monfried, a painter and friend of Gaugin's. Both women were seamstresses by profession, and worked in the same tailor shop. It may be that Juliette also repaired Gaugin's clothing, but her main occupation was posing for his pictures – and not only that, as in November, 1891 she gave birth to a little daughter, Germaine, whom Gaugin acknowledged as his child. One must grant that the artist behaved a gentleman, as even before leaving for Tahiti, he bought Juliette a sewing machine and left her some money, so that mother and daughter would not starve to death. I took the word *gentleman* out of quotation marks, even if this seems unfair, as this type of behavior of men with respect to their out-of-wedlock children was considered unusually decent. The majority of children out of these relationships, such as between Juliette and Gaugin, were handed over to the mother's family, who lived in the country, most commonly, or placed in orphanages, thus supplying successive ranks of future Parisian prostitutes.

Gaugin's stay in Paris this time was taken up, not only by discussions with colleagues on the subject of new directions in art (and in chasing their wives), but also, and maybe primarily, in striving to procure of funds for his travel to the tropics, which had been planned for some time. At first, Gauguin planned to travel to Tonkin (currently Vietnam), counting on co-financing of the trip by the French government; however, as nothing came of this, he wanted to travel to Madagascar, where he dreamed of founding an artists' colony, similar to van Gogh's, who planned to establish his in Arles. As this idea also did not work out, Gaugin started to gather funds for a trip to Tahiti, as there appeared to be some hope of obtaining a significant discount for the voyage, granted to persons traveling officially to the French colonies. Gaugin, thanks to the patronage of his acquaintances, obtained a document entitling him to a major discount on the ticket price, saying that Mr. Gaugin, artist and painter, was travelling to Tahiti on an official mission. This document allowed Gaugin not only to undertake the travel for a small sum, but, after his arrival on the island, caused the authorities to treat him as someone important, at least in the beginning, suspecting that he was a person whose unofficial mission was to inspect their efficiency.

The first weeks of his stay in Papeete, the capital of Tahiti, were very promising. Received with respect by the local elite, the painter expected lucrative orders of portraits, which would allow him to live at a high level. He even had the promise of audience with King Pomare V, which unfortunately, did not occur, as the monarch had suffered a long time from alcoholism, and died before the day of the planned visit.

After some time, the painter felt rather disillusioned with Papeete, in which strong European influences could be recognized. In one of his letters, he wrote, "It was Europe – the Europe I thought I had finished with, in a form even worse, with colonial snobbery and aping of our customs, fashions, vices and crazes in a manner so grotesque that it bordered on caricature." (54) Bored with the snobbishness of the French settlers, as well as with the staff of the colonial administration, Gaugin began to visit places frequented mainly by the natives. One of these was the district of nighttime recreations, where dances were held twice weekly. Being a good dancer, he quickly gained the liking of the local women, proof of which was the fact that they began to ask him to dance. It is hardly surprising that he did not refuse the invitations, as the beauty of the local women, their dresses, and customs were unusually tempting for him. It was actually for this that he had come to Tahiti, to find himself in a different civilization, in a different world than that, which he had experienced in France. So this is what a description of the diversions in which Gaugin took part looked like, seen through the eyes of another Frenchman living there:

> On all sides are groups of native women in long white dresses, with thick black hair worn loose; eyes as dark as their hair, and sensuous, inviting lips. All wear a showy white gardenia in their ebony-black hair, and, reclining comfortably on their mates, fan themselves

and smoke long cigarettes. Barely visible in the half-light, which lends itself so admirably to flirting and intimate talk, they receive the tributes, compliments, and jesting approaches of the men with a delightful charm peculiar to these tropical women, which always has a touch of piquancy, owing to their immorality, incredible candour, and uninhibited *joie de vivre.* (55)

Another French writer added, "What these women chiefly desire, quite simply, is to intoxicate themselves with singing, dancing and drinking and loving (56), while Gaugin added, "All Tahitian women have much love in their veins that it is always love, even when it is bought." (57) After the dances ended, their participants, generally couples already, dispersed to the district's parks or groves, where they occupied themselves with each other until dawn, or sometimes longer.

Gaugin was delighted, and it appeared that he had finally found in Tahiti what he had longed for. After years of poverty and restrictions, he had some money, was surrounded by young and beautiful women – for whom, as a European, he provided a certain attraction – far from European civilization, and surrounded by tropical nature, he found himself in seventh heaven. Unfortunately, awakening came more quickly than he had expected.

In September 1891, Gauguin fell ill, and found himself in a hospital. This was a military hospital, one of those in the town where mainly Europeans were treated. The cause of the hospitalization was hemorrhage from the respiratory tract, and heart problems. (58, 59) Not all biographers agree as to the date of this occurrence, providing various versions, among others that of March 1892 (59). Unfortunately, almost all of them indicate that the cause of the illness was syphilis, with which the painter had supposedly been infected at age 17 or 18, during his first travels to Rio de Janeiro. (60) I do not agree with this diagnosis and consider it of very low probability.

Commenting on the painter's stay in the hospital, adherents to the syphilis theory of his illness suggest that the cause of the hemorrhage from his respiratory tract was heart disease caused by syphilis. The patient was treated with mustard plasters applied to his chest and legs, and also with preparations containing digitalis. I will add, however, that none of these measures are ever used in the treatment of syphilis! The signs of the illness, as well as the method of Gaugin's treatment, do not indicate that Dr. Chassaniol, under whose care he was, considered that the patient was ill with lues. It is true that in late syphilis changes in the circulatory system can occur; one of the most frequent are lesions in the large vessels, most often the aorta, in which aneurysms appear (*cf.* Alfred de Musset). Sometimes, syphilis causes changes in the heart valves, while stenosis of the mitral valve, which causes high blood pressure in the lungs can cause not very great hemorrhages. Just as, in Gaugin's time, syphilis was the cause of heart ailments more often than currently, it certainly was not one of its causes. There are many causes of mitral valve defects, and one of these is rheumatic fever, caused by β-hemolytic streptococci, which also frequently cause sore throat. Here, I would like to remind the reader of a certain episode in Gaugin's life, when the painter was hospitalized in Paris with a diagnosis of tonsillitis, and stayed there for close to a month. It would appear that Gaugin was ill with something more than tonsillitis, as putting a patient into the hospital for this cause is quite rare. It is probable that the cause of the Paris hospitalization was not just a throat infection, but also one of its serious complications, which could have been rheumatic fever caused by β-hemolytic streptococci. A frequent complication of the latter disease includes changes in the valves of the heart to cause a derangement in their function. In Gaugin's case, we are dealing with yet another damaging phenomenon, namely his habitual smoking and excessive use of alcohol.

Gaugin was a habitual smoker and as Bengt Danielsson writes, "He did not have a cigarette in his lips only then when he was smoking a pipe, and also had the habit, calling it absentmindedness, of filling his empty coffee cup with cheap brandy." (61) I do not have to explain that this type of lifestyle is a huge burden on the body and a frequent cause of diseases of the heart and circulatory system. The cause of Gaugin's heart-lung problems during his stay in Tahiti did not have to be lues, and most probably was not. Another, very important argument speaking against a syphilitic etiology of Gaugin's heart-lung derangements is the fact of his putative infection with lues for a second time, several years later. The same authors, who maintain that Gaugin was infected with syphilis in Rio de Janeiro, write about a second infection, forgetting or not knowing, about so-called premunition or intercurrent infection immunity, which does not permit reinfection with syphilis by persons who had once been ill with it. Thus, if not completely cured from a first luetic infection – which, in Gaugin's time, would have been impossible – a second one would have been equally so.

After remission of his symptoms, Gaugin quickly left the hospital, mainly due the high costs of the stay and of treatment. The painter returned to his hut in Mataiea, on the southern edge of the island where he had lived from the time of his leaving Papeete. His life gradually returned to normal. During the day he painted, fished, and gathered fruit, while evenings he spent in the company of young women from the village, who considered it an honor to sleep with a white man. None of them considered this as something immoral or disgraceful, because this type of behavior in the social code of the local population was equated to eating, taking a walk, laughing or singing, and was not treated as being in a category of sin, despite the activity for quite a time there, of Christian missionaries. (62) Gaugin himself was not sure whether he was acting morally, sharing his musings on the subject in his journal (the so-called *Journal for Aline*):

In Europe, intercourse between men and women is a result of love. In Oceania love is a result of intercourse. Which is right? The man or woman who gives his [or her] body away is said to commit a small sin. That is debatable, and in any case sin is wholly redeemed by creation, the most beautiful act in the world, a divine act in the sense that it continues the work of [the] Creator. The real sin is committed by the man or woman who sells his [or her] body. (62)

Sleeping with his young neighbors, Gaugin certainly did not consider himself to be a sinner, yet he lacked a woman with whom he could not only go to bed, but who could make the bed, clean house, and cook a meal. Just before his health failed, he had established a relationship for a short time with a young girl named *Titi* (Breast), but the young woman was not of pure Polynesian blood (her mother was a Tahitian, but her father, an Englishman), and was *very playful*. She liked to dress well, loved dances, and often went to Papeete in order to play. She was not the type of woman that the painter wanted, and he set about looking for a *vahine* (partner/wife) in a different region of the island. When in Faaone, a small village, and invited for a meal by a family he met there by accident, he confessed that his goal for the trip, among others, was to find himself a *vahine*; his host proposed a 13-year-old girl by the name of Teha'amana (Tehura) (Fig.5c.8). The young woman came from the island of Tonga, and lived in Faaone with her foster mother. After a short conversation, which is reminiscent of marriage vows ("Are you frightened of me?" No." Do you want to live with me in my hut for ever?" "Yes." "Have you been ill ? No."), the girl's foster mother interrupted, asking that Teha'amana, after a week's stay with Gaugin be allowed to return home and make her own decision as to her future. And that is what happened. After staying a week with Gaugin, the girl returned to her foster mother, but only to announce that she was going to stay with the painter permanently. (63)

Teha'amana is one of the best recognized of Gaugin's *vahines* (the painter had more), testifying to which is the large number of paintings for which she posed. Similarly to Gaugin, Teha'amana did not treat the marriage very seriously. Brought up in the Polynesian culture, she did not have a sense of fidelity to her *Koke* – as she called him. In the course of her stay with the painter, she had many lovers, with whom she met in the surrounding forest, when Gaugin thought that his *vahine* was occupied with gathering fruit or gossiping with her girlfriends, and soon became pregnant. We do not know who the child's father was, nor what happened to him, as there is no record of Teha'amana giving birth. (64)

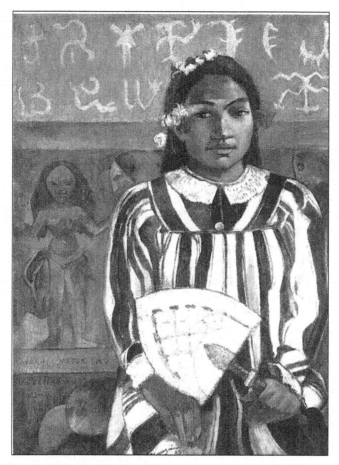

*Figure 5c 8 The Ancestors of Teha'amana. Portrait of
Teha'amana by Paul Gaugin (1893)*

After the passage of about a year, Gaugin's Tahitian idyll began to fade, mainly for financial reasons. The painter needed money, but that was not forthcoming. Gaugin was counting on his friends in Paris to be able to sell at least a part of his paintings or ceramics, but not much came of it. To repair his financial state, the painter took a poorly paid job with the civil administration of Papeete, but was not satisfied with it, and more and more frequently thought of returning to France. An additional reason for a decision to leave was the state of his health. (64) His heart problems returned (attacks of tachycardia, or rapid heartbeat), but fortunately without hemorrhages from his respiratory tract. The causes of these problems Gaugin attributed to a diet rich in fruit, vegetables and fish, and tried to supplement it with "European food" that reached the island exclusively in the form of preserves. It was expensive, poor in taste, and evaluating it from today's point of view, unhealthy.

Following unsuccessful attempts at obtaining a free ticket, Gaugin returned to his country on his own money. After a longish voyage undertaken in none-too-luxurious conditions, the painter landed in Marseilles on August 30, 1893, with only four francs in his pocket. On the other hand, he had a trunk full of paintings and sketches done on Tahiti, which he judged he would be able to sell. It quickly became apparent, however, that there were no takers for his paintings, while appreciation by a wider public for his art was far from what he had anticipated. As often happens in such situations, a change in luck was decided by accident. His 75-year-old uncle, who had lived in Orleans, died without issue, and left his entire fortune to Gaugin and his sister. Because testamentary formalities lasted a long time, the painter availed himself of the help of friends and of loans that he was able to make on the basis of his inheritance. He was also able to persuade the owners of the Durand-Ruel gallery to organize an exhibition of his works from Tahiti. Despite a special guide written by the already famous August Strinberg, in which that author clarified the principles of this new style in painting cultivated by Gaugin, the public was not in a state either to understand or appreciate his work. His unnatural colors were made fun of (yellow ocean, purple trees), while one of the English women, looking at a dog of a crimson color, even shrieked with emotion at the effect. (65)

However, the artistic elite in Paris, with the known poet-symbolist Stephen Mallarme at its head, reacted completely differently at a Gaugin exhibition; Mallarme wrote, "It is extraordinary that so much mystery can be put into so much brilliance." (66) A certain solace for the painter was the fact that although it was possible to sell only eleven canvases, one of the few purchasers was Edgar Degas, who bought two paintings and six drawings. From the financial standpoint, the exhibition was a failure; however, the artist retained a good opinion of himself, and in a letter to his wife boasted "For the moment many people consider me the greatest modern painter." (67) Having the appreciation of the artistic elite, Gauguin began to invite other creative artists, not just painters, to meetings that he organized every Thursday in his new home. After returning to Paris, Gaugin rented a not very large apartment on the first floor, where he also had his studio. In the same house, on the ground floor, lived the Molards.

Ida Ericson-Molard was a Swedish woman, who occupied herself with sculpture, while her husband William Molard, was a composer. The Molards had a daughter, 13-year-old Judith, who was the issue (whom William had adopted) of a short-lived relationship of Mrs. Molard with a singer in Stockholm. The Molards belonged to the Parisian bohemia, and their frequent guests received on Saturdays were such known people as Maurice Ravel, Edward Grieg, Claude Debussy, and Frederick Delius. For their Saturday meetings, Gaugin was also invited, and he quickly became friends with the Scandinavian marriage, and, in particular, with their 13-year-old daughter. On Thursdays, a similar group met at Gaugin's apartment, although, among his guests there were more painters. Among those were Alphonse Mucha, a painter of Czech origin; the Pole, Wladyslaw Slewinski; his old friend Schuffenecker; as well as others. One of the last was the well-known author and dramatist, August Strinberg, who wrote the guide for Gauguin's art exhibition. Strindberg, who suffered from eczema on his palms, occupied himself with amateur chemistry; during the course of one experiment, he burned his already affected hands, causing him to land in the hospital. Here is a short account of what he saw there: "he was surrounded by what he called a company of spectres... a nose missing here, an eye there, at third with a dangling lip, another with a crumbling cheek." (68) This fragment from Strindberg's account is interpreted as an account of patients hospitalized there with syphilis, which disease, it has been attempted to attribute to Strindberg. However, the patients described by him did not have to be ill with syphilis, as these types of skin lesions could have been the result of tuberculosis, or malignancies, or other systemic diseases, and not necessarily of venereal origin.

Gauguin's marriage to Mette had been in a state of falling apart for a long time, and the chances of the couple growing closer were ever less. Their mutual communications during this time concerned mostly financial matters, which separated them even further. The painter behaved as a free person, while around him many women circulated, fulfilling or wanting to fulfill the role of a *vahine*. Shortly after returning to Paris, Gauguin met with Juliette Huet, the mother of his daughter, who did not want to live with the painter this time, being concerned that Gaugin could obtain paternal rights to her only child, whom she loved very much. This does not mean that she did not want to meet with him, but here, she met with a certain problem, as in the painter's life there now appeared a new 13-year-old girl of oriental beauty, who was called, "Annah the Javanese." (5c.9). Annah was offered to Gaugin as a model, and pleased him, as she reminded him of Teha'amana, left on Tahiti, although Annah was much different than Tache'amana. She did not like taking care of the house, was meddlesome and talkative, and appeared at Gaugin's house with a small monkey that she kept as a pet. It was Annah and her monkey that became the cause, pregnant with consequences, of a mishap that befell Gaugin in Brittany.

In April 1893, upon the invitation of the Polish painter, Wladyslaw Slewinski, Gauguin left for Brittany. Slewinski rented a small house in Le Pouldu, in which he organized an artists' studio. A group of painters who were friendly with Gaugin were already there; during the day, they spent their time painting, the evenings in local restaurants, and the nights in the arms of girlfriends, whom they had brought with them. The cheerful company often visited surrounding villages, and one day a larger group traveled to a small fishing village, Concarneau situated not far from

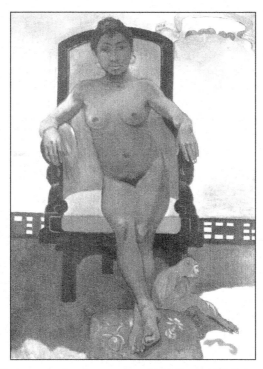

Figure 5c 9 Annah de Javnesse (1893 or 1894) as painted by Paul Gauguin

Pont-Aven. While the company walked along the main street, the attention of the people, mostly of the children, turned toward Annah and her monkey. At a certain moment, comments regarding Annah were heard, and then stones were thrown. When the painters tried to stop the boys from throwing stones, their fathers came to their defense, and this, as a consequence led to a fight among the adults. Gaugin, similarly to the other men, joined the brawl, which ended terribly for him, because he experienced a break in his right calf. This was an open fracture of the shinbone (69), although others write that it was a "compound fracture of the malleolus with dislocation of the foot." (70) Gaugin was transported to the hospital, where doctors informed him that the process of healing would be long and painful. After several days' stay, he was allowed to return to the hotel, where he was bed-bound in the company of ever-more-bored Annah. He was prescribed strong medications for pain, including morphine, whose action the painter enhanced with a larger amount of alcohol. In the meanwhile, an additional problem appeared. His landlady from his previous visit to Le Pouldu, Marie Poupee, refused to return the paintings and sculptures left with her, something on which he had counted, so Gaugin took her to court. Then he was informed that he would soon be needed at the trial brought by those injured in the fight in Concarneau. Annah lasted with him until the end of August then, left for Paris, while Gauguin stayed in Brittany as a result of the slowly healing leg and the court procedures. During this long and idle stay at the seashore, the painter became more and more settled in the conviction that his stay in France made no sense, and that only a return to one of the southern islands – this time he was dreaming of Samoa – was the only solution for him.

After his return to Paris, Gaugin found himself in an almost empty flat, as Annah, upon moving out, had taken the bulk of the furnishings – although, in contrast to Marie Paupee, she did not take the paintings hanging there. Annah, as one can guess, was not particularly tied to Gauguin, and had romances with many other men, among whom were Stanislaw Wyspianski, whom I have already mentioned, for whom she posed, and whose mistress she was for a time. In a drawing by Wyspianski, Annah is presented somewhat differently than by Gauguin, namely as a pugnacious girl with an unruly tuft of hair falling onto her face. (71)

Gauguin did not like loneliness, and after Annah left him, consoled himself with the company of Judith Molard, the 13-year-old daughter of his downstairs neighbors. Young Miss Molard had a crush on the painter, who, from time to time, gave her painting lessons. The 45-year-old Gaugin treated the 13-year-old as something between a daughter and a pretty doll, with which one could play. He perceived the infatuation of the young Miss, but did not try to take advantage of it. Judith often sat in his studio watching how he worked, and was a witness to other of Gaugin's women – Juliet Huet and Annah, when both, meeting at the painter's, did not avoid spiteful comments. Completely in love with the painter, as she wrote in her memoirs, Judith would not have had anything against a greater aggressiveness from Gaugin, whose occasional caresses were restricted to fondling the growing breasts of the young girl. Judith lived through Gaugin's next trip to Tahiti with difficulty, and when on the day before he left, the painter invited her to the theater, she held his hand in her palms with feeling, looking steadfastly at his greying hair, not daring to touch it in a theater full of people. (72) Several days earlier, Judith asked the painter for a lock of hair as a memento; this was recounted as:

> She asked him for a keepsake and he gave her a lock of hair vaguely gold coloured, in a malachite pendant, he asked for a lock of hers - but not from her head – [from] the beard as he delicately put it, telling her he would keep it under his pillow to bring him beautiful dreams. (72)

Despite a clear consent, and maybe wishes from the developing young woman, Gaugin did not take advantage of her. He understood that it was not appropriate to take advantage of the youthful feelings of an inexperienced teenager, or, perhaps he did not want to incur the disfavor of her parents, with whom he was on friendly terms. Another reason for such a decision may have been the fact that at the time when he was saying good-bye, it was just after anti-luetic treatment, and it is more than likely that his doctors forbade him sexual contact because of the possibility of infecting his partner.

Gaugin became infected with syphilis most likely in January 1895, as Henri Perruchot reported in the following words:

> In January when accompanying Sequin (a friend of the painter's) to a dance hall near Avenue du Maine one night, he had been accosted by a prostitute. A policeman had warned him of the danger he would run in the arms of that particular girl, but he had merely shrugged his shoulders: 'At my age, one never catches anything!'

However, that night he caught syphilis. At the beginning of March, Gauguin went to Brittany for a few days, no doubt to finish off some last –minute business. Sequin, who was there with him, wrote to O'Connor (another painter) on the 7th, "The poor old chap is very ill. He has a syphilitic rash all over his body, and particularly on the wounds in his leg." (73) A generalized rash, which appears usually after 6 weeks from the time of infection, implies that, in March 1895, Gaugin was in the second stage of syphilis, in which skin changes may appear practically in every place on the body, characteristically including the palms and soles.

The disease and its cure delayed Gaugin's voyage to the other hemisphere by several months. The purpose of the trip also changed, as he decided not to go to Samoa, but, rather, to Tahiti again, recognizing that he would need medical help, that only the military hospital in Papeete could assure. The wound on his leg did not want to heal, and the frequent return of symptoms of secondary syphilis did not help. Treatments for this disease at the end of the nineteenth century were less toxic than earlier, but were still of little effect, and relapses of skin lesions were observed in many patients.

Gaugin arrived in Papeete at the beginning of September 1905, and his first impression was not the best. Just after arrival, he realized that in the time he had been in France, Tahiti had undergone further Europeanization, which led him to the conclusion that, in order to find himself in a region of Polynesia untouched by civilization, he should travel farther and, concretely, to one of the islands of the Marquesas archipelago. He was unable to do this right away as a result of the state of his health, which required frequent visits to the doctor. The wound in his leg was not healing while on other places on his skin, there appeared ulcers and rashes, most probably associated with lues, which can continue usually for two-three years from infection. That the painter was not in his best state is attested to b the behavior of his former *vahine*, Teha'amana, who appeared when she first learned that *Koke* had returned to the island, and was prepared to continue the interrupted relationship. After Gaugin's departure for Paris, Teha'amana married, or, to say it more accurately, bound herself to some young man, with whom she had lived for some time.

Teha'amana remained with Gaugin for only one week, and it was said that she was with him that long only because the painter bestowed many presents on her. The girl was frightened by, and with difficulty hid her aversion to this once adored man, who, as described, was covered all over with running sores. (74) I will permit myself to remind the reader again that skin changes in secondary lues can mimic other diseases, such as ecthyma, psoriasis, smallpox or pyoderma.

In recurrent secondary syphilis, there are symptomless periods when the patient appears normal, and it is most probably thanks to that that Gaugin was able to find himself another *vahine*. She was a 14-year-old girl, whom the painter named Pahura, although her full name was Pahura a Tai. Pahura was neither as attractive, nor as intelligent as Teha'amana, and it is probably for that reason that she agreed to stay with Gaugin. The painter built a house not far from Papeete, doubtless counting on a need for availing himself of the hospital. He found himself there in July of the following year, as a result of the bothersome, non-healing ulceration on his leg, and major pains associated with it. Notes from Gaugin's stay on the general ward have been preserved in hospital documents from this time.

We know that Gaugin had many health problems during this time, including ulceration over the calf associated with (concurrent) eczematization, bilateral conjunctivitis, inflammation of the joints, a post-traumatic wound on the right calf, as well as syphilis. In the hospital entries, the following information was found: "The patient weighed 71.5 kg, had a shoulder joint dislocation, and ... was treated [with]: sulphur baths, zinc oxide salves, mercury ointment and injections of sodium cacodylic sodium as well as morphine." (75) Treatment did not last very long, as he was unable to pay the costs of his stay, but it probably helped, as Gaugin felt better, and began to paint again. Many of his significant paintings appeared during this time, including one showing Pahura in a pose reminiscent of Manet's "Olympia." In December 1896, a check from Paris arrived, which improved how he felt even more, as it allowed payment of his debts and the purchase of indispensible necessities for painting and furnishing of his house. Unfortunately, this positive state did not last long, as in April of the following year, he received a letter from Mette with the information that his beloved daughter, Aline, had died of pneumonia, as well as a notice that he would have to leave the house in which he lived, because the lot on which it stood had been sold. Whereas the death of Aline affected the painter very deeply, the fresh news that his newborn daughter had just died did not have any great effect on him at all. Not many biographers mention this incident, although, in my opinion, it is worth noting they described Gaugin as a syphilitic.

So, shortly before Christmas 1896, Pahura bore him a new daughter. The child was weak, and died in a few days. (76) This news came from a cousin of Pahura, M. Poarai a Tai, and has its corroboration in January 1944 article by Eric Ramsden, "Death of Gaugin's Tahitian Mistress" (*Pacific Monthly*, Sydney). Knowing Gaugin's state of health at this time, one can wonder about the cause of the child's death. Did she die, as many other newborns, of one of variety of possible causes, of which there was no lack then, or did Gaugin perhaps infect Pahura with syphilis, and she then gave birth to a child with congenital lues? There is no information available to say that Pahura had symptoms of syphilis, nor that she was treated for it. All that we know is that Gauguin experienced a resurgence of skin lesions, which in secondary syphilis are very infectious.

One speaks of oozing ulcerations, which are commonly swarming with treponemes, being a huge danger for a sexual partner. However, one could have questioned a hypothesis of congenital syphilis in Pahura's child, by presenting as evidence the fact of her having borne a healthy son. That, however, is not an argument for excluding such an illness in Pahura, as Gaugin's son was born three years later, at a time when the chance of giving birth to a healthy child by a mother sick with lues was far greater.

The year 1897 was not a happy year for the painter. The news about his first daughter's death drove him into a depression, which deepened by the recurring skin changes, now difficult to hide from friends and neighbors. Some of them gossiped and wondered if Gaugin might not be suffering from leprosy. His skin problems were joined by problems with his eyes, and in November, the painter experienced a mild heart attack. Gaugin began to think about death: "My journey to Tahiti was a mad adventure, but it has turned out to be sad and miserable. I see no way out except death, which solves all problems ...." (77) Despite being depressed, however, during this difficult period, Gaugin painted one of his best-known paintings, entitled, *Where do we come from? What are we? Where are we Going?* after which he decided to finish himself off; equipped with a box of arsenic, he climbed up a mountain, on which he intended to commit suicide (Fig.5c 10) However, as he had little experience in this area, he took too big a dose of the arsenic, which caused violent vomiting, thus emptying his stomach of the poison.

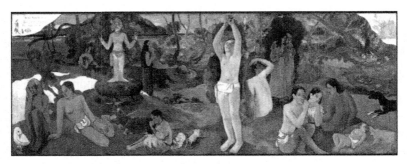

Figure 5c 10 Where do we come from? Who are we? Where are we going? Painted by Paul Gauguin (1897).

After more than a dozen hours of lying in the bushes, the unsuccessful suicide returned home on his own legs. He began to paint again, while to repair his small budget, he undertook journalism, writing mainly for satirical periodicals. This also was not enough for living expenses, and he obtained employment in the Public Works department in Papeete. In March 1900, the Ambrose Vollard auction house in Paris signed a contract with him, in which it obligated itself in return for a certain number of regularly conveyed paintings to pay him a monthly stipend. From this, one can get the impression that Gaugin's painting slowly found buyers, which would indicate that having a constant income that could possibly increase with time. The artist would then be able to devote himself entirely to painting and to lead a peaceful life in Tahiti. Additionally, his age and worsening health could have suggested that the painter would settle down, but Gaugin would not have been himself were he not to try something new.

For some time, Gaugin had intended to move to a region of Polynesia less touched by civilization than Tahiti; the choice fell to the Marquesas archipelago, and, concretely, to the island of Hiva Oa. The painter hoped to find new vistas to paint and new models, which he began to lack in Tahiti. According to a befriended neighbor to whom the painter unburdened himself of his problems, it was actually a lack of women that was one of the most important reasons for relocating: "It was in fact the sores which made him leave Tahiti, because no woman there would sleep with him any more. The women of the Marquesas were poorer and more primitive and he would have better opportunities." (78) According to this same source, Gaugin was said to have replied that he had been told that in the Marquesas one could rent a model for a handful of sweets (candy). When he proposed to Pahura that she leave with him, she declined, and it is hard to be surprised. She was by then twenty-years-old, had a 2-year-old son, and did not intend to devote herself to an ageing and sick painter. The fate of her son appeared to be of little consequence to Gaugin, as he judged, appropriately, in fact, that Pahura would have no problems with eventually giving him up for adoption, should she wish to arrange her life differently.

Gaugin left Papeete on the September 10, 1901, and after a voyage of six days landed at the small port colony of

Atuona on the island of Hiva Oa. Even at the moment of disembarking, Gaugin realized that his hope of finding a civilization untouched by European influence was unrealistic. Among those greeting the ship's passengers was a French gendarme in uniform, some Catholic missionaries clad in dark cassocks, and also natives, who, as he imagined, should have presented themselves in half-naked attire, but were clothed in long dresses reaching to the ground. What hurt him the most was that the local women, who, as he expected would greet him in scanty costumes, were dressed in long dresses, closely covering their bodies. It shortly became apparent that the inhabitants of the island lived in a certain cultural vacuum and, although there were people among them who remembered the taste of human flesh, a large part of them took full advantage of the accomplishments of European civilization, which did not go well for them. In the course of 50 years from the appearance there of Europeans, the population of the Marquesas was reduced by close to 80%, largely due to the introduction there of formerly unknown infectious diseases such as smallpox, measles, tuberculosis, leprosy, and venereal diseases. One of the later plagues owed to Europeans was the appearance of alcohol and an epidemic of alcoholism among the adults. (79)

Gaugin decided to stay in Atuona, as it was the only place in the Marquesas that maintained regular contact with Tahiti, as well as being the place where the only doctor on the island lived. The last was very important, as the painter's health was failing ever more frequently.

Gaugin bought a lot and built a house covered with palm leaves, which was large for the local conditions; it had large living quarters, a large patio, and a studio workshop where he could paint. Very quickly he established contact with his neighbors, mainly women, organizing parties abundantly sprinkled with alcohol. Amusements would last until midnight and often longer, with at least one of the lady participants usually staying until morning. His house, on which he hung a sign reading *Maison du Joie* (The House of Pleasure), was frequently visited by old and boring (female) neighbors, whereas, as we may remember, the painter rather preferred young women who had not exceeded fifteen years of age. In a short while, he found a family that had a 14-year-old daughter, *Vaeho*, and, with the help of gifts and bribes, managed to persuade her parents that it would be better for their daughter to leave school and to live with him. Besides Vaeho, there appeared in Gaugin's house a cook and a gardener (we don't know of what sex), employed for a small amount of money, which he now did not lack. (80) Gaugin began to employ models, among them one with red hair, which was rarely encountered among the inhabitants of this region of the world. Her name was *Tahotaua* and she had a husband, whom it bothered not at all that his wife not only posed, but also slept with Gaugin. On the Marquesas, and generally throughout Polynesia, polyandry was a quite common phenomenon, and husbands had nothing against other men taking advantage of their wives, as long as it suited those wives. Tahotaua appeared in one of Gauguin's portraits, entitled *Young Girl with Fan*, as well as on a photograph probably taken at the same time. Both the painting and the photograph are currently in the Folwang Museum in Essen, Germany, and show a young woman of very original beauty. (81, 82)

In July 1802, Gaugin found out that his steady partner, *Vaeho* was pregnant, and in mid-September, he became the happy father of a little girl. Vaeho moved back with her parents, and Gaugin was left by himself. Accustomed to the company of young girls, he started to curry the favor of young students attending a school run by Catholic mission located near his house. This naturally did not please the school's administration, and its director, Bishop Martin, forbade the students to go to Gaugin's house. The painter considered this a declaration of war.

Bishop Martin reportedly did not observe all of the commandments, himself, including the one obligating him to celibacy. He had a servant named Teresa, about whom everyone *knew* that she was his mistress, and Gaugin contrived to embarrass him. He sculpted two life-sized figures, which he placed at the entrance to his property. One of them represented the Bishop, the only difference being that in place of the hat on the clergyman's head, there were horns; the second was a naked woman, looking for all the world like the Bishop's supposed mistress. It need not be added that neither Bishop Martin nor his subordinates were delighted with this, and it was a moment in which the war axe between Gaugin and the influential bishop was bared for good. This happened at the least advantageous moment, as just at this time, his health started to fail, whereas he should have been able to depend on having the greatest number of friends around him. In addition, the entire row, caused by the painter's appetite for young girls, made no sense, because his health had deteriorated to such a point that he would not have been in a state to play with them anyway. In autumn of 1902, severe leg pains appeared, associated with ulcerations. Gaugin could not sleep; he gave himself injections of morphine and took large doses of laudanum, which caused him to be constantly drowsy. (83) Unable to work, and not seeing any end to his sufferings, he began to consider a return to Europe. The friend with whom he corresponded, recommended against returning to Paris, explaining that "a return could damage his status as an already legendary artist working on the antipodes." (84)

Unable to paint, Gaugin began to write, and finished a book entitled *Before and After,* which is something of a type of diary. Additionally, he engaged in a polemic with the town administration, standing in defense of the original inhabitants of the island, supposedly taken advantage of by the authorities, and concretely, with one of its components, the local gendarmerie. It all ended with Gaugin being sentenced to payment of a fine, as well as three months in jail. The painter filed an appeal of the sentence, but it no longer had any meaning. The legal skirmishes with the authorities' representatives were not without significance for his health. He was losing his balance, and after one of his court rows, began hemorrhaging from his respiratory tract. (85)

Gaugin was already a very sick man, practically an invalid. Ulcerations on his legs were oozing pus, the skin around them was itching, and he could neither walk, work nor sleep. The painter lived on morphine and laudanum. On the day of his death, the local pastor appeared at his bedside; he was called by a neighbor who had been taking care of the patient for some time, playing the role of nurse and physician, because the only doctor who had been on the island had gone to Tahiti. When the pastor appeared, Gaugin had experienced two bouts of unconsciousness. He lay helpless in his bed, not knowing what was going on around him. After examining him, the pastor-turned-physician, found a large abscess at the base of Gaugin's spine. He lanced and drained it, apparently providing relief to the patient. (86) After a short conversation, he left the painter, who appeared to be in a better state. When called again a few hours later, he found Gaugin lying in his bed, dead. Next to his bed was found an empty morphine syringe, as well a laudanum box, equally empty. To his surprise, he also found Bishop Martin and several monks from the Catholic mission there; despite the contentious relationship, they had managed to compose themselves for a friendly gesture, and came with the Church's last sacraments.

The last picture that Gaugin painted in the Marquesas bore the title, *Snow Scene in Brittany*. Could it be that the painter, who so often fled from European civilization, was homesick for Europe during the last months of his life?

VINCENT VAN GOGH (1853-1890)

Vincent van Gogh, one of the most famous European painters of the nineteenth century, did not have luck with women. He longed to love and be loved, but none of the women to whom he declared that love wanted to return it. Everything that he did in life, he did with passion. First, as a Protestant lay preacher and evangelizer among miners working under conditions that defied any norms and suffering great poverty, he passionately voiced the word of God; then, later, he devoted himself to painting, to which he gave himself up exclusively, working from morning till night. His paintings currently adorn the greatest museums on earth, or are the pearls in private collections, despite the fact that, during his life, he was able to sell only one. He yearned for love, but did not meet a woman who wanted to return it. He sought consolation in the arms of prostitutes, but there, also, found none. On the other hand, he did find something he was not seeking, namely two diseases: first, gonorrhea, then syphilis. However, the supposition that the latter was the cause of van Gogh's death is, in my opinion, unfounded, as, long before he became infected with lues, the painter had symptoms of mental illness, and it was the consequences of that, which led him to suicide.

Vincent Willem van Gogh was born in March 1853 not far from Breda in southern Holland. His father was the pastor of the Reformed Church of Holland, while his mother occupied herself with the home. Vincent was the second by birth, but the first healthy child born to the van Goghs, as their first son was stillborn. Vincent received the name of his grandfather, who, like his father, was occupied with theology. In the family home, two professions dominated: the van Goghs occupied themselves either with serving God or with art. Vincent's paternal uncle was a sculptor, while other family members either traded in works of art, or were pastors. Vincent tried all three occupations. First, he worked as an art trader, next he dedicated himself to serving God, and finally he undertook painting.

Vincent began to draw while at school, and despite a later variety of undertakings, never stopped. In school he did not distinguish himself in anything, yet at age sixteen, and thanks to one of his uncles, he obtained employment in the firm *Goupiel et Cie*, which was occupied with the art trade (Fig. 5c. 11). Van Gogh must have discharged his duties well, as, after four years working at The Hague, he was sent to London, where the English branch of the company was located. It was in London, at age twenty that the future painter fell in love for the first time, the object of his affections being a Miss Eugenie Loyer, the daughter of the housekeeper where he lived. Unfortunately, Vincent was too late, as the young lady had already given her heart – and perhaps not only her heart – to the previous tenant, to whom she was secretly engaged. Vincent nonetheless tried to fight for Eugenie's favors, but was not successful. Jo Bonger, later his sister-in-law, felt that the young man was greatly affected by this first romantic failure, that he lived through this first disappointment with difficulty, and that this could have negatively affected his character. Supposedly, from this time onward, Vincent became very quiet and very religious, and began to show a tendency toward depression. (87) In a letter to Anthony van Rappard, written a year after this incident, van Gogh wrote: "It remains a wound which I carry with me; it lies deep and cannot be healed. After a year it will be the same as the first day." (88)

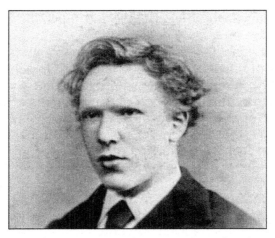

Figure 5c 11 Photograph of Vincent van Gogh (ca 1872)

At the end of 1876, Vincent returned to Holland, and after a few months of work in a bookstore in Dordrecht, he left for Amsterdam, where he began theological studies. During his stay in that town, he managed to become known as an eccentric and misanthrope, avoiding any entertainments of student life, and devoting his free time to translating the Bible into various languages, or to drawing. It is difficult to say whether this was the result of his romantic disappointment or of interest in theology, but during his time in Amsterdam, he did not seek the favors of any women. His studies did not go very well, and at a certain point, he rejected the study of Greek and Latin, considering these languages to be dead and not of any use to his intended further missionary work.

As van Gogh did not pass the required examinations, he was sent to do evangelical work in the mining center of Borinage in Belgium without a diploma. He found himself there in an environment of underpaid, hard-working miners, living under conditions defying any standards. He joined in with them, and tried to live as they did. He also did a lot of drawing, and from this period comes a series of sketches representing miners and their difficult life. The nature of his missionary work, and attempts to live at the level of his parishioners did not please his church's superiors. Likewise, the miners, with whom he attempted to live in solidarity, and to whom he professed the Bible, considered him a crank. (89) In a short while, he was recalled, and returned to his parents, who were living in Etten, in Holland. It was then that his parents, probably for the first time, came to the conclusion that their son was ill, and needed psychiatric care.

During Vincent's stay in Etten, a cousin, Kee von Stricker, older than he by seven years, visited his parents. She was the daughter of Madam van Gogh's sister, and had an 8-year-old son. Kee had been widowed not long before, and sometimes accompanied Vincent during his trips out of town, watching him as he drew. The poor widow was shocked when van Gogh, without warning, proposed marriage to her. She answered, as cited by all biographers, with the words, "No, nay, never" (*nooit, neen, nimer*), after which she quickly returned to her parents. Even while Kee's husband, was alive, Vincent had visited the von Strickers in Amsterdam, and remembered the idylls represented by the picture of a loving family, about which he wrote in one of his letters: "When one sees them sitting together in the evening ... They are devoted to each other and one can readily see that where love dwells the Lord commands his blessing." (90) In asking for Kee's hand, he surely saw himself in the role of her late husband, taking care of his wife and child. Vincent had long thought of establishing a family, and it had appeared to him that fate had provided a solution of which he had long dreamed. He was convinced that Kee was a woman he loved, and would always love. "She and no other," he would say, and could not understand why Kee had refused his proposal. In correspondence with his brother, with whom he exchanged hundreds of letters, he bewailed his fate, and sought advice and consolation. (91, 92)

Not discouraged by the refusal, he sent a letter to Kee's father, Pastor Stricker, in which he announced his coming to

Amsterdam, with the intention of meeting with his daughter. He emphasized that his intentions were serious, and that he would be an ideal husband for Kee. During his visit with the Strickers, Vincent found out that, upon learning of his coming, Kee had left the house, while Pastor Stricker explained to him in no uncertain terms, that he could not count on marriage with his daughter, whereas he considered van Gogh's pressing for a change in this decision to be improper and loathsome. In response, Vincent put his hand over the flame of a kerosene lamp, declaring that he wanted to see Kee, if only for the time that he was able to hold his hand over the flame. Reportedly, the Pastor, acting by reflex, quickly blew out the flame, Vincent, having instead demonstrated that his mental state needed treatment. (93)

The visit in Amsterdam and flat refusal on Kee's part radically changed the future artist's perception of the world, particularly his relations with women. In a letter to Theo, he wrote:

> That dammed world is too cold for me; I need a woman, I cannot, I may not, I will not live without love. I am only a man, and a man with passions; I must go to a woman, otherwise I shall freeze or turn to stone – or, in short, I shall have let events browbeat me. (94)

The consequences of this transformation were noticeable just two months later, when, in his next letter to his brother, he wrote that he had met a woman who suited him, and with whom he wanted to become involved, and next described her.

> She was fairly tall and strongly built; she did not have the hands of a lady like Kee, but the hands of a woman who does a great deal of work; but she was not coarse or common, and had something very feminine about her. She reminded me of some quaint figure by Chardin or Frere or perhaps Jan Steen.

Well, what the French call "*une ouvriere*" (a prostitute). She had had many careers, you could see, and life had ben hard for her. Oh, nothing refined, nothing out of the ordinary, nothing unusual ... It is not the first time I was unable to resist the feeling of affection, aye affection, that special affection and love for those women who are so damned and condemned and despised by the clergymen from the lofty heights of the pulpit. I do not damn them, I do not condemn them. I do not despise them. (95)

The text of this letter witnesses to the fact that van Gogh had started to take advantage of the services of prostitutes, that he looked upon their profession with understanding and compassion, and even condemned those (clergymen) who condemned them. His attitude during this period clearly shows that nothing linked him with his church any longer, and that he did not agree with its opinions; he even criticized the lack of compassion in its representatives.

Not long afterwards, van Gogh met Clarise Marie "Sien" Hoornik, a homeless prostitute and alcoholic, with whom he began to live under one roof. When Vincent met her, Sien already had a 5-year-old daughter, and was expecting another child (about which Vincent most likely did not know), who was born six months later. This time, the painter's partner was neither tall, nor well built, nor strong. Older than Vincent by three years, she was a pale, thin woman of mistrustful look, a raspy voice and a sharp tongue. Nevertheless, through Vincent's eyes, Sien was "beautiful" – although the drawing representing her does not confirm such a judgment. Drawing Sien, van Gogh wanted to present the appearance of a weak woman fighting for her place in life, a scorned woman, toward whom compassion is due. This drawing, he named *Sorrow*.

Involvement with a prostitute was met with criticism from Vincent's family and friends. Acquaintances of the time began to avoid him; Theo tried to persuade him to end the relationship, while his father did everything possible to separate Vincent from Sien. The older gentleman voiced his opinion this way and that, saying that the behavior of his son was proof of his lunacy, and that he should get himself to a psychiatric hospital as quickly as possible. Vincent did, in fact, land in a hospital, but not in a psychiatric one, rather on a ward for the treatment of venereal diseases. He had become infected with gonorrhea, and the source was Sien, who was then in an advanced stage of her pregnancy. This fact was kept from the family, although Theo was informed of it. "I am in the hospital ... I have what they call the 'clap'," wrote van Gogh in a letter to his brother. (96) The Doctors assured him that his state was not serious, but that treatment would take a few weeks. I want to remind the reader that, whereas currently gonorrhea is treated with a single dose of antibiotics its treatment was neither easy nor totally effective at that time. It was long and painful, and complications were a daily affair, with one of the more common being narrowing of the urethra, causing difficulty in urination. Many patients suffered from gonococcal arthritis, mainly of the large joints (knees, ankles, or hips), which often ended in permanent crippling. Vincent was treated with urethral irrigations containing sulfates, which were among the most painful, as well as with tablets of quinine, doubtless for fever, which could have indicated that the infection was not limited to the urethra, but that he could have had what we would now call "disseminated gonococcal infection (DGI)." During his stay in the hospital, van Gogh was visited by friends, and also his father, who, finding out about all this, decided to reunite with his son. Sien also visited him, and, before long, found herself in the hospital, where she gave birth to a healthy son.

After returning home, Vincent felt completely well, but Sien's state of health, particularly her mental state, began to awaken many reservations in him. Their relationship worsened, while he feared that Sien wanted to return to her previous occupation. Additionally, the painter himself began to come to the conclusion that taking care of an ill woman suffering from alcoholism was beyond his strength, particularly as he discerned that his work as an artist-painter was suffering as a result. After almost a year of living together with Sien and her children, Vincent decided to move out, and for a short time rented an apartment in Drenthe – a locality situated near the border with Germany. He did not feel well there, and soon moved back with his parents living now in Nuenen in southern Holland. There, he also did not feel comfortable, as his parents were putting pressure on him to get some type of paying occupation that would allow him to continue his artistic interests. This state of frustration potentiated his feelings of guilt about abandoning a sick woman and her children, to whom the artist had become accustomed, had taken a liking to, and somehow yearned after.

More or less a year after breaking up with Sien, a new woman appeared along his path – Margaretha (Margot) Begemann, who was his parents' neighbor. Margot was 12 years older than Vincent, and she first became interested in him. She lived together with her mother and three sisters, among whom was a distinct rivalry, based on which among them could find a husband first. Margot often was in Vincent's company, going for walks in the area, and conversing on a variety of subjects. It appears that she expected some initiative on his part, as she was still a young woman, quite pretty, and with a warm character. Yet, it was said that it was she who first expressed her love for Vincent, and the young pair began to dream about plans for marriage. This idea did not appeal to either Vincent's family or to Margot's sisters or mother. Margot's family considered him unsuitable for a husband, that he was too young for her, and that he was encumbered by his recent relationship with a prostitute; additionally, he had no stable source of income, and was, generally speaking, an irresponsible person.

Vincent's family, for their part, felt that their son should first find a stable occupation, and only then think about marriage. In such a setting, Margot took strychnine during one of their walks ; this was a poison favored by suicidal women at the time. Vincent tried to save her by inducing vomiting, then took her to a physician, who gave the unsuccessful suicide an antidote. Margot recovered after a time, but there was no further talk about marriage.

The interpretation of Miss Bergemann's behavior, similarly to its being a motive for suicide, was not clear to the end. It was said that Margot could have been expecting a child by Vincent, something that he categorically denied, asserting that he had never slept with her. Another version said that the doctor who saved her confirmed the presence of opiates in her stomach, which could be evidence that the lady was treating herself "for nerves." Vincent knew something about the subject, as, when writing about Margot, he spoke of her "critical nerve disease ... her neuritis, her encephalitis, her melancholia, her religious mania." (97) He did not feel very well after these happenings, while his father wrote to Theo, "We have had difficult days again with Vincent ... He is very irritable and over-excited ... sad and unhappy ... Melancholy had led to drink and drinking led to violence ... There is a question whether we can go on living together." (97)

Nine months after the affair with Margot Bergemann, the senior Theodorus van Gogh died, the cause of his death most likely being a stroke. Despite the many things that differentiated them, Vincent was greatly moved by his father's death, and experienced a guilty conscience, the more so because his mother kept reminding him that it was his behavior and the problems he had caused that accounted for that death. She made up her own mind as to the psychological state of her son, and continued to maintain that the most appropriate place for him was a psychiatric hospital.

Due to the difficult atmosphere at home, Vincent moved away from his mother, and took up residence in the suburbs of Nuenen, from where it was closer to the locations where he was painting, where he could paint rustic landscapes and scenes of the lives of the villagers. It is from this period that came one of his better-known early paintings, titled *The Potato Eaters*, and representing the peasant de Groots family during their evening meal. One of the figures in this painting is a woman by the name of Stien (Gordina de Groot), sitting at the table wearing a wide, white bonnet (Fig. 5c.12).

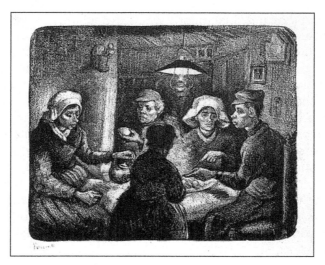

Figure 5c 12 Vincent van Gogh. The Potato Eaters, Lithograph (1885)

Stien often posed for Vincent, a fact that was noticed and appropriately interpreted by the neighbors and friends of the girl. One day, the local minister appeared before Vincent (some biographers say that there were two), and notified him that the local community was opposed to his actions, and that he should not expect any of the parishioners to pose for him any longer. Van Gogh was accused, although not immediately, of romancing his models, and this certainly referred to Stien, who as it soon became apparent, was expecting a child. After a while, it became clear that the father of the 17-year-old Stien's child was someone else, whereas the friendship of Vincent with Miss de Groot was of a purely platonic nature.

The unfavorable atmosphere that now prevailed in the area caused Vincent to leave Nuenen. In November 1885, van Gogh arrived in Antwerp with the intent of studying painting at the local Academy of Fine Arts (*Academie des Beaux Arts*). Very quickly, however, he got into a conflict with the director of this institution, whose teaching, in Vincent's opinion, was rather conservative. Vincent endured no longer than six weeks at the Academy, and later, on his own, started to study the works of the great masters, mainly Rubens, whose paintings he found in the local museum. Despite the fact that studying the works of the great masters was time-consuming, Vincent managed to find some free time, which he devoted to drinking absinthe and visits to the local bordellos, of which – Antwerp being a port town – there was no shortage. The consequences of such a lifestyle were not long in coming. Vincent became infected with syphilis, most likely at the end of 1885. Not all agree as to the diagnosis, some believing that the treatment used does not indicate lues. (97a) In none of the biographies available to me did I discover in which stage of the disease Vincent was when he went to a physician for the first time. I can only suppose that the first visit to Dr. Amadeus Gavenaille took place during an early stage of disease, that is, primary or secondary, in which the first skin manifestations of this lues appear, i.e. painless ulceration on the genitals in first-stage syphilis, or easily noticeable rashes on the skin or mucous membranes in secondary syphilis. Suggestions that van Gogh could have become infected in January 1882, I consider rather unlikely. They are based on the text of a letter that he sent to his brother, in which he wrote that he had headaches and a fever, and felt terrible. (98) This is not the first time that I have met suggestions considering the moment of infection with syphilis to be based on the fact of development of fever, headaches and malaise. The truth is that in the early stage of secondary syphilis, usually after several weeks from infection, these types of symptoms can appear, but they are rare and described as unusual, which indicates that they can also be found in many other diseases. In the course of my multiyear medical practice, I have taken care of many patients ill with syphilis, and only a small handful presented at the clinic with these types of ailments. The majority of patients presented themselves with skin changes, which appeared on the genitalia or the skin of the trunk or extremities, or on the face. Here, I have to add, however, that there is a certain group of patients in whom skin changes either do not appear or are not very noticeable, and who find out about their illness by accidental (or intentional) blood testing for lues. This form of the disease we call latent syphilis, and one can only detect it with the help of appropriate laboratory tests. In van Gogh's time, such tests were not available, while patients with latent syphilis learned of their disease only in its late stage, when signs and symptoms of *tabes dorsalis*, general paresis, or the skin manifestations of third-stage disease appeared. A large proportion of patients with latent syphilis were completely unaware of their lues, and people died happily from other causes, unaware of the fact that they had once become infected with the pale treponeme.

Returning to van Gogh, it appears that he noticed some symptoms that inclined him to a visit to Dr. Cavenaille, who was a venereologist. Vincent was treated in accord with principles then in force, namely with mercury or, perhaps, iodine preparations. Vincent was also admitted to the Stuyvenberg hospital in Antwerp, where, as he noted in his sketchbook, he took *bain de siege* (seated bath or hip bath).

Mercury preparations, he took orally and/or in the form of rubs, whereupon, as he informed his brother, he suffered from almost all possible side effects that this type of treatment produced. Vincent wrote of "greyish phlegm in [my] mouth, which was so filled with sores that [I] couldn't chew or swallow food." He had stomach problems, and felt very weak. His teeth loosened and began to fall out, and, just before leaving Antwerp, van Gogh had to pay a dentist 50 francs, a large sum for his means, to remove about a third of his dentition. (99) It was at this time (January 1885) that Vincent painted a skull with a cigarette in its teeth, which according to some biographers, was supposed to indicate that he felt like a dead man. Looking at this picture, I came to the conclusion that he probably did not have himself in mind, as the skull, from the teeth of which a cigarette sticks out, has a surprisingly full dentition, something that cannot be said of his own jaw – from which one-third of its teeth had been removed.

In March 1886, persuaded by Theo, Vincent moved to Paris. The capital of France was then the cultural capital of Europe, if not of the world, a city that attracted all kinds of intellectuals, artists, painters and scientists. The two brothers lived together, which, knowing Vincent's character and his frequent pretensions against his brother, boded no good. Vincent enrolled for a course in painting with Fernand Corman, where he met many fellow painters, whose works currently hang in the world's best museums. Among the students at Corman's school, were his later friends, Emile Bernard and Henri de Toulouse-Lautrec. (100) Besides these, van Gogh met many other painters there, including Paul Cezanne, Edgar Degas, Camille Pissaro, Claude Monet, Edouard Manet and Paul Gaugin. Many of them were just beginning their artistic careers, while some, such as Manet or Toulouse-Lautrec developed infections with syphilis similarly to Vincent, either before him or later. Vincent and Theo lived in Montmartre, an area inhabited mostly by artists, a place where there were many small cafes, nightclubs, cabarets and of course, bordellos. A certain Italian woman, Agostina Segatori, many years older than Vincent, and one with a past, also had a club there. There, van Gogh exhibited then popular works of Japanese art which he had collected, as well as some of his own paintings. He arranged with Signora Segatori that, for the opportunity of boarding at her club (named The Tambourine) and an option to exhibit his own works there, he would pay her with paintings. Vincent not only ate there, but also may have slept with the proprietress. The arrangement functioned up to the moment when the owner declared bankruptcy, and closed the restaurant. As it turned out later, Agostina was mixed up with some clandestine activities. When they broke up, van Gogh had to break in to the already-closed club in order to reclaim the things he had left there. However, during this time, Vincent painted a picture of a naked woman with skin changes resembling syphilis. For many years it was considered to be a representation of Signora Segatori, but recent examinations have proved that the painting is of an unknown prostitute whom Vincent met on the street. (101) This painting is now the property of the Barnes Foundation in Philadelphia.

In one of his letters to Theo from summer, 1887, Vincent wrote about Agostina warmly, sympathizing with her about her bad state of health caused, presumably, by a recent miscarriage or abortion. Vincent was very forbearing about it, suggesting that he understood why she had behaved that way, although this could have had more to do with the fact that the woman did not know who the father of her child was. One also cannot exclude the possibility that Segatori herself could have been ill with syphilis, or that the child's father (could it have been Vincent?) had recently had the disease, which, in van Gogh's opinion could have justified the performance of an abortion. (102) These are only speculations, as the content of this letter can be interpreted in many different ways.

Residing together with Theo led to frequent conflicts, and the brothers, while having enough of each other, also were somehow needed by one another. Theo helped his brother financially (and not that alone) during the whole time, while Vincent tried to support his brother in his difficult moments. Both brothers had untidy sexual lives, and both took advantage of paid sex. At one point, Theo fell in love, and went through a difficult time when his offer of marriage was rejected. His chosen was Johanna (Jo) Bonger, the sister of Andries Bonger of the Goupil firm, at which both Theo and Andries worked. During the time when they were lodging together, the brothers mutually confessed the secret hidden for a time, that they were both ill with syphilis. As some biographers suggest, both consulted the prominent Parisian doctors, Louis Rivet and David Gruby, whose practice included, among other things, the treatment of those ill with lues. Theo became infected with syphilis from an unknown prostitute, similarly to Vincent, but the former's disease ran a difficult course and it was that, unlike in Vincent's case, which led to Theo's death.

The stay in Paris turned out to be the turning point in van Gogh's painting career. Thanks to Theo, who dealt in works of art, Vincent landed in an environment of artists rebelling against then-current modes in painting, and belonged to the so-called impressionists or neoimpressionists, who exhibited their works in the "Salon of Independents." Vincent changed his former customs regarding color, and his paintings became brighter. He was one of the first to begin using the technique of *pointilism*, otherwise known as *divisionism* or *chromoluminarism*, the originator of which was Seurat. This was a technique in which a multitude of small colored dots is applied to the canvas, which when seen from distance, creates an optical blend of hues. The style stresses the value of complementary colors – including blue and orange – to form vibrant contrasts that are enhanced when juxtaposed. It was during this part of a two year stay in Paris that van Gogh completed close to two hundred paintings among which are found many masterpieces.

By the end of the year, the brothers had enough of each other to such an extent that Vincent moved away from Theo, and went to live in Asnieres, which was then a suburb of Paris. At the end of November 1887, Theo and Vincent met Paul Gaugin. Gaugin had worked on the building of the Panama Canal for a time, then lived on Martinique, before arriving in Paris to nurse his debilitated health. Gaugin appealed to van Gogh, who wrote about him that he had "savage instincts" and that for Gaugin, blood and sex prevailed over ambition. He added, "Gauguin interested him very much as a man – very much." (103) Vincent praised Gaugin saying that he would like there to be more men like he, "men with the hands and stomachs of women ... Men with more natural tastes – more loving and more charitable temperaments – than the decadent dandies of the Parisian boulevards have." (103) Tired of his almost two-year stay in Paris, van Gogh decided to leave for the south of France, where, as he put it, "There is more light and space, and more clean air to breathe." At the time, he had problems with his health, and coughed a lot, something that was probably connected not only with the smoked-up atmosphere of Paris, but also with his own excessive smoking of tobacco. Yet another reason for leaving the big city was the new idea that took possession of him, that of organizing a Utopian, idyllic colony for painters, who could create their works far away from the city noises and in peace.

After arriving in Arles, Vincent became friends with the Danish painter, Christian Mourier-Petersen, and awaited the arrival of Gaugin, whom Theo invited to his house. It was this fact that gave rise to the oft-repeated gossip that something other than friendship connected Vincent to Gaugin, something more than simple friendship and interest in

385

painting. His stated interest in Gaugin "as a man," the description of his visit to the bedroom of the sleeping Gaugin, and his fury and disapproval when the latter decided to leave Arles, are supposed to attest to homosexual tendencies in van Gogh. Two paintings that appeared in this period are also used by some to support this idea. One represents Vincent's chair, on which lie a pipe and a bag of tobacco, and is supposed clearly to manifest such a need and Vincent's masculinity, while the other, also of a chair, but one belonging to Gaugin, and taken to be more affected, is plush, with a divan, suggesting a woman's boudoir to some, and is supposed to attest to effeminate tendencies of the latter. (104) The entire concept concerning putative homosexual tendencies of the two gentlemen appears to me to be too stretched and rather nonsensical, as both were unable to do without women, being frequent guests at local bordellos, and both were in love – if one can describe it so – with the same young prostitute from Arles.

Mutual work and being under the same roof augured nothing good for two people with strong personalities and explosive characters. Daily quarrels and discussions on artistic matters, together with the consumption of large amounts of absinthe, were transformed into frequent fights between the two. After one such, just before Christmas, an agitated Gaugin left the house. In his footsteps followed Vincent, with a razor in hand, but when Gaugin, ready for an attack, took a defensive posture, Vincent backed away and returned into the house. Gaugin spent that night in a hotel; Vincent, on the other hand, in a fit of rage, cut off a part of his own ear, after which he made for a bordello, where he handed it to a prostitute, favored by both men, named Rachel. After this event, van Gogh found himself in a hospital in Arles, where, after a few days, he had another attack of delirium, at which time he had to be dressed in a straitjacket and placed into isolation. Given the alarm by Gaugin, Theo traveled to Arles and spoke with his physicians. He could not stay very long as he was on his way to Holland in order to pay a visit to the family of Jo, who, in the end, agreed to become his wife. In fact, he was no longer needed, as the mental state of the patient began to improve, and already by the end of the year, Vincent had calmed down, and began to paint once again

In March, Theo married Jo Bonger, which upset Vincent a bit, and he began to worry about the stipend paid him regularly by his brother. Here, I have to explain that, for a long time, Theo had been sending Vincent money for his upkeep, and the costs associated with his painting, in exchange for the pictures that Vincent executed, which both hoped would begin to sell. Van Gogh's concerns regarding further financing by his brother became unnecessary, as his new sister-in-law turned out to be a person friendly to the artist and an admirer of his talents, and had nothing against adding to the financing of his creativity.

Vincent's mental state gradually improved, although the painter was aware that he was not entirely well. In April, he wrote to his sister:

As for myself, I am going to an asylum in St. Remy, not far from here, for three months. I have had, in all, four great crises, during which I didn't in the least know what I said, what I wanted and what I did. Not taking into account that I previously had three fainting fits without any plausible reason, and without retaining the slightest remembrance of what I felt. (105)

The content of this letter testifies that Vincent had improved from the physical standpoint, but was aware that his mental state did not yet permit him to return home; he saw that his place, at least for some time, was in a psychiatric hospital. It is significant that he made such a decision knowing that the local community was expressing its antipathy toward him in an ever-clearer manner, considering van Gogh to be a person dangerous to his surroundings. After four months had passed since his first attack of delirium, Vincent was accepted to the ward of the psychiatric hospital in St. Remy, situated less than 15 minutes from Arles. On the information card, a physician from the hospital in Arles wrote:

> I, the undersigned medical superintendent of the hospital in Arles, declare that six months ago Vincent van Gogh, 36 years old, was affected by complete mania and general mental derangement. At the time he cut off his ear. At this moment his state of mind is much improved, but he nevertheless thought it useful to have himself treated in a mental institution. (106)

In the hospital in St. Remy, Vincent had at his disposal two rooms, of which one was a bedroom, and the other served as a studio. Almost from the first day of his stay in his new place, Vincent threw himself into a whirlwind of work, asserting that it was the best medicine for the state of his nerves. He was not mistaken, although the therapies ordered for him by the local physicians would be difficult to call treatment, from today's point of view. The institution specialized in hydrotherapy, and Vincent underwent frequent baths overseen by nuns. During recurring attacks of delirium, he was placed into special containers of water, such that only his head protruded and was doused with water cold as ice – which, as was explained, was to evoke a thermal shock that was supposed to act therapeutically. As the patient calmed down, warm water was added gradually, with the aim of consolidating that state. Baths were given daily, with the belief that they had a prophylactic effect. Endeavors such as this, to tell the truth, neither helped not hurt the patients; their real advantage was that they were subjected to a good washing, something that could not be said about patients in other medical institutions!

During his stay in St. Remy, Vincent was treated very well, equally so by the hospital personnel and the director of this institution, as the latter considered van Gogh's case unusual; other than the attacks of delirium, the patient gave the impression of being an intelligent person. (107) During times of remission, Vincent was allowed to move about the hospital freely, and even to leave the grounds, although with a male guardian. He could then paint the area of St. Remy, whereas when he felt worse and was in isolation, he painted only what he saw from the windows of his room. It was during this period that a series of his masterpiece paintings appeared – which the painter had hopes of selling, in order to cover the costs of his hospital stay. Unfortunately, despite help on the part of his painter friends, and attempts by his brother, he did not succeed in turning any of his paintings into cash.

In July 1889 Vincent received a letter from his sister-in-law (Jo), informing him that she was expecting a child. This news electrified him, as he liked her very much, and could not wait until he became an uncle. The approaching arrival date was anticipated with great joy, but also with great anxiety. Those in the know remembered the baby's father's syphilis, for which he had had treatment not too long before. Complications in pregnancy caused by syphilis occurred very frequently then, while stillbirths and premature births with congenital syphilis were not rarities. Theo's general state of health still wasn't the best: he would have strange episodes of paralysis of the facial muscles, during which his face would swell; he had coughing fits, and frequent mood changes were noticeable. (108)

Vincent also was ill, and this period (September, 1889) is considered the worst during his entire stay in St. Remy. The painter experienced periods of deep depression, and had several attacks of lunacy and suicide attempts. On one occasion, Vincent ate some paint and drank methylated spirits, which he found in the lamp that stood in his room.

During his hallucinations, he imagined that someone wanted to kill him, and did not want to leave his room, even in the company of his guardian. It took a long time for him to recover, and even when he had again started to paint, remained mistrustful of his surroundings. During this period, he painted a series of pictures of religious content, such as *Pieta* and *The Raising of Lazarus*. (109, 110)

On the last day of January, 1890 Jo gave birth to a healthy boy, to whom was also given the name, Vincent. Van Gogh was delighted and could not wait for the moment when he would see his namesake and godson with his own eyes. The state of his health improved so much that he started to plan a trip to Paris. At about this time, he received a letter from Jo, in which she wrote about her little son, and also informed him that she had had an opportunity to admire his paintings exhibited in the "Salon of Independents." This news built up Vincent's faith in himself, and confirmed his conviction that his mental state was so good that he could leave the hospital and visit his brother. Jo, likewise, encouraged him in this, although Theo did not share his wife's opinion, remembering the problems he had had with Vincent during their mutual residence under one roof. He did, in fact, agree to invite Vincent to his home, but for a limited period of time, and while actually trying to persuade him to move closer to Paris to live together with another painter, Camille Pissaro in Auvers-sur-Oise. Vincent appeared in Paris in a short while, and after a stay of several days at his brother's, moved to Auvers, although not with Camille Pissaro; rather, he moved close to the home of Dr. Gachet, a physician who occupied himself with homeopathy and the treatment of mental illness. (111)

Doctor Gachet was a widower, had a 15-year-old son and a 20-year-old daughter, who would play a certain role in Vincent's life. It appears that both the doctor and the painter were quite satisfied with their neighborhood. Vincent had a specialist at hand who could help him when he felt an attack of his illness approaching, while Dr. Gachet, a lover of art and collector of artwork, met a new painter whose work he appreciated, and on whose advice he could count. Dr. Gachet was a painter himself, but, first of all, did engraving. He moved in a circle of artists, was not a stranger in the artistic community, and his frequent patients were Renoir, Cezanne and Pissaro. Vincent occupied himself in getting started with painting, again, and often took advantage of Dr. Gachet's garden, in which Marguerite, the doctors' daughter, took care of the flowers.

Dr. Gachet himself lived to see several portraits of him done by van Gogh. In one of these, he is sitting on a chair, propped up on his elbow on a table, on which, as appropriate to a physician, is found a plant called the "foxglove," from which is obtained digitalis, an alkaloid used in medicine until the present, mainly for diseases of the heart (Fig.5c.13). This painting was sold at auction in 1989, one hundred years after it was painted, for the sum of $80 million.

Van Gogh painted not only the doctor and his garden, but also his daughter, the 20-year-old Marguerite. The young woman was of middling beauty, but was able to play the piano, facts that Vincent immortalized on canvas. There are those who claim that this acquaintance with Marguerite may have been the beginning of the end for the artist. Supposedly, Gachet's housekeeper (actually the mother of his son) informed her employer that something more than just a friendly relationship linked Vincent and Marguerite; this is supposed to have induced the doctor to declare that he did not wish to see Vincent in the role of his daughter's paramour. (112) The gentlemen doubtless had a man-to-man talk, after which Vincent felt insulted and denigrated by a man whom he had until then considered a friend. Apparently, after this incident, van Gogh's mental state deteriorated dramatically, and he is said to have visited the doctor's house uninvited, creating rows and threatening his family. Finally, on July 27th in the afternoon, Vincent shot himself with a pistol, and died the next day. It is unclear to what extent Dr. Gachet's reaction to van Gogh's romance with his daughter caused the latter's death, and to what extent it was a consequence of the painter's illness. The fact is that, according to the reaction of a witness to the incident, when Dr. Gachet was called to the mortally wounded artist, Vincent did not want to look at nor speak with him. (113)

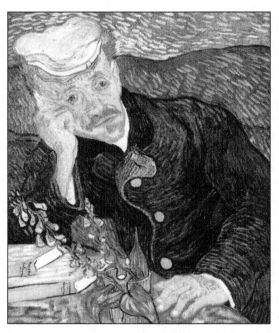

Figure 5c 13 Dr. Paul Gachet paited by Vincent van Gogh (1890)

Almost from the day of Vincent van Gogh's death, his biographers have wondered about the cause of his illness, and then, what the cause of his death was at the young age of thirty-seven. One of the hypotheses speaks of syphilis, but in my opinion, this disease should rather be found at the *end* of a long list of illnesses which might have destroyed the painter's health. We know that van Gogh did suffer from syphilis; he was treated for it, not only in Antwerp, but also later, when, together with his brother, he visited Parisian physicians who took care of luetic patients. In no biographies available to me, in which are described the psychiatric signs or symptoms suffered by van Gogh, did I find signs of late syphilis of the nervous system, that is, of general paresis or *tabes dorsalis*. In the case of general paresis (GP), an increasing mental dulling of the patient appears as a dominant sign, whereas Vincent was blessed with high intelligence until the end. In *tabes dorsalis*, neurologic signs – impairment of movement coordination, ataxia, paresthesias, shooting pains, gastric crises, urinary bladder dysfunction, fecal incontinence, and decreased sexual potency – dominate. Aside from this last problem, which could have had a completely different cause, none of the above signs or symptoms occurred in van Gogh.

One sign, which can suggest syphilis of the nervous system is that of epileptoidal attacks (often described by physicians as "epileptic attacks"), which can be a sign of meningeal or meningo-vascular syphilis, but in these forms there are also other signs and symptoms – which the painter did not have. It should be remembered that Vincent van Gogh was unbalanced mentally from early youth, something that his parents had already observed. In other members of the van Gogh family, and particularly in his youngest brother, Cor, signs of depression occurred at an early age. Cor later went to South Africa, and there, ten years after Vincent's death, committed suicide himself. Vincent's sister, Wilhelmina (Wil), with whom the painter corresponded regularly, began to show signs of mental illness not long after his death, and spent the last forty years of her life in a psychiatric hospital in Holland. She made two suicide attempts during this time: one, during which she tried to drown herself by immersing her head in the toilet, and the second, when she tried to drive a crochet hook into her head.

Two of van Gogh's mother's brothers suffered from mental illness, while his mother, herself, had periods episodes of protracted depression.

The most likely diagnosis, although not encompassing all of the signs appearing in the artist, would appear to be bipolar disorder, (manic- depressive psychosis), in which patients in manic or submanic states can create wonderful works, while in the depressed state, they undertake suicide attempts. To the general deterioration of the painter 's health – who, by nature, was as strong as an ox – contributed his poor and irregular nutrition, overwork, abuse of alcohol (mainly absinthe), and maybe even contact with oil paints, of which many contained lead. It is said that Vincent had a habit of licking the tip of the brush that he used for painting, but this was doubtless not his main problem.

Just as Vincent almost certainly did not die as a result of lues, so his brother certainly did become its victim (Fig.5c.14). Theo experienced his brother's death with great emotion, and one can be tempted to state that the stress associated with the loss of a person so near to him exacerbated his own health problems, both physical and mental. Signs and symptoms that gradually began to appear had the characteristics of *taboparesis*, attesting to the "taking over" of his central nervous system by syphilis. In contrast to Vincent, who had mental problems almost exclusively, in Theo, in addition to mental symptoms, there appeared neurologic problems. After a row at the firm, in which he had worked for many years, Theo was hospitalized in a private hospital in Passy, while taking care of him was the doctor already mentioned by me in accounts of other famous, French syphilitics, Antoine Blanche. In addition to attacks of delirium and periods of lunacy, during which he would tear his clothes and throw furniture, van Gogh was calmed by the use of chloroform. Theo also had neurologic disturbances: he could not walk, had trouble speaking, was incontinent of both urine and feces. During those difficult days, Jo Bonger visited him almost daily. Adoring her husband, she did not want to accept a diagnosis of syphilis, and questioned the methods of treatment. She talked herself into believing that her husband was having a nervous breakdown as a result of the loss of his beloved brother, and that his troubles would pass with time. She succeeded in transferring her husband from the hospital in Passy to the Willem Arnstz Clinic in Holland, not far from Utrecht. Due to his bad mental state, Theo undertook the train trip in a straitjacket, in the company of his wife and two male nurses. As Steven Naifeh and Gregory White-Smith wrote:

They arrived at the asylum on November 18th in a wretched state: bubbling in a mash of languages, disheveled, incontinent, and barely able to walk. He could not answer questions about who he was, where he was or what day it was." (114) Later accounts of his worsening state of health appear, as well as signs typical of *tabo-paralysis*, known to readers from descriptions of this form of lues in other syphilitics discussed earlier. For the next month Theo lived the same life of confinement in Utrecht that his brother had lived in Arles and Saint-Remy. Long days of delusions, delirium and drug-induced stupor were followed by long nights of restless, haunted sleep, or no sleep at all. He sat for hours in his padded cell, conducting fevered, incoherent monologues – arguments with himself – in multiple languages. His mood swung wildly from "cheerful and boisterous" to "dull and drowsy," according to the asylum reporters. At other times, a sudden fury possessed his delicate body. He shook with tremors from head to toe in paralytic attacks indistinguishable from epileptic seizures. The look of his eyes, the timbre of his voice, his whole character, changed as if commandeered by some other entity. In these transformations, the cultured art dealer of refined sensibilities clawed at his underclothes, ripped up the sheets on his bed, and tore the straw from his mattress. The warden had to wrestle him into a straitjacket to [calm] him." "Speech became increasingly difficult, as did walking, as the tremors invaded every part of his body. The muscles of his face twitched uncontrollably. He had trouble swallowing. Eating was a torment, and he vomited up most of what he ate. His bowels malfunctioned. Urination was painful, and attempts to insert a catheter failed. He couldn't feed himself or dress himself. After he was found asleep in the bath, he wasn't allowed to bathe himself for fear he might accidently drown. He had to be placed in a covered, padded "crib" at night so he could not harm himself. (114)

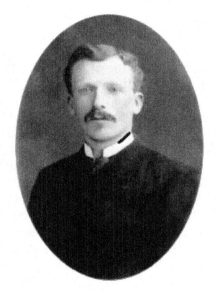

Figure 5c 14 Theo van Gogh (1888)

Theo van Gogh died on the 24th or 25th of January, 1891, half a year from the date of Vincent van Gogh's death. By today's criteria, this above, rather lengthy, yet detailed account of Theo's last days corresponds well to a diagnosis of general paresis, with elements of *tabes dorsalis*.

Differing courses, as also different clinical pictures of the disease in the two brothers illustrate how much we learned just in the tw^{entieth} century, including from the infamous experiments in Tuskegee and in Oslo. The results of those experiments clearly showed that the course of syphilis in different people, even brothers whose genomic structure overlaps by 50% can be different, and depends on many still unknown factors. Some, syphilis killed in a relatively short time, others lived with the disease for a long time, often dying from other, unrelated causes.

HENRI de TOULOUSE-LAUTREC (1864-1901)

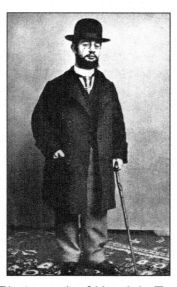

Figure 5c 15 Photograph of Henri de Toulouse Lautrec

The reader of this book will readily notice that the majority of the well-known artists described by me became *heroes* of this book only because they frequented bordellos or became infected with syphilis from a street prostitute. Henri de Toulouse-Lautrec, a French painter from the end of the nineteenth century, who became infected with lues from a Parisian prostitute by the charming name, Rosa La Rouge, belongs among them.

That venereal diseases are connected with prostitution, every adult person knows, and it is difficult to understand why intelligent and well-educated people, who had to have recognized the imminent danger to themselves, were unable to overcome the temptations of easy, paid sex. I will remind the reader, however, that we are speaking of the end of the nineteenth century, when the prevalence of syphilis was unusually high, while its diagnosis (detection) was unusually low. The disease was practically incurable, and ended in death in every third infected person – a death, often with great suffering, which fanciers of easy sex could observe in members of their own families, and among friends, acquaintances and neighbors. Taking advantage of the services of prostitutes reminds one of Russian roulette, in which participants in the game (should) know that every few bullets in the pistol are real, and that one of the players can lose his life.

Toulouse-Lautrec was one of those fanciers of sex for money. It can be said that he even surpassed his friends in that respect, inasmuch as he not only frequented bordellos, but went a step further and took up residence in one; he treated the institution as a boarding house in which he not only slept and took his meals, but also worked there, painting scenes of the everyday life of his surroundings, of the women working there, and of their visiting clients. Among the prostitutes he had more-and less-favorite models, which he presented in a variety of poses, not excluding a painting of prostitutes getting ready for a medical examination, most probably by a venereologist . Many paintings by Lautrec deal with pornography, presenting without restraint erotic scenes between men and women, and even exclusively between women. In addition to such erotic scenes, among his works are paintings representing scenes from the daily life of such institutions, full of appreciation and sometimes sympathy for the women employed there.

Henri de Toulouse-Lautrec was physically handicapped, but this did not decrease his intelligence or talent in any way. He had a specific sense of humor, while his behavior was often – let us call it eccentric, for want of another term. Lautrec abused alcohol, and this, combined with syphilis, led to his mental degradation; the artist died very young, not attaining thirty-seven years of age.

Henri was born November 24th, 1864; his parents were Countess Adele and her husband, Alfonse de Toulouse-Lautrec-Monfa. The Count and Countess were the owners of an expansive estate, which included the castle Malrome, near Alba, where Henri, their firstborn son came into the world. The painter's parents were first cousins, as their mothers were sisters. (115) This doubtless influenced the fate of their first child, as Henri was the victim of a genetic disease, which had appeared periodically in the family. Its first signs were manifested at age thirteen, when Henri broke his right femur, and a year later, his left. Both fractures healed poorly, and shortly it became apparent that the boy was a victim of a disease that today's specialists called *pyknodysostosis*, or Toulouse-Lautrec syndrome. Among other causes of this type of crippling disease are listed derangements due to *osteoporosis*, *achondroplasia* and *osteogenesis imperfecta*. The genes responsible for the disease had circulated in the family for some time, as at least three close cousins of Henry suffered from dwarfism or congenital skeletal defects; one was wheelchair-bound all his life, because he could not, for some reason, move around on his own legs. (116)

After breaking both femurs, Henri stopped growing, or, speaking precisely, his legs stopped growing, although he retained normal development of other parts of his body. In many commentaries, it is stressed that nature compensated him for the lack of development of his lower extremities in a way, by endowing him with abnormally large genitals. (117, 118)

Not being able to participate, as a result of the disease, in the typical amusements of boys of his age, young Lautrec began to draw; his first works showed that he had a lot of talent, probably inherited from his forebears, as his grandfather, father, and also an uncle were talented draftsmen. As long as we are speaking about the influence of genetics on the painter's life, maybe I should add that Henri inherited a tendency to eccentric behavior from his father, which tendency became readily apparent in his later life.

Henri's father, occupied with hunts, travel, and other activities that can be called passing time pleasantly, paid little attention to his ill son, leaving him to the boy's mother, who took care of him practically his entire life. It was she who helped her son while he was studying in Nice, and it was she, who, at the suggestion of a painter friend, travelled with him to Paris, where Toulouse-Lautrec began to study painting, first under the direction of the famous Leon Bonnat, then, afterwards, at the artist school of Fernand Cormon, where many well-known artists of this period studied.

One of Toulouse-Lautrec's friends from this school was Louis Aquetin, a handsome and well-built man, who enjoyed favor with women. Seeing his successes, Henry developed a complex, which he tried to overcome with intensive work at the easel. With some help in this regard, along came another painter friend, who persuaded one of the models to "take care" of Lautrec. This was Marie Charlet, a girl of 16-17 years, who "ate at more than one restaurant," and about whom much could be said, but not that she was an innocent girl. It was even said that she was a nymphomaniac, and slept with anyone who might be a novelty in sexual matters. And here, one can say, Henri found his own, or, as Henry Perruchot wrote:

> Marie Charlet found piquancy in the adventure; Lautrec's monstrous constitution filled her with delight. She went about boasting happily of the dwarf's qualities as a lover and nicknamed him *'Portmanteau.'* This publicity attracted the attentions of the abnormal and of nymphomaniacs to Lautrec. With Marie Charlet he felt disgust and contempt. Was this love? Was this what women were like? Or, at least, the sort of love and the type of woman he was destined to have? But he had no illusions. The vicious loves were but a new aspect of his wretched life. He was afraid of exciting pity; he inspired sadism. He could do nothing but acquiesce. 'One must know how to bear oneself' he said sometimes. Besides, Marie Charlet had revealed to him the strength of his instincts, which once freed, now no longer knew restraint. (119)

In the arms of Marie Charlet, Henri confirmed to himself that, beyond art, there were other pleasures in life, which he did not intend to forego. He moved out from his mother's home, and moved in with friends in Montmartre, then a new, but already fashionable district in Paris. This was the place where a variety of artists gathered: painters, sculptors, poets and writers, philosophers and students, but also every manner of crank, model and prostitute. At this time, also, there began to appear in Montmartre new coffee houses and bars, dancing halls, little theaters and cabarets. The atmosphere of the new district enchanted the new painter, who tried to take part in every attraction it offered. Although he continued to study at Cormon's, he distanced himself more and more from the master's advice, developing his own style. He constantly needed new models, and so chanced upon his next model-mistress, Marie-Clementine Valadon. Mademoiselle Valadon was a young woman of unique beauty, who also occupied herself with art (she drew well), of which not many people were aware. She was brought up only by her mother, who was unable to determine whom the child's father was. Marie, from an early age, earned her living as a seamstress, a nurse assistant, a waitress and a seller of vegetables at a nearby market. As a 15-year-old girl, she had tried a circus career, but after an accident she had during one of the rehearsals, had to resign from that profession. Lautrec was not the first painter for whom she had sat, while among masters of the paintbrush who had something to do with her, was Pierre-Auguste Renoir, who placed her in several of his paintings. Even as a model, Marie bore a son, to the fatherhood of whom no one wanted to admit. Among the candidates to the title were named a popular cabaret singer, a certain aristocrat-painter, and also the subsequenty famous, Spanish painter, Miguel Utrillo, who eventually (after eight years) decided to acknowledge the boy as his son. One cannot be too surprised at the hesitation of these gentlemen, as there was not yet any genetic testing then, whereas in today's times, DNA testing can prove or exclude paternity with virtually 100% accuracy. In the late 1800s, one of the criteria taken into consideration was the physical similarity of a son to his father, but only after attainment of a certain age by the child. In Utrillo's case, another criterion confirming fatherhood might also be talent, as both Maurice Utrillo and his father, Miguel, were famous painters. Marie had no objections when it came to sleeping with Lautrec, compensating the painter's physical frailty by other merits with which nature had reportedly endowed him. Their relationship went through various trials, as neither Lautrec nor Marie had vowed fidelity to one other. Henri "painted" other models besides Marie during this time, while Marie, who behaved very independently, working with or having sex with him only when she, herself, wanted to. She did not react when Lautrec organized group meetings plentifully seasoned with alcohol, and willingly took part in rather specific jokes or amusing situations organized by the painter. One evening, Lautrec invited Marie to his flat for supper, and decided to make fun of his housekeeper, who had the reputation of being a woman of principle. He asked Marie to take off her clothes and to sit at the table only in her shoes and stockings, then burst out laughing at his maid, when she acted as though she didn't notice anything. The next day, the indignant housekeeper complained to Bourges, a friend and co-boarder of the painter, saying, "Monsieur Henri had insulted her." (120) Bourges, who was a student of medicine and rented the flat together with Lautrec, tried to explain to her, seriously, that, after all, nothing wrong had happened, as, during the aforementioned supper, Lautrec had had his own clothes on, and that, being a woman, the sight of a female body should not shock her. The relationship between Lautrec and Marie lasted some time, all the way to the moment when, for unclear reasons, Marie announced that she intended to kill herself. When it turned out that the entire story had been hatched, together with Marie's mother, with the aim, probably, of taking advantage of the painter, he immediately broke off with her.

Despite the fact that evenings and nights spent with friends in theatres, cabarets and bars took a lot of time and energy, Lautrec found time for painting. He painted scenes from places that he frequented, as well as the people he met there, beginning with famous artists appearing on the stage, such as, for example, Aristide-Bruant – the owner of the *Mirliton Cabaret*, creator of then-current hits – and ending with prostitutes, who took refuge there from raids arranged by the "morals police." One of these latter "girls" particularly caught his eye, probably as a result of the fiery redness of her hair; she soon became the painter's favorite model, and he painted her portrait several times. When one of these portraits was hung on the wall of the *Mirliton Cabaret*, someone, who knew the woman well, tried to warn the artist, saying that too much intimacy with this "model" could end with a serious illness, Lautrec's reaction was a smile and a reply that, unfortunately, the warning came too late. This was 1888; Henri Lautrec was 24, and the model was *Rosa la Rouge* (Fig.5c.16).

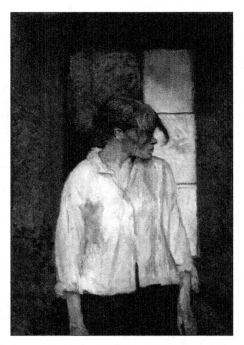

Figure 5c 16 Rosa la Rouge (1866-1887) painted by Henri de Toulouse-Lautrec

We do not know with what, or for how long Lautrec underwent treatment. Medications used at that time, mainly mercury preparations and iodine, were noted for their poor efficacy, while those ill often interrupted or stopped treatment as a result of the unpleasant side effects. Henri Perruchot wrote, "In obedience to Bourges, who looked after him, the painter submitted himself to energetic measures. He could be [in] no doubt that the life he led was much unsuited to his condition." Bourges constantly warned him that "More than anyone, the syphilitic requires a sufficient numbers of hours of sleep ... he cannot overwork his intelligence and abuse his mental activity with impunity." (121)

After the treatment, which probably took place during the second half of 1888, Lautrec left Paris, and spent three winter months in Villier-sur-Morin in the company of a friendly married couple, the Greniers. Bourges inclined him toward this, after noting signs of depression in the artist, caused by the awareness that the disease that he had contracted would accompany him until his death. Another cause of depression could have been the secondary effects of treatment, which did not belong among the most pleasant. I am convinced that Bourges used all therapeutic methods available then, as he was personally interested in syphilis, as witnessed by the publication of a scientific work, entitled, *"L'Hygiene du Syphlitique."* (121) We also have evidence that Lautrec himself was aware of the seriousness of the situation, as evidenced by the comment he is said to have made upon seeing the painting by Andre Gill, entitled *Le Fou* (The Fool). This painting shows a man in a straitjacket with the expression of a madman with eyes wide open and fearful. After seeing this painting, Lautrec is said to have told a friend, "That's what's in store for me." (122)

In the first weeks of 1889, Lautrec returned to Paris. Very clearly, he felt better, as he quickly returned to his former lifestyle, i.e. having good time, intensive work, and large quantities of alcohol. He painted women from shady society *(demimonde)*, including Rosa la Rouge, as though he wanted to show that he was not displeased with her; painted a known actor from the *Comedie Francaise;* and also decorated the hall in one of the cabarets with very original painting. In autumn, he participated in the "Salon of

Independents," where he exhibited three of his works, while, at the beginning of November, he took part in the famous event that was the opening of a new dance hall in the Montmartre district called the *Moulin Rouge*. From then on, this name would be inextricably associated with the Toulouse-Lautrec, who became as though an icon of this cabaret. Fascinated by its atmosphere, Lautrec was its permanent guest, almost from the opening. Every evening, he had a table that awaited him there, and also a cluster of loyal friends and unlimited access to alcohol. In just a short while, several of his paintings appeared on the walls of the cabaret, among them *L'Ecuyere du cirque Fernando* and *La Dance au Moulin Rouge*.

Frequenters of the Moulin Rouge, when describing scenes that remained in their memories would remember a small person, consuming drinks, sparkling with wit, surrounded by a gathering of friends and well-wishers, who appeared to be an inseparable attraction of the place. Lautrec in the Moulin Rouge, not only had a good time there, but derived inspiration and material for his work as well. Scenes from the Moulin Rouge constitute a significant portion of paintings that came from his brush during this period. (123) The greatest stars of the cabaret competed for his friendship. Among these were Louise Weber, better known as *La Goulue,* and Jane Avril – her real name was Jean Beadon – for whom Lautrec created posters; he also painted several canvases, for which they willingly posed. (124)

La Goulue, who had been on stage long before the appearance of the Moulin Rouge, acquired her nickname, "The Glutton," from her excesses (Fig.5c.17)

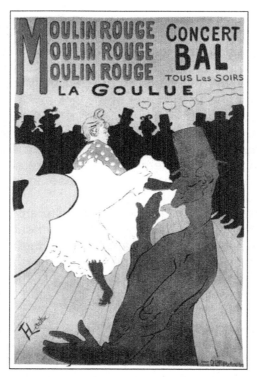

Figure 5c 17 Moulin Rouge: La Goulue (1891) by Henri de Toulouse-Lautrec

She was so greedy that, on occasion, she would even empty the dregs of the glasses on the tables. La Goulue was a foul-mouthed guttersnipe, whose conversation was a stream of obscenities; but as soon as she started to dance, to perform one those improvisations that were her secret, she was transfigured. She was not merely a dancer; she was the dance itself. (125)

La Goulue found herself in many of Lautrec's paintings, including the one called *The Quadrille*, in which, together with another dancer, she demonstrated the "High Kick," so typical of her. This dance figure was appealing mostly to the male component of the audience, due to the exposition of intimate undergarments, which were seen under her upflung dress. I will remind the reader that even until not long ago, showing a bare leg to the level of the ankle was considered an act of uncommon bravery, while what La Goulue showed was a signal of ebullient sexuality. The higher the dancer raised her legs, the more popular she was. La Goulue and, later, Jane Avril were masters at this, and were able to knock the top hats off the men ogling them; these, in turn, hid their arousal with difficulty.

Jane Avril was of a somewhat different style than LaGoulue. Thin and tall, and of with movements filled with grace, she was as though an antithesis to the forceful and not rarely vulgar La Goulue. Jane's mother was a courtesan while her father was an unknown foreigner, supposedly an aristocrat, as sometimes rumored, and creating, by this means, a nimbus of mystery around her. Highly paid and valued by the cabaret's owners, Jane was the public's favorite for a long time. It was she, next to LaGoulue, who popularized the CanCan dance, fashionable since that time, which she presented, among others, in guest appearances in London. The character of Jane Avril has appeared in at least two films about *Le Moulin Rouge*. One comes to us from the 1950s the person of Jane being incarnated by Zsa Zsa Gabor; the other from 2001, in which the role of the dancer was played by Nicole Kidman.

Toulouse-Lautrec, also an admirer of her talent, made a poster, showing the dancer with a leg raised high, most probably dancing the CanCan. In addition, he executed a series of paintings showing Jane in various situations: dancing on the stage, leaving the cabaret, putting on gloves, wrapped up in an ample coat with her hands in its pockets, always remembering to portray her facial expression as melancholic i.e. that of a person absorbed in her own thoughts. Jane did not hide her sympathy for the painter, and never refused him when he asked her to sit for him. They were often seen together in restaurants in Montmartre, where they would meet for coffee or lunch.

Dancing was not the only thing seen at the Moulin Rouge. Well-known singers and musical ensembles, circus acts and illusionists (magicians), and even an "artist" whose shows depended on making sounds, in various tones, from the rear end of his body – which would appear to show that the owners of the cabaret tried to meet the tastes of the most "sophisticated" portion of the public. Officially, *Le Moulin Rouge* shut down its activities at midnight, but that did not mean that the cabaret became empty at that time. Regular customers, like Lautrec, knew that was when the fun and games really started. Artists appearing for their own pleasure let loose the reins of fantasy, allowing themselves far more than they could do with open curtains. Lautrec took advantage of this, trying to immortalize these performances on the pages of his sketchbook. When everyone was already very tired and longed to go to bed, Lautrec would persuade his friends to continue the good times in other places, yet unclosed. During these escapades, the painter drank greater quantities of alcoholic drinks, slighting practically not a single one of them.

Unfortunately, these were the beginnings of his addiction to alcohol, as Henri now drank not just in the evenings or at night, but began in the morning, after having barely arisen. His biographer, Henri Perruchot described it thus:

"From being a pleasure, drink had become a necessity. He had hardly got out of bed in the morning before he started drinking. Vermouth, rum, white wine, Armagnac, champagne, cocktails; he would drink at any hour of the day." (126)

In autumn of 1891, Gabriel Tapie de Celeyran, Toulouse-Laytrec's cousin, appeared in Paris. Gabriel was a physician, who specialized in surgery, and who had obtained an assistantship with the already famous French surgeon, Jules-

Emile Pean. Dr. Pean, after whom a surgical instrument is named (he developed haemostatic forceps), headed a department at the Saint Louis Hospital in Paris. This is the same one in which, to this day, one can find a collection of *mulages,* representing currently unseen cases of skin diseases and, specifically, skin manifestations of 3rd stage syphilis. Tapie de Celeyran and Lautrec appealed to one another. Celeyran admired the artistic talent of his cousin, and was very sympathetic toward the latter's physical infirmities and his extravagant behavior, whereas Lautrec valued the physician's good nature, his agreeable character, and, what is germane here, his contacts in the medical world. Lautrec became interested in surgery and thanks to his cousin's help, obtained permission to observe surgical operations as performed by the famous surgeon.

Dr. Pean was a pioneer in certain categories of surgery, performing probably the first resection (removal) of the spleen, the first removal of a portion of the stomach, and removal of the ovary (oophorectomy), thus instituting, in some measure, a new division in surgery. (127) Lautrec treated his own presence in the operating room almost like a visit to the theater, observing and drawing in his sketchbook, not only the operations themselves, but also scenes accompanying them, such as the wiping away of sweat from the surgeon's forehead, describing in detail the washing of hands before an operation, as well as examination of the patient. In addition to numerous drawings, Lautrec completed two paintings dedicated to Dr. Pean, *Une Operations de Pean* and *La Tracheotomie.* His fascination with surgery and with the famous surgeon withstood the test of time, as, after several years, when Pean retired and funded the "Hospital Internationale" with his own money, Lautrec completed several works of art there, still astonished at the surgeon of whom it was said that he would "rummage in stomachs as if he were looking through his pockets for change." (128)

Halfway through 1892, Lautrec was still very active professionally, painting his beloved dancers from Le Moulin Rouge, and traveling to London and Toulouse, where he supervised the printing of one of his posters, until at a certain moment, he disappeared without a trace. He fell like a stone into water, while his friends and acquaintances did not know what happened to him. He was not seen at Le Moulin Rouge, nor in any coffeehouse in Montmartre, nor in the studio where he worked. The puzzle was solved after several days, when one of his acquaintances met the painter in one of the bordellos. Lautrec had simply moved in there. He slept, had his meals and painted there without leaving it. Asked for an explanation, he indignantly said "Bordel? What do you mean bordel? To the disapproving, he would exclaim, "They are the houses of the bord de l'eau. They need a lot of water, eh? Technique of ablution." (129)

Regardless of jokes on the subject of bordellos, of which there are many, it is worthwhile wondering what it was in them that was so alluring as to incline Lautrec to install himself in one. In the second half of the nineteenth century, the relationship of society to these institutions was different than in either later or earlier times, while the subject of prostitution at one point became fashionable, particularly among artists. Prostitutes became the heroines of theatrical works of such authors as Guy de Maupassant, Edmond Goncourt, or Huysmans. Courtesans were likewise the heroines of opera, as, for example, *La Traviata* by Verdi, or *Manon Lescaut* of Puccini, while many painters, not just Lautrec, immortalized their likenesses on canvas. Lautrec, nonetheless, outdid his colleagues in painting scenes from the bordello, which presented prostitutes in their natural environment, if not to say at work. According to him, these women were better models than the professionals.

Models always look as if they were stuffed, while these women are alive. I wouldn't dare pay them to pose for me, yet God knows they are worth it. They stretch themselves out on divans like animals ... they are so lacking in pretension, you know! (130)

Another explanation for his liking bordellos and their workers could be the fact that Toulouse-Lautrec – who, as a result of his lameness was discriminated against and made fun of, and not just once – found soulmates in women who had been discriminated against and ridiculed, even if for a far different reason. Nevertheless, one cannot exclude that Lautrec was an erotomaniac to some extent, and that the atmosphere predominating in bordellos excited him, and that he experienced pleasure looking at scenes of perversion or strange forms of sexual relationships. Yet another explanation of his behavior could be the fact that the painter loved practical jokes and shocking his friends in very varied, often strange ways.

Despite the fact that Lautrec had to pay for living in a bordello, (not excluding payments for sexual services), the painter felt himself to be a part of the institution, sharing his daily life with the prostitutes. He ate meals with them, played cards, took part in their conversations, and imparted his advice. He remembered birthdays, offering gifts, and inviting some of them to the circus or theater. He paraded on the streets with the women, or invited them to his loge at the opera, treating them like married men treat their spouses or girl friends.

But, above all, he painted them. He executed portraits of prostitutes or made paintings of their activities. In these there are prostitutes waiting for clients, in the course of their services, during their baths or asleep, often two in one bed. There are women in unmistakeable lesbian relations, which were not rare in bordellos, and scenes bringing to mind venereal diseases, which were the plague of these institutions, as evidenced by the painting already mentioned, i.e. the one representing prostitutes getting ready for examination by a doctor (Fig.5c.18).

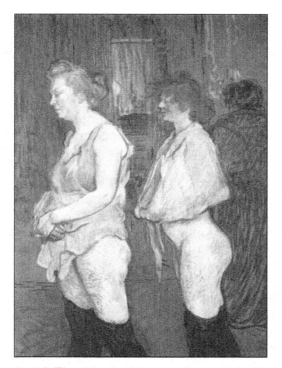

Figure 5c 18 The Medical Inspection painted by Henri Toulouse-Lautrec, 1894

Lautrec painted not only what he saw in bordellos, but also the bordellos themselves – that is, he decorated the walls of these institutions with his productions. Being friendly with him, the Madam owner of the one on Rue d'Amboise asked Lautrec to decorate her salon and several other rooms, to which the painter readily acquiesced, painting leaves and garlands of flowers on the walls, as well as sixteen medallions in the rococo style and with portraits of women.

Henri's mother and his friends were equally alarmed at his new lifestyle, and tried, by various methods, to lead him onto a better path. Friends invited him to meetings and social get-togethers, or even to their own homes for weekends, while his very religious mother engaged several nuns to pray for her son. She also asked priests for help, but Lautrec got rid of their sermons in a less-than-polite manner, telling one of them, "Oh yes, *Abbe*, don't worry; I am digging my grave with my cock." (131) Taking into account the painter's health, the reply cited could have had a deeper meaning, as Lautrec was aware of the fact that his syphilis could lead him to his death.

The extravagant (to say the least!) lifestyle of Lautrec had no greater influence on his creativity than that the majority of his works are of scenes from the life of a bordello, or portraits of the prostitutes working there. At the same time, his posters grew in popularity, and the painter received orders for them, mainly from cabaret artists with whom he was friendly. Supposedly, they were so popular that they would disappear right after being hung, stolen by admirers of his talents, or taken by the artists' fans. In addition, a new passion appeared in his life – lithography – thanks to which his work could be copied in any quantity.

At the start of 1893, Lautrec took part in an exhibition organized by Maurice Joyant, a friend of the painter's, at which were displayed thirty of his works, not only paintings, but also posters and lithographs. Reviews by the press were very flattering, while the known painting authority, Edgar Degas, is said to have remarked, "Well, Lautrec, it is clear [that] you are one of us." (132) The same Degas could also be less polite to his younger friend, at another time saying, "The gentleman is wearing trousers that are too big for him," while many years later, just after Lautrec's death, in commenting on his creativity, he is said to have remarked, "It all stinks of the pox." (133) This does not speak well for the author of these words, who, despite his well-known misogyny, also was interested in life in the bordello. (Reported by Joyant). (132)

Lautrec had a different relationship with women than Degas; he was understanding of their weaknesses, saw their problems, was sympathetic, and often helped them. One day, he and friends visited a woman who, as he expressed it, "Was more famous, in her time, than the President of the Republic." This was Victorine Meurent, a former model who, thirty years earlier, had posed for Manet's *Olympia*. Old and now in ill health (she was an alcoholic) Victorine supported herself playing the guitar and dancing "monkey dances" on the terrace of a coffee house. Some maintain that Lautrec visited her, not only to help her, but equally, to see how she, a person sick with alcoholism looked, aware that his dipsomania could one day lead him to a similar state.

At one point in his life, Lautrec befriended a group of literary figures gathered around the periodical, *Le Revue Blanche,* established by the Natanson brothers, Alexander and Thaddeus. They were Poles living in France who moved about in artistic-literary circles. Thaddeus Natanson particularly appealed to Lautrec, but his wife Misia, who was half-Polish, even more so. Misia's father was the famous sculptor, Cyprian Godebski, monuments of whose work stand in Krakow and Warsaw to this day, (134) while her mother, Sophie Servais, was the daughter of the famous viola-cellist, Adrien-Francois Servais. Brought up by the parents of her mother, who died in childbirth, Misia, from her youngest years, also moved about in the company of artists, mainly musicians. Among them was Franz Liszt. Later, in school, her teacher was Gabriel Faure. (135) At age twenty-one, Misia married Thaddeus Natanson, and it was in his house that Lautrec met her. The Natansons would frequently hold receptions for artists, such as Claude Monet, Pierre-Auguste Renoir, Claude Debussy, Marcel Proust, Steven Mallarme and Andre Gide. Lautrec, who also would take part in these receptions, felt best in the role of bartender, serving cocktails of his own recipes. Misia, unusually pretty and possessing sex appeal, was a precursor for literary figures in the novels of many writers, or posed for paintings, while the composer, Maurice Ravel, dedicated several of his works to her. Lautrec put her in several of his own paintings, e.g. *Misia reading a book*, *Misia at the piano*, as well as on a poster advertising *La Revue Blanche,* published by her husband. Pierre-Auguste Renoir, for whom she dared to expose her breasts (while not doing such a favor for other artists), also executed a portrait of her, which, of course, gave rise to gossip.

Among Russians who benefitted from Misia Sert's hospitality or assistance was Sergei Diaghilev, the founder of the Ballet Russe, but he was not the only one. Another famous artist helped by Misia was Igor Stravinsky, an episode about whom Artur Rubinstein, the famous Polish pianist, recorded in his memoirs. (137) One evening, Stravinsky telephoned Rubinstein with a request for an immediate meeting in regard to an unusually important matter. When the latter proposed a meeting the following day instead, the famous composer indicated that he had to meet with him that same day, as this was a matter of unusual importance for him. When the two gentlemen met later at a restaurant, Stravinsky announced that he had no money for living, and that he needed immediate financial help, as well as rapid medical help, since he had just discovered that he was impotent! Hearing the details pertaining to both problems, Rubinstein declared that, in the first matter, Misia Sert could help him, since, as he put it, "She is a woman of great resources ... and he had no doubts that when he talks to her, she will find a way to give him solid financial help." (138) As concerned the second problem, however, he didn't believe that Stravinsky's self-diagnosis was accurate, and suggested a visit to the bordello on Rue Chabanais, to which Stravinsky expressed agreement.

At this famous institution I said to the *sous-maitress*: 'Call Madeleine.' And when this beauty arrived I told her, 'Madeleine, take care of this gentleman.' It was the first time that I did not participate, but simply waited. After half an hour, Stravinsky appeared in triumph and said appreciatively: *Cette femme est genial.* So ended a difficult day. (139)

I cited this fragment from the memoirs of the famous pianist to show that Misia befriended not only famous people of her epoch, but could also be a direct help to them. In Stravinsky's case, this role was later taken on by her friend, Coco Chanel, foundress of the Chanel perfume brand, who invited Stravinsky, together with his family, to her villa in Paris; there, she ensured everyone room and board, and assured the composer that "Madeleine's help" would no longer be needed by him! Another reason that I cited this fragment from Rubinstein's memoirs is to show yet another role that bordellos played in those times, namely of an institution providing diagnostic-therapeutic services in a then-poorly-known field of medicine that sexology is today.

During her friendship with Lautrec, Misia was the wife of Thaddeus Natanson, which did not interfere with Lautrec's adoration of her, something he did not hide. Misia played the piano for him – Beethoven's "Ruins of Athens," his favorite work – while during her rests in the garden, they would sit under the tree, she with book in hand; Lautrec would tickle her bare feet with a paintbrush, explaining that he "noticed imaginary landscapes there." (140) Misia had nothing against posing for Lautrec, but once, irritated by something she saw, asked him why the women in his pictures, not excluding herself, were so ugly. "Because that is the way they are," the painter was said to have replied. (140) The women remembered the slight, and took their revenge with a similar "compliment" describing the painter's appearance during a visit to one of them (the singer, Yvette Guilbert):

'A puppet,' the maid exclaimed as she hurried to warn her mistress of the unexpected visitor. And Yvette

Guilbert was herself taken [a]back. She could find nothing to say at the sight of the huge, dark head, the red face and black beard, the greasy oily skin, the nose broad enough for two faces, and a mouth that gashed across the face, from cheek to cheek, with huge, violet-rose lips, that were at once flat and flaccid (*"Le Chanson de Vie,"* Yvette Guilbert memoirs). (142)

It must be added, however, that, despite her first impression, Yvette and Lautrec became friends, and the painter made well over a dozen lithographs of her, which appeared in an album dedicated to the singer. Similarly to other women, Yvette was portraited as unusually unattractive, while her mother, after seeing the album, encouraged her daughter to go to court with a citation for defamation.

The growing popularity of Toulouse-Lautrec as a painter, poster artist, lithographer and illustrator gathered an ever growing circle of admirers; he, however, if it can be put so, gathered with other admirers of drinks around the coffee houses and bars where alcohol was served. The favorite places to which the painter invited friends were the *Cosmopolitan* and *Weber* coffeehouses, and the *Irish and American Bar*, on Rue Royale. In the latter two, Lautrec started to appear in the company of two new admirers, the English dancer, May Milton, a friend of Jane Avril's, as well as the Irish singer, May Belfort. May had a more girlish appearance, and the painter named her the Orchid, although Maurice Joant called her the Frog. Looking at her portraits, one can conclude that both gentlemen were right; however, depending on which painting, one can have various appraisals of the beauty of the model. Lautrec painted five portraits of May, as well as a series of lithographs, and a "splendid crimson" poster, which, as a result of its vivid color, attracted the attention of the inhabitants of Paris well. (141) The painter attempted to bed May several times, but apparently the lady was steadfast and remained just his model.

His frequent presence in bars and coffeehouses where alcohol was served did not serve the artist well; Taddeus Natanson observed that "the hair of his moustache had little time to dry." Yet even though Lautrec was merely drunk in the full sense of the word, it was said that even the smell of a coctail would suffice to restore him to the "magic enchantment of alcohol." (143) During receptions at the homes of friends, Henri especially liked the role of barman, preparing in the course of a single night hundreds of drinks for guests - not forgetting himself, of course.

Overwork, lack of sleep, and excessive alcohol and sex began to affect Toulouse-Lautrec's health. There began to appear sudden mood swings, such as one in which, following an amusing episode at which the painter laughed himself to tears, then fell into a deep depression and didn't speak to anyone for a long time. He was able, without any reason, to twist the fingers of the person whom he was greeting – which was forgiven by his friends, but not always by people newly met. There were periods when his utterances would become incomprehensible, not only to strangers, but also to friends, who knew his manner of expressing himself. Time spent with wineglass in hand as well as periods of alcoholic intoxication, during which he was unable to paint, began to reflect on his productivity, causing the number of paintings, lithographs and posters executed by him to diminish.

This was not yet the worst period of his life; despite clear signs of alcoholism, the artist could become interested in new things. This was a time of resurgence of bicycling, which fascinated the painter. Although wanting to be, he was not himself a bicycle rider, yet was a frequent guest at bicycle contests, immortalizing scenes of races in his paintings, as well as executing portraits or lithographs of their winners. I will add that the popularity of bicycling influenced a change in fashions for women, in that they began to wear trousers, called "Zouave trousers" – which was an unusual occurrence at that time, and about which Parisian newspapers commented, comparing the new fashion to the arrival of a "third sex." (144)

In mid-1895, Lautrec, together with Joyant, traveled to London. Henri enjoyed England and felt very well in that country. He had many friends there, among them the painter Charles Conder, who belonged to a group of artists associated with Oscar Wilde. (145) This was not a good period in the life of that British poet and dramatist, as in March of the same year, Wilde was accused of sodomy and awaited the trial, which, as we may remember, ended in his being convicted and sentenced to prison. Lautrec was impressed with Wilde during his meetings with him; although the latter refused to sit for him, Lautrec painted his portrait from memory. After returning to Paris, he submitted a drawing representing Wilde, seated on the bench of the accused, to *Le Revue Blanche*. The painter belonged to a large group of French intellectuals who expressed their solidarity with followers of Wilde in England, and who considered the judgment of the London court to have been highly unfair. The figure of Oscar Wilde also found itself in decorations done of *La Goulue*, by Lautrec, which significantly increased the interest of viewers of her performances.

Toulouse-Lautrec was not only full of understanding and sympathy toward male homosexuals, but was equally interested in women "loving differently." This was the period during which he did a series of lithographs for Cha-U-Kao, a dancer from Le Moulin Rouge, who passed for a lesbian. Lautrec had already painted her earlier, dancing a waltz in the arms of another woman. (146) His interest in lesbians caused him to be a frequent guest at the bar, *La Souris*, situated near Place Pigalle, where women of persuasions similar to that of Cha-U-Kao would meet. Henri Perruchot described it thus:

Here at "La Souris" – "La Touris," as he pronounced it – he [Lautrec] mingled with his accustomed ease among these women, some of whom were strapping and manly types with short hair and high stocks, while others were languorously and exaggeratedly feminine, and dressed in the brightest of colors. Wearing their vice like flowers in their hats ..., [c]ouples fondled or quarreled. Some play cards, some dice, and they all chattered. They all smoked too. The ashtrays overflowed with the lipstick-stained butts of Turkish cigarettes and even big cigars. To the odour of alcohol, musk, amber and patchouli were added the ether and morphine of the drug-addicts. (147)

Although men were not entirely welcome in *La Souris*, Lautrec, as a result of his physical defects, or maybe because of his rising popularity, was tolerated, and even liked. Many regulars of the place willingly posed for him, while some of them found in him a confidante for entrusting their problems to him. Just being in a lesbian environment did not entirely satisfy the erotic interests of the painter, to which testifies the following citation from his biography:

From time to time he organized 'lascivious spectacles ... sapphic occasions.' And on one occasion he took a lesbian, nicknamed *Le Crapaud*, from La Souris to a brothel in the Rue de Miromesnil. There he threw her into the arms of the other women, and, as a passionate spectator, watched their gambols. (147)

This type of behavior on the part of the painter may appear to today's reader – who has access to the Internet – to be difficult to understand, but at the end of the nineteenth century, nobody dreamed that such scenes could be watched by clicking on an appropriate computer key.

From among the three passions of Lautrec – painting, sex, and alcohol – the last was the most dangerous. The painter drank ever more frequently, and always more. His friends saw this, and tried to help. Misia and Thaddeus Natanson, who bought some property outside Paris, invited Henri for short, and for longer stays, organizing the plan of the day so that the artist had as little occasion to drink alcohol as possible. All drinks containing alcohol were removed from the house, leaving only small quantities of wine served for lunch. Excursions around the area were organized, including swimming in the river and boating. Discussions on literature, invitations to interesting friends, in a word, everything, was done to minimize the painter's contact with alcohol. To everyone's surprise, Lautrec handled the absence of alcoholic drinks very well, while the hosts were happy that they were helping their friend to escape the bad habit. Unfortunately, it turned out to be a delusion, as, at the garden's end, the Natansons had a small gate leading to the street, near which there was a small inn with a well-furnished bar.

After returning to Paris, Lautrec no longer had to steal through a gate in the garden to satisfy his thirst for alcohol. More and more frequently, he was seen in the local bars, heavily drunk, making a row with the guests, or simply dead drunk and sleeping on a bench or under a table. One of his friends saw him in such a state at *La Souris* "among a crowd of women dressed in men's clothes. It was a distressing sight. Saliva trickled down the thin cord of his pince-nez, and fell drop by drop on to his waist coat." (148) His friends did not cease in their efforts to turn the painter's attention away from alcohol, organizing business trips to other towns or abroad, something that began to irritate Lautrec.

> This behaviour was more than ever marked by irritation, ungovernable range, and certain wildness. His eccentricity was becoming comparable to his father, and he was liable to fall heavily asleep

anywhere and at any time for two minutes or for two hours. This restlessness was no longer due to excessive vitality. Alcohol and the disease he had caught from Rosa La Rouge, which had been completely neglected during the last four years, were corroding and undermining him ... His friends were anxious. But what could they do? Lautrec was becoming more intractable and more difficult to manage every day. Bourges, who had published his "*Hygiene de Syphilitique*" that very year, advised a long cruise; it would afford, so the doctor thought, a sedative, tonic and restorative treatment. (149)

It was difficult to dismiss the lack of logic in this type of advice, although one can sympathize with the doctors for having so little to offer their patients. Lautrec tried travel, considered treatment under conditions of confinement, stopped drinking cocktails, and limited himself to port – all of which some attribute to the painter's short-lived ardor toward his young cousin, Aline, who had just left the convent. Unfortunately for him, the girl's father quickly put a stop to all hopes for romance, and Lautrec quickly returned to his previous habits. To changes in the painter's psychologic state were added neurologic problems. Lautrec, who already had been a weak walker, now moved about with difficulty; disturbances occurred in his speech, he began to stammer, and became incomprehensible. In the winter of 1898, his state of health clearly deteriorated. Visual and auditory hallucinations appeared; he imagined that he was being attacked by flies, and genuinely feared that they could cause him harm. He went to bed at night in "button hook" out of concern that insects could attack him at night, and ordered that the painter's studio in which he worked had to be sprayed with "paraffin" (oil) out of concern, not only for insects, but also unseen microbes. A person was hired to look after Henri 24 hours a day, and whom the painter, as evidence that he had not lost his sense of humor, called "commissioner of his district." Unfortunately, this "keeper" also liked alcohol, which resulted in Lautrec – who had a stronger head – leaving the drunken "keeper" in one bar, while he, himself, would make his way to another

Lautrec tried to work, and friends like Jane Avril ordered paintings and posters from him attempting to occupy him in some way in order to weaken his attraction to alcohol (Fig. 5c.19). Unfortunately, in this area of the artist's life, the disease caused a disruption, as the works that came from his hands during this time are clearly strange – as though marked with the stamp of mental illness. Hallucinations appeared ever more frequently: "He tried to fight a cardboard elephant; a pack of terriers yapped at his heels; and monstrous, headless animals prowled about the room trying to drive him against the bed and crush him. In a sweat of terror he would hide under the bedclothes." (150) At this point, one can ask to what extent, and for which symptoms alcohol was responsible, and which of these one can attribute to long-untreated syphilis. I fear, however, that it is not possible to divide them, as the majority can appear equally in third-stage syphilis (general paresis) as in the disease of alcoholism, *delirium tremens.*

All wondered how to help the ill Lautrec, and in the end, his family and friends came to the conclusion that only treatment on a closed ward could give him a chance for recovery. After consultations with many specialists, the artist was placed in a psychiatric institution in Neuilly, near Paris. The hospital was very expensive, located in a seventeenth century building surrounded by a beautiful park, and, for the patients, there were expensively appointed flats with several rooms, private bathrooms and a private garden. Lautrec arrived there at the end of 1899, and even after a few days' stay, his health began to improve. Hallucinations ceased, and it began to reach him that he was in a closed institution, and supervised by a personal attendant (male nurse) 24 hours a day. Upon realizing this, he was shocked, scared and desperate. He collected his thoughts with difficulty and wept frequently, but, not having a choice, quickly resigned himself to his new situation. Lautrec's health, however, continued to improve, the return of his psychotic symptoms was ever rarer, and approximately a month later he was already so calmed that he could go out for walks in the garden in the company of his attendant.

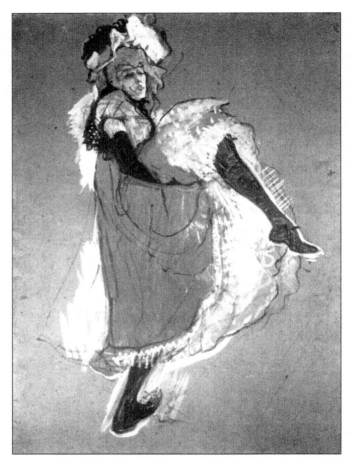

Figure 5c 19 Painting of Jane Avril by Toulouse Lautrec

Along with improvement of his mental state, the fact of Lautrec's compulsory isolation became increasingly painful to him. He tried to paint, sketched patients as well as hospital staff, and quickly fell upon the idea that the fact that he was able to work would be an argument, which could convince the doctors that they could let him go home. These were in no hurry to decide, however, probably considering that a longer period of convalescence was needed to give the patient a better guarantee of return to good health. In letters to his friends, as well as to people visiting, Lautrec tried to give them to understand that he was already completely well, and would ask for their intervention in the matter of leaving the hospital. Finally, as a result of pressure on the part of the family, as well as of the endeavors of the painter himself – who was painting more and more, wanting to prove his return to health – and after a council that took place in mid-May, Lautrec was permitted to leave the asylum. However, a *caveat* was noted that,

> Owing to his amnesia, the instability of his character and lack of will-power it is essential that Mr. Henri de Toulouse-Lautrec should be subject in his life outside these premises to material and moral conditions of continual supervision so that he may not have an opportunity of relapsing into alcoholic habits and so pave the way to a relapse of a more serious nature than his previous symptoms. (151)

Happy for his recovered freedom, Lautrec agreed, without objection, to an "overseer," employed by his mother, who was to take care that the painter would not fall back into bad habits. He was a distant cousin, a person of gentle nature, delicate and tactful, understanding of Lautrec's difficult situation, and full of desire to help him. A great merit of the new guardian, in comparison to the former one, was a stomach problem that allowed him to drink exclusively tea. Lautrec liked him almost from their first meeting, and, with a sense of humor typical for him, called him "my bear leader." After a short stay at the seashore, the painter returned to Paris in the autumn, where he began to paint and make lithographs again. It appeared that he had fully regained his strength, equally physical as psychologic, although his friends noticed certain changes. Maurice Joyant wrote, "In this human mechanism there was something 'broken.' Lautrec's curiosity was destroyed. He could laugh and joke but it was no longer with the laughter and the vitality of the past. It was as if he were forcing himself to resemble the old Lautrec." (152).

The period of convalescence after hospitalization lasted about five-six months, during which it appeared that the painter had a chance to return to normal life. He painted a great deal, and experts maintain that after leaving the hospital Lautrec changed his style, paying more attention to colors, which now became more subtle and warmer.

This state did not last too long, however, as Lautrec again started to drink. His kindhearted guardian, who was full of good intentions, did everything to eliminate Lautrec's contact with alcohol, but the latter turned out to be crafty. The painter had long used a cane, but now acquired a new one with a silver pommel, which he bought at an Italian antique dealer's. He made no mystery about this, but did not reveal to anyone that the cane had been hollowed out in the middle, so that he could put a half-litre of a liquid of his choice inside. Similarly, the silver pommel was not a simple decoration; after unscrewing it, could serve as a liquor glass. I do not have to add that the liquid with which the painter filled the cane was not mineral water, but any alcoholic drink that he desired! The situation began to be dangerous, because Lautrec treated his return to his bad habit as something that had to happen, and consoled himself with the thought that this was the beginning of the end. His family and friends tried to convince him that not everything was lost, and Joyant began to make efforts to obtain the medal of the Legion of Honor for him, judging that maybe this prestigious distinction could change his attitude toward life. When both friends appeared at the office of the appropriate minister, who was a fan of Lautrec's works, and began to talk on the subject of the distinction, Lautrec interrupted the conversation saying, "Have you considered, Monsieur le Ministre, how odd the red ribbon will look when I go to paint a brothel?" (153) Lautrec did not receive the medal, and it was not because he didn't fulfill all the criteria named by Andre Gide (he was under forty years of age), but because it was of no special consequence to him.

The year 1900 and the beginning of 1901 marked a period of decline in the painter's life, both from the point of view of art and of his health. Lautrec painted less and less, and ever more slowly, while the quality of his paintings underwent a distinct deterioration. His creativity during this period became average, one could no longer see what was there formerly, i.e. the talent of a true artist. And, in regard to his health, it was even worse. Lautrec did not eat much, lost a lot of weight, and his clothes hung on him as though on a hanger. Visits to the bordellos became limited, but not because of any disturbance in potency, as one could have imagined, but, rather, for financial reasons, as his family greatly reduced their material assistance, while his income from the sale of his paintings significantly declined.

In March 1901, the painter underwent a greater crisis. Signs of paranoia appeared, while his legs, already poorly functional, completely ceased to obey his commands. The treatment that he undertook – electrical stimulation and certain doses of *nux vomica* – seemed to help a little, but his physicians forbade him alcohol and sexual relations, which did not help his psychologic state. A month later, in mid-April, Lautrec appeared on the streets of Paris, shocking those people who knew him. He was but a shadow of his former self, frighteningly thin, and moving with difficulty. He tried to work, but probably saw that this no longer made any sense. Losing his desire to paint, the artist lost his desire to live. He closed his studio and left Paris. In mid-1901, as his biographers write, an "attack of paralysis" occurred. His mother, whom his guardian informed of this fact, took her son to Chateau de Malrome, where she lived. After a short period of improvement of the state of his health, during which Lautrec again tried to paint, deterioration appeared anew. "The paralysis gradually spread through his body. He could neither walk nor eat. He was taken out in a carriage into the park. At meals, he was brought to the table in a wheelchair. "(154) Periods of loss of consciousness appeared, and the painter did not really know what was happening. Henri Toulouse-Lautrec died on the morning of September 9, 1901.

As always in this book, I put the question to myself of how much syphilis, with which the painter became infected at the age of 24, caused his death, and how much other diseases were responsible. The answer, particularly in the case of Lautrec, is very difficult to determine with certainty, as the painter was a cripple from his early years, and then, for a long time, suffered from alcoholism. The gamut of manifestations of the latter disease is very wide, and in many ways can overlap with those of tertiary syphilis (general paresis, *tabes dorsalis*, or meningo-vascular lues). Also, one cannot exclude that the "paralysis," which afflicted the painter in the last year of his life could have been the result of cerebral attack or stroke (hemorrhagic, thrombus, etc.) related neither to syphilis, nor to prolonged alcoholism. So, what the immediate cause of the painter's death was, I have to leave without any definitive answer.

CHAPTER 6

A CHANCE DISCOVERY

It is said and written that had Alexander Fleming been more mindful of tidiness, he would not have made his discovery. There is much truth in this statement, but also some exaggeration. Fleming was not at all as untidy as some assert, whereas the discovery he made was not only the result of chance, but, in large measure, the result of the developed intellect of this Scottish scientist (Fig.6.1).

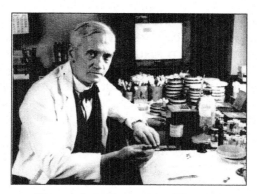

Figure 6.1 Alexander Fleming

The summer of 1928 was rainy, and the air over London was saturated with moisture. Dr. Alexander Fleming, a bacteriologist at St. Mary's Hospital, was conducting experiments on *Staphylococcus* bacteria. He cultured them in Petri dishes, which, after completion of the experiment, were supposed to be discarded. One day he did not do this and left for a short vacation to a summerhouse he had near

London. Upon his return, he began to clean up the Petri plates left on the table, and noticed that on several of them, among the overgrown cultures of staphylococci, large blue colonies of mold had appeared, a mold, which is a type of fungus, that appears on food kept under improper conditions. There would not have been anything unusual in this, had there not been an unusual phenomenon accompanying the mold on the plates. Specifically, around the blue mold there appeared an open area caused by the disappearance of the yellow colonies of staphylococci. It looked as though the mold had clearly inhibited the growth of the bacteria, and the scientist began to wonder about the cause of this phenomenon. Fleming took a sample of the blue mold, and, examining it through the microscope, noted brush-like growths characteristic of a mold of the genus *Penicillium* – one of the most commonly encountered types. Next, he took the remaining mold off the plate and transferred it into a boullion broth used to culture a variety of microorganisms. After a couple of days, a luxuriant growth of mold could be noted on the surface of the liquid, with a yellow and clear area underneath. As it turned out later, the clarity of the solution was due to a substance produced by the mold, the same as that which had hindered the growth of bacteria on the Petri plates. Next, Fleming conducted several similar experiments, using other genera of fungi, but only those of the genus *Penicillium* produced substances that inhibited bacterial growth.

In order to determine whether the bouillon broth on which the mold was found was toxic to animals, Fleming injected various amounts into rabbits and mice, all of which survived the tests without any problem. The scientist gradually began to realize that, thanks to a fortunate accident, he was possibly the author of a discovery that could change the face of medicine, as, until that time, the only substances known to have an antibacterial effect were toxic to humans and animals, and intended almost exclusively for external use.

Fleming called for consultation a colleague whose laboratory was situated in the same building, but on the floor below. This was Professor J.C. La Touche, a specialist in fungi. The famous professor, after examining the "blue mold," determined that it was *Penicillium rubrum* (others maintained that it was *Penicillium notatum*) that had arrived on Fleming's Petri plates, together with the air from a window open onto the street below. Gwyn McFarlane, one of Fleming's biographers, was of the opinion that the mold got to his plates, not from the street window, but through a door open onto the staircase, most likely from La Touche's mold (mycology) laboratory, which was situated on the floor below. (1) Hence, had Fleming's laboratory not been above La Touche's, or in a different part of the building, we would have had to have waited for the discovery of penicillin a while longer. So, how can one not believe in a fortunate accident? Scientifically, this is called serendipity.

In regard to Fleming's academic career, that also swarms with happenstance. Alexander Fleming, "Alec," came from a poor Scottish family, working in farming. At age fourteen, he arrived in London, where his older siblings already lived. One of them was Thomas Fleming, an ophthalmologist, who enrolled Alec as well as his younger brother in the Polytechnic Institute in London. Alec attended this school for two years, after which he decided to undertake work with a shipping company as junior clerk. Resigning from an education and undertaking employment was dictated by his wanting to reduce the costs borne by his brother for educating the family, and, eventually to save funds for a later continuation of his studies. And here, again, a happy accident occurred. One of Fleming's uncles, an old bachelor, died without issue, leaving an estate to the family, which, in Alec's case, came to 250 pounds, a considerable amount in those times. Receipt of these unexpected funds opened up new possibilities for Fleming, who, after a four-year administrative career, began, at age of 20, to think about further studies. He did not know on what field to decide, but, at the persuasion of his doctor-brother, as well as of his sisters, who had doctor-husbands, chose medical studies. (2) After passing entrance examinations, he became a student at St. Mary's Hospital's School of Medicine in London. He chose that one, perhaps – and here we again are dealing with a happy accident – because, as a member of a water polo team at one time, he had played against the St. Mary's team and had met several of its members.

Alec was an able and hard-working student, proven by the prizes and stipends he obtained. He took part in sports, being a member of the water polo team, as well as of the rifle team. This latter passion is not without significance, as it is thanks to it that Fleming became a bacteriologist, despite the fact that all the while, he thought of devoting himself to surgery.

A friend, probably the leader of the rifle team (who wanted the good rifleman that Fleming was to stay with the St. Mary's team), talked him into bacteriology, and arranged a job for him with Sir Almroth Wright's group, which was occupied with vaccines. Alec, with a certain degree of hesitation, accepted the proposal, with the hope that it would not collide with his plans to become a surgeon. And so, at the age of twenty-five, began Fleming's adventure with bacteriology, an adventure that changed the face of medicine. It must be added that, in addition to his discovery of the bactericidal action of penicillin, Fleming also has several other significant accomplishments to his credit. It was he who first recognized that there is a bactericidal substance in saliva, which was later named lysozyme. Fleming also worked on a vaccine against acne, as well as – and here, I stress with satisfaction – occupying himself with venereology, specifically the testing of the then-new medicine for syphilis, called Salvarsan.

Co-creator and proponent of treating lues with Salvarsan, about which I wrote earlier, was the German physician, Paul Ehrlich. Fleming's chief was a friend of Ehrlich's, and it is no surprise that St. Mary's Hospital was one of the first foreign (to Germany] medical centers that received Salvarsan with the aim of trying it in patients with syphilis. Alec Fleming found himself in the group testing the new medicine, and was one of the first English physicians who used the "magic Bullet," as Salvarsan was then known, in treating patients with syphilis in England. Salvarsan was one of the first chemotherapeutic agents that worked bacteriocidally against the "pale spirochetes," *Treponema pallidum*, with greatly reduced toxic effects on the human organism as compared to other agents, used from the end of the first decade of the twentieth century and later in association with bismuth preparations, it was considered the first effective treatment for lues.

His discovery of the antibacterial action of penicillin changed the object of Fleming's scientific interest, and he then devoted himself almost entirely to testing "the miraculous mold." A serious problem became the isolation of a pure chemical substance, the one that had the antibacterial activity; another was the testing of this activity in patients ill with diseases caused by bacteria. Work on the first of these took Fleming many years, but the experiments of other scholars were themselves of great help. Among the latter were two immigrants working at Oxford, the pathologist Howard Florey from Australia, and Erst B. Chain, a German-Jewish chemist and a refugee from Hitlerian Germany. Working independently of Fleming, the group was able to obtain a yellow-brown powder, thanks to the then-new process called lyophilization (freeze-drying), which was the almost pure form of penicillin (3). After numerous trials on animals and, later, on humans, it turned out that the substance obtained by them is the same antibiotic as we know today. All three researches, Fleming, Florey and Chain received the Nobel Prize in 1945 for their work.

In addition to the Nobel Prize, Alexander Fleming received many prestigious awards, among them that of the French Legion of Honor. It is possible that he knew the famous saying of Andre Gide regarding the criteria for receiving this prize, as in the speech he gave upon receiving the Nobel award, he apologized, saying, "I have been accused of having invented penicillin. No man could invent penicillin, for it has been produced from time immemorial by a certain mold." (4) Despite Fleming's insisting that he was not the "inventor" of penicillin, he accepted the prize standing in the same row of laureates (including those suffering from syphilis) from whom many could have been saved if Fleming's "invention" had appeared earlier.

Here, one must remember that Alexander Fleming was not the first person who had noted the antagonism between molds and bacteria, as not many years before the discovery of penicillin, publications on this subject had already appeared (Ernest Duchesne, 1897; Codomiro Picado from the Pasteur Institute, 1923). Nevertheless, Fleming was the first person able to confirm this experimentally, while his later work opened the door to studies thanks to which the substance named penicillin was obtained.

From the first tests until the common use of penicillin in the treatment of bacterial diseases, many years passed. A burning problem became the procurement of adequate quantities of the "brown powder" that would allow its use on a larger scale. However, when it was discovered that penicillin was concentrated by the kidneys, in order to help with the purification of penicillin early during World War II, agar cultures of the mold were fed to London Bobbies, and their urine was collected for further processing. With fewer of many complex contaminants, the active material could be purified more readily from that source for use among wounded soldiers. (W. A. K., quoting UCLA Professor Ruth

A. Boak, M.D., Ph.D.). In 1944, Florey and Chain opened a mini-factory for producing penicillin in Oxford, only to have to cope with many problems. One of these was the necessity of maintaining the appropriate sterility, in which penicillin had to be produced. The investigators hired so-called "penicillin girls" dressed in white overalls, scarves and gloves to keep themselves warm in the frigid condition. Benches and floors were soaked with oil to prevent dust from rising into the air' as germs, carried through the air by dust, could destroy an entire batch of penicillin. Unfortunately, the oil created slippery conditions that caused more than one penicillin girl to take a spill in the line of duty. (5)

The mini-factory produced small quantities of penicillin, and Florey, upon the invitation of the Rockefeller Foundation, went to the U.S.A. with the hope that he could obtain some help. After arrival, he went to Peoria in the state of Illinois, where a laboratory was located the work of which increased production of penicillin to a significant degree. This increase was obtained thanks to use of a new strain of the mold, which appeared in the laboratory thanks to one of its female workers.

Mary Hunt, known as "Moldy Mary," was a laboratory worker, whose assignment was going daily to the produce market to examine rotten fruits and vegetables with the aim of finding and pre-testing the molds found on them. One day, "Moldy Mary" had a bit of luck, and brought to the laboratory a very rotten cantaloupe, from which was isolated *Penicillium chrysogenum*, that turned out to be 200 times more productive of penicillin as species discovered by Fleming.

Positive experience with penicillin used among wounded soldiers during World War II produced an interest in the new medicine among people in authority. At a rapid rate, there appeared in England and the U.S.A. large institutions to produce penicillin, which, at least at the start, was destined for the needs of the Army. It was mainly due to penicillin that it was possible to save the lives of many wounded soldiers, who, without the new antibiotic had no chance to survive. In due time, and with ever increasing production of the antibiotic, this medicine became available for ever larger groups of patients, not just the military, and it began to be used for ever expanding groups of diseases caused by bacteria.

That penicillin could be an effective medicine against syphilis, we discovered also thanks to serendipity. John Mahoney, of the Venereal Disease Research Laboratory in New York, obtained a small amount of penicillin from the National Research Council, with the aim of confirming earlier information saying that the new antibiotic was effective in treating sulphonamide-resistant gonorrhea. Gonorrhea was a real plague, particularly in the military forces of the U.S.A., and the authorities were very anxious for as rapid a control of this disease as possible, as it had begun to reach epidemic levels, due, among other causes to the appearance of gonococci resistant to sulphonamides. Mahoney, acting to some extent in violation of regulations, decided to find out if penicillin might also be effective in the case of syphilis. After a positive test in rabbits, from which it turned out that penicillin acted against the treponemes, Mahoney decided to give the antibiotic to four patients with early syphilis, counting on the fact that in case of failure, the patients would be subjected to arsenotherapy, the then-standard form of syphilis treatment. Mahoney's patients received intramuscular injections of penicillin daily for eight days, and these caused a rapid remission of the symptoms of the disease. (6) Subsequent observations on the advantageous action of penicillin in early syphilis encouraged investigators to experiment further with penicillin, this time in its various stages.

News of the rapidly acting, non-toxic medication for syphilis made it to the press, and shortly, Time Magazine, in an article entitled "New Magic Bullet," published information about the appearance of a new treatment for syphilis. This increased interest in penicillin enormously, and caused the start of testing of antibiotics on much larger groups of people suffering from lues, which confirmed the high effectiveness of penicillin in all stages of the disease. After the publication, in 1944, of the work of Mahoney and his co-workers (7, 8), penicillin began to be routinely used in the treatment of syphilis and gonorrhea, beginning with the Army, and then among the civilian population.

Enthusiastic, positive opinions about the new medicine among physicians and their patients notwithstanding, other opinions, presenting negative consequences of the use of penicillin in the treatment of venereal diseases were also heard. Various moralizers began to give voice to theories that their rapid and painless treatment would itself increase the promiscuity of patients, which would produce a rise in the morbidity due to venereal diseases, and accusing medical science of ignoring sociologic and moral aspects of the new discoveries. Similar opinions were also aired by some representatives of the U.S. Public Health Service. (9) Fortunately, the prognoses of the naysayers did not materialize, as after the introduction of penicillin, morbidity due to syphilis in the U.S.A. during the '50s of the last century fell to the lowest point in the history of this country. (10) Skeptics of the use of penicillin did not take into account a very important aspect of the action of the new medication, namely the fact that a rapid cure caused the patients to cease being infectious for their partners, which is particularly pertinent for persons who frequently change partners, and for women engaged in prostitution.

The greatest enthusiasm resulting from the introduction of penicillin to the treatment of venereal diseases reigned among patients and the physicians treating them. I have been told that at one of the post-war international venereology conferences, a well known British venereologist is said to have asserted that when the use of penicillin, became widespread, specialists taking care of venereal disease patients would have to find another occupation, as these diseases would disappear from the face of the earth. I would remind the reader that, in those days, European physicians had practically to deal only with lues and gonorrhea, and did not know that such diseases as genital herpes, genital warts, NGU (non-gonococal urethritis) caused by chlamydia, some types of hepatitis, and, later, HIV/AIDS, are also venereal, or, in current terms, sexually transmitted diseases.

After a huge drop in syphilis morbidity in the '50s, a gradual increase in its prevalence was observed in later years. This was a signal for epidemiologists, who said that a fall in infectious diseases was not decided exclusively by the ease of treatment. It became clear that the morbidity of venereal diseases was decided by other factors, such as early detection, attained by, among other things, mass screening examinations, easy access to a physician, use of prophylactic measures (condoms), prophylactic treatment of contacts, public education, and many other sociologic and cultural factors.

Recognizing the elements that influence the morbidity of syphilis ever better, organizations responsible for syphilis control began to consider the introduction of complex actions having as their goal its elimination. I remember how, in the '70s, when I worked in the VD Control Division of the CDC (Centers for Disease Control and Prevention) in Atlanta, there were discussions of plans for the elimination of syphilis in the U.S.A. These plans acquired a realistic form in the '90s of the last century, when a program to eliminate syphilis in the country by the end of the twentieth century was formulated. Unfortunately, despite the efforts of many persons and organizations involved with this problem, it turned out not to be possible to attain the intended goals. The global morbidity of lues, according to data from the World Health Organization (WHO) at the beginning of the twenty-first century reached about 12 million cases, (11) the number of illnesses in particular regions of the globe being dependent on very many factors, not only medical ones.

So, despite the introduction of penicillin for treatment, and the huge reduction in number of cases, syphilis is alive and well, and the chance of its complete elimination is not in sight. A comforting thought, however, is that, despite the fact that, from the introduction of penicillin for the treatment of lues over half a century ago, this antibiotic is still the number one effective remedy. Penicillin is cheap and generally non-toxic, and it can be used in pregnant women, the only contraindication being occasional allergic reactions, although even these can usually be managed by desensitization. Many other bacteria have become resistant or less sensitive to penicillin, a fact that has resulted, for example in the treatment of gonorrhea, in a need to increase the dose of antibiotic several fold, or to replace penicillin with another antibiotic toward which the gonococci have not yet acquired resistance. (12)

Despite the fact that, in the treatment of syphilis, other antibiotics, such as tetracycline, erythromycin, or, more recently, azithromycin, are effective, these are used mainly in cases in which the patients cannot be treated with penicillin. Their use is associated with a number of problems, as, except for azithromycin, they have to be taken several times over a period of 2-3 weeks, while, except for erythromycin, one cannot use them in pregnant women. A most recently appearing problem has been associated with the detection of spirochetes resistant to them. Thus, despite the existence of other forms of therapy, penicillin, discovered by accident close to 90 years ago, is still the most effective treatment for syphilis. (13)

Concerning just how effective a weapon penicillin is against the *Treponema pallidum*, (pale treponeme), is evidenced by an old joke that I have told while giving lectures on the treatment of syphilis. A spirochete meets a pale treponeme, and asks, "Why are you so pale?" The one asked replies, "I caught penicillin." This old venereologic joke was proved didactically, as it has not yet happened that a single one of my students, during an examination in venereology, did not respond correctly to the question of what is the most effective treatment for syphilis.

CHAPTER 7

FEAR, SHAME ... AND MORE

From the beginning of the syphilis pandemic, the disease evoked fear, about which it is hard to be surprised. Its then-unknown cause, violent course, skin changes that disfigured the patient's appearance, and severe pains, as well as a lack of response to all attempts at treatment were a sufficient reason to produce fear in patients, and panic around them. This consternation was also communicated to physicians, who were helpless in regard to the new disease, and, not knowing the method of its spread, fled from the sick, fearing infection. The renowned humanist of the time, Erasmus of Rotterdam considered syphilis as the worst and most damaging of the diseases that had befallen mankind at the time, as it "concentrates in itself everything that was appalling in other diseases: pains, contagiousness, danger of death, difficult and loathsome treatment, which does not bring a full return to health." (1) Erasmus, himself the grandson of a physician, was fearful of syphilis, and refused a meeting with his friend and intellectual contemporary thinker, Ulrich von Hutten, who was ill with lues. Von Hutten, who was involved in the Reformation, had to leave Germany, and had difficulty in finding a place where he could live and work. These difficulties resulted not only from the fact of announcing himself to be sympathetic to the Reformation (and was therefore looked at askance by the Catholic majority), but also, perhaps mainly, because he was ill with lues, and, despite multiple treatments, had reached the stage of frequent recurrences of the disease. Zwingli, one of the Reformation leaders in Switzerland, came to his help, allowing him to settle away from the city, on the lightly inhabited island of Ufenau in the Zurichersee, where von Hutten died at age thirty-five, and where, to this day, is found his grave, frequently visited by tourists (Fig.7.1 and 7.2).

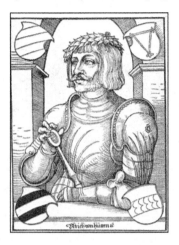

Figure 7.1 Ulrich von Hutten

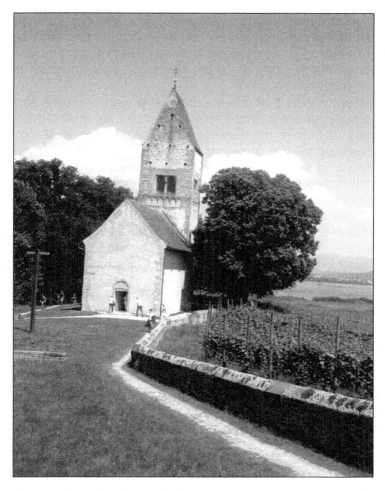

Figure 11.2 Ulrich von Hutten is burried to the right of the chapel on the Ufenau Island. Photo: E. Mroczkowska

The first observations indicating that syphilis could be transmitted sexually added feelings of shame to the fear of the disease. The sphere of human sexuality had always been one of bashfulness and great privacy, while infection with

445

syphilis or other venereal disease was proof of breaking certain moral maxims, i.e. marital infidelity, utilizing paid sex, loss of virginity or abandoned celibacy. Shame accompanied lues from the beginnings of the pandemic, and much of this remains to this day.

An early view that disease can be a sign of God's anger and a punishment for not keeping his commandments added a sense of guilt to the feelings of fear and shame. Many of the diseased tried to appease the Creator for sins committed, by practicing self-flagellation or by taking part in processions or pilgrimages to holy places or by offering generous gifts to the Church. The belief that syphilis could be a punishment meted out by God underlay the bases of the name given to this disease, for the genesis of which we are indebted to the sixteenth century poem authored by the Italian poet, Girolamo Fracastoro, under the title of "Syphilis sive Marbus Gallicus" (Syphilis, or the French Disease). The protagonist of the poem is a shepherd named Syphilus, who broke his word to the god, Apollo, for which he was punished by a terrible disease. It is worth noting that from the time of appearance of the aforementioned poem, until use of the term syphilis became common, 100 years passed, although the term really did not begin to be commonly used until the eighteenth century. Girolamo Fracastoro is a figure of interest in the history of medicine as he was not only a talented poet, mathematician, astronomer and geographer, but, first of all, a physician. His work from 1546, under the title of *De Contagione* (On Contagion), is the first serious description of typhus fever, while this author of the poem about the shepherd, Syphilus, also undertook treating the disease, which owes its current name to him. The recent discovery in the collection of the National Gallery in London of a portrait of Fracastorius by Titian, known for his numerous portraits of sovereigns and representatives of the higher aristocracy of this period, gave impulse to suppositions that this sixteenth century painter also was a patient of Fracastoro, who was supposed to have treated him for syphilis, the portrait mentioned supposedly payment for services bestowed. (2) This hypothesis, however, appears to me to be of little probability, taking into consideration the long and productive life of Titian, who died at close to 90 years of age.

As I already mentioned, fear of syphilis was associated not only with the disease itself – which had a significantly more stormy course initially than now and often ended in death – but equally, with the fact of little effectiveness in its treatment, which, not uncommonly, was worse than the disease. People were afraid of those ill with lues, while centers that undertook their treatment – I do not want to call them hospitals – were usually located outside the perimeters of towns, in order not to infect their inhabitants through contact with the sick. The average period of stay in such an institution did not exceed two months, although some patients were held longer there, even over a year, while the mortality among patients with syphilis was 16-24%, which is not at all a bad outcome for those times. (3) It seems that, by the end of the sixteenth century and in subsequent years, syphilis had an apparently less dramatic course than at the beginning of the pandemic. This could have been related to a lesser virulence of the germ, which, as the result of multiple passages from patient to patient, was becoming ever less aggressive, as well as of a certain tidying up of methods of treatment, which were becoming more varied and less toxic for the patient.

To the same extent that fear of lues was no longer the same as earlier, feelings of shame and the accompanying wish to hide its signs, plus the fact of the disease, became that much more important. Many ill persons manifesting skin lesions on exposed parts of the body did not leave their houses until they had remitted. Tons of powder masked blemishes on the face, while huge hats covered lesions on the head. At the cusp of the sixteenth and seventeenth centuries, there appeared in France a mode for wigs, which permitted hiding signs on the head, such as rashes or balding associated with secondary syphilis, or of subsequent treatment with mercury. Not all are of the opinion that the mode for wigs was the result of constantly increasing numbers of those ill with syphilis, and stress that usually famous and influential persons dictated what is *en vogue*, styles that the rest of the people then tried to imitate. Examples of monarchs from this period who wore wigs were Elizabeth I, Queen of England, and the King of France, Louis XIII, the latter starting to wear a wig when he lost his hair while very young. The mode for wigs was supported by Louis XIV, who not only had poor hair, but even worse teeth, which he lost completely even before completing age 40. In several places, I found information that the last-named monarch could have lost his hair and teeth as the result of anti-syphilitic treatment – this was not confirmed in more serious works, however. Besides the mode for wigs, which sovereigns and those suffering from syphilis made popular, there were also other reasons for wearing them; let us call them of a hygienic nature. One of these was the need for getting rid of the then very common, head lice, as well as of pubic lice (the latter of which are currently on the list of Sexually Transmitted Diseases). Shaving the head and wearing a wig allowed its owner to save a lot of the time associated with combing out or catching lice, while if any of these parasites were found in the wig itself, one could get rid of them by immersing it in boiling water. In the battle with pubic lice, loin (pubic) wigs, popularly known as "merkins," turned out to be very practical. Apparently, they were known even from the mid-fifteenth century, while from the time of the beginning of the syphilis pandemic, they were used mainly by prostitutes, who by this means were able to hide from their clients the signs of syphilis in the genital region. This type of wig (merkin) is also in use today, mainly by women of the Far East, and treated as genital adornment, with the goal of heightening the sexual attractiveness of their wearers. Somewhat different merkins, are used by male actors taking part in erotic scenes, in order to hide signs of arousal that cannot be shown on the screen.

Returning to head wigs, this mode ended at the end of the eighteenth century, mainly as a result of the French Revolution and its condemnation of everything associated with the aristocracy. In England, however, extinction of the wig mode is associated with the introduction, by the British government, of drastic increases in taxes on the powder with which they were sprinkled. If that, in fact, was the case, it would be yet another proof that the syphilis epidemic had little connection with the mode for wigs, although in the nineteenth century the number of cases of lues did not decrease; on the contrary, they rose.

Writing about the fear of syphilis, one cannot close one's eyes to the fact that it was unscrupulously taken advantage of by charlatans taking care of the sick, but also – and I acknowledged this with shame – by some physicians. It had to do, first of all, with obtaining patients, on whom unnecessary procedures were performed, or to whom were sold useless medicines produced by the culprits. For this purpose, they published hair-raising accounts of the sufferings of those ill with syphilis, while simultaneously telling people that they possessed medicines, which in an almost miraculous manner would relieve them of their sickness. The authors of this type of texts took advantage of the need to maintain private the fact of having the disease, underlining that, inasmuch as the medicines recommended by themselves could be taken in the quiet of the home, the patient's full privacy would be guaranteed. One of such authors was J. Smyth MD (about whose qualifications there can be doubts), who, in his publication, lauded a substance patented by himself, called "Smyth's Specific Drops," as a tested treatment for venereal diseases as well as those of nervous origin. (4) Another businessman advertising his products was the French physician, Nicholas Christier de Thy, who sold his medicine in England under the name of "Water of Safety," advertised as being effective even in the most advanced manifestations of venereal diseases. (5) To patients who did not fancy treatment with mercury, Dr. Isaac Swainson recommended an alternative treatment with a "Velnos Vegetable Syrop" that lacked this metal, asserting that he "could cure the most extreme cases of penis ulcerations in patients who had been condemned ... to the knife by surgeons." (6)

A great deal of knowledge on the subject of venereal diseases in eighteenth century London we owe to the memoirs of James Boswell, a Scottish lawyer and intellectual, whose stay in the capital of the British Empire was associated with multiple infections, most likely only with gonorrhea (Fig.7.3). Boswell wrote about himself that "I am of a warm constitution: a complexion, as physicians say, exceedingly amorous, and, therefore suck in the poison more deeply." (7) Regardless of any apparent inborn susceptibility to venereal diseases, Boswell did everything to infect himself multiple times! As he wrote in 1760-69, he had sexual contact with three well-born women, four actresses, romanced the mistress of J.J. Rouseau while having three of his own, and also added relations with at least 60 street prostitutes in between. (8) Boswell is said to have been infected with gonorrhea, and that, from 13-19 times, which appears to me rather exaggerated, although some of these infections could have been relapses or complications of the same infection. Testifying to this is the fragment of his memoirs cited earlier, in which he wrote:

I have had two visitations of this calamity. The first lasted ten weeks. The second, four months. How severe a reflection is it! And, O, how severe a prospect! Yet let me take courage. Perhaps this is not a very bad infection, and as I shall be scrupulously careful of myself. I may get rid of it in a short time. (7)

Boswell's reaction regarding the course of the disease may indicate that its author most likely had gonococcal epididymitis (note from memoir dated February 4, 1763): "I had been very bad all night, I lay in direful apprehension that my testicle, which formerly was ill, was again swelled." (9)

Complications of gonorrhea in the pre-antibiotic era were very frequent and, most probably, Boswell was a victim of them, although manifold infections with gonorrhea as are attributed to him may have been re-occurrences or complications of the same infection. Boswell was lucky, as he probably, did not infect himself with syphilis, something indicated by the methods of treatment used by his physician, a Dr. Douglas. Boswell himself, as an experienced patient, was able to diagnose his gonorrhea, writing, for example, that he "had a meeting with Signor Gonorrhea," (10) not calling his ailments syphilis or the then still popular alternate name for syphilis, "the pox." Another thing, though, is that in Boswell's time, the two diseases were not differentiated well, and gonorrhea was often considered to be a milder form of syphilis.

Boswell, in opposition to other authors of the time, was aware of the fact that, if ill with a venereal disease, one could infect a sexual partner. (11) Not all were as smart, while some frankly considered that the source of the infection were exclusively women, first of all prostitutes for whom "venereal disease is a permanent state, while for men it was something foreign and temporary." Some went even farther in their misogyny, suggesting that women are capable of regenerating syphilis and conveying it to men:

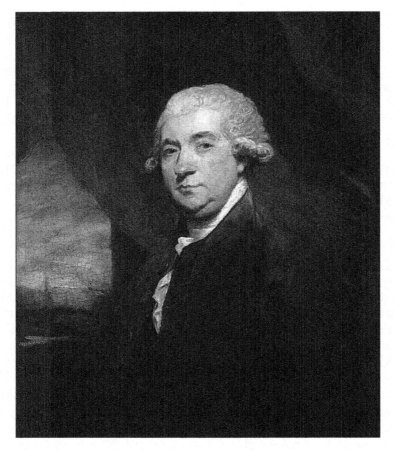

Figure 7.3 Portrait of James Boswell of Auchinleck (1785)by Joshua Reynolds

Women's sexual passivity and the 'delicate' nature of their sexual organs both of which were governed by nature and determined by the biology of their bodies, were thought to make them actually capable of generating syphilis and transmitting it to numerous men. The uteruses of loose women naturally labored to produce disease rather than progeny. (12)

In addition to this sort of fantastic ideas, there also appeared, at the same time, completely sensible opinions declaring that infected women were symptomlessly ill (asymptomatic) more often than men – which recommends that men be particularly careful in contacts with prostitutes.

Such opinions Boswell voiced also, publishing maxims of the type: "To avoid the 'plague of Venus', men need to be more careful consumers." (13,14) Unfortunately, despite the fact that he himself used condoms (made from animal intestines), he did not protect himself against numerous possible infections—luckily for him probably only with gonorrhea.

The first half of the nineteenth century did not bring any major changes in the perception of syphilis, either among those infected or the public at large. About how those ill, their families and friends reacted to the news of having become infected with syphilis, I wrote especially in the biographies of the nineteenth century artists who were sick with the lues. Some of them accepted the fact with blusterous resignation or reacted with dark humor at the news of what they were ill with. Although, among their closest friends they did not hide – or could not hide – the fact of their infection, very scant information about their health reached public knowledge, and everywhere, referring to the illness by its name was avoided like fire, euphemisms being depended on instead. I will only recall the journal of the brothers Goncourt from the nineteenth century, whose many objects of description suffered from syphilis, and in which are found accounts of its signs or symptoms – yet the name of the disease, which would have informed the reader of what a described person suffered from or died of, is nowhere to be found. Avoidance of the name, syphilis, itself applies not only to literature or letter writing, since, I will remind the reader, even in private letters written about an ill person, the name of the disease was avoided. The same applies to medical documentation, in which a diagnosis of syphilis was usually not given or was in time removed, so that in medical records available today, one can rarely find the name of this disease, despite everyone knowing of what a prominent artist suffered or died. Even in death certificates, the name, syphilis, was not always used, rather being limited to formulas saying that the cause of death was cessation of heart function, or a cerebral hemorrhage, thus avoiding the name of the underlying disease.

Physicians treating those sick with lues tried to protect their patients from defamation, of which the best proof was the custom of not bowing to patients on the street, in order not to expose them to gossip. This was particularly important in small communities, as everyone knew what illnesses a physician would be treating. An example of a physician who was concerned about the good name of his patients was Dr. David Gruby, mentioned earlier, who treated Guy de Maupassant, and, even before that, Heinrich Heine, the German poet living in Paris (Fig.7.4). Dr. Gruby, who first diagnosed syphilis in Heine (the poet had been treated earlier for something else), visited his patients travelling in a carriage without windows, with but one opening in its roof. (15)

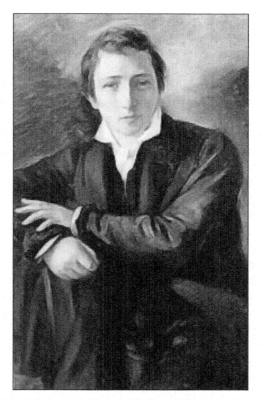

Figure 7.4 Portrait of Heinrich Heine (1831) painted by Moritz Daniel Oppenheim

During the second half of the nineteenth century, several bits of new information about syphilis appeared. Thanks to the work of Alfred Fournier, patients with *general paresis* and *tabes dorsalis* learned that their symptoms and signs were caused by syphilis. At that time, almost every 5th patient in psychiatric hospitals was there as a result of *general paresis*, while signs of *tabes dorsalis* were attributed to such diseases as rheumatism, gastric ulcer disease, a variety of diseases of the visual apparatus or neurologic problems not associated with syphilis. Confirmation of syphilis as the etiology of general paresis and *tabes dorsalis*, in association with the mistaken concept of "genetically transmitted congenital syphilis," increased the already great fear of the disease. At more or less the same time, there appeared a new theory, which, had it been shown to be accurate, could have produced true panic among those sick with lues. This theory stated that leprosy was the fourth stage of syphilis! It gained adherents during the second half of the nineteenth century, mostly in America, and produced a certain degree of consternation, equally in the medical world as among patients. Both syphilis and leprosy belonged among diseases stigmatizing patients, who not only feared and were shamed by them, but were also the objects of a certain type of harassment. Particularly leprosy, known from biblical times, was a disease that engendered a general fear, which caused those with leprosy to be banned from society and isolated in closed facilities, often on distant islands, the so-called leprosorias. In the 1980s, I was a member of a group testing the effectiveness of a trial vaccine developed with funding by the World Health Organization (W.H.O.). As a result, I received additional education and training at the National Hansen's Disease Center in Carville, Louisiana, where I saw cases of the disease (which is rare in the U.S.A.), and learned about its history, methods of treatment and prevention. On the grounds of the Carville Center, there still lived long-term patients of this institution under a *de facto* form of voluntary isolation, which was a help to sick people discarded by society. That even modern society greatly fears, yet knows very little on the subject of leprosy (Hansen's disease), I learned from my own experience. Thus, having as an assignment the testing of the value of a new, trial vaccine containing killed leprosy bacteria, we were to evaluate whether giving it to selected volunteers would increase resistance to the disease, as measured by the so-called lepromin skin test. The first volunteers were physicians taking part in the experiment, which required mutual injection of the appropriate dose of test vaccine into the skin. The local reaction to the injection was the appearance of discoloration and small scars on the upper arm, which, with time, would become reduced, or completely disappeared. By chance, at the time, I was invited with my family to lunch at some friends, who lived in an apartment complex with a large swimming pool. While swimming in the pool, which had a large number of people in it, I was asked by one of the swimmers where I had got three small, but easily visible scars. I replied truthfully that they were scars from a vaccine against leprosy, which evoked a certain degree of consternation. After a short time, I noticed that my daughter and I were the only ones swimming, while the people sunning themselves on lawn chairs all around had started to leave. After a few days, my friend who invited us telephoned me with the information that he had received a visit from the manager of the apartment house, to whom one of the tenants had turned with the complaint that people who had contact with leprosy were being invited to the pool that was used by both adults and children! I cite this story only to show how badly, even in the tw[entieth] century, people feared leprosy – and do so still – despite the fact that the disease has been curable already for several decades, while also acknowledged as one of the least infectious of the bacterial diseases.

The idea that leprosy is the fourth stage of lues, I came upon in a film that I saw on a religious television channel. There was a scene, in which a priest undergoing medical examination was ordered to raise his habit and lower his trousers, while the examining physician looked for signs of some disease – one can conclude venereal – in the area of the genitals. This intrigued me, and I then saw the film in its entirety, thanks to which I learned about the concept that leprosy is or could be the fourth stage of syphilis! I am overlooking an error in the scenario, which probably had not had the benefit of a consultation with a venereologist, suggested by the fact that looking for signs of third or fourth stage syphilis in the area of the genitals makes no sense, as only in early syphilis do signs of the disease appear in this area, and they remit without leaving any trace. Regardless of the apparent error that I mentioned, the film brought to my mind a certain truth, which could have been very alarming for those with lues, who could have felt threatened by the prospect of being isolated in a manner similar to that imposed on those ill with leprosy. The film that I mentioned was *Father Damian*, which described the history of the work of the Belgian priest, Joseph de Veuster (Fr. Damian), who devoted his life to those suffering from leprosy and isolated on the Hawaiian island of Molokai. Working closely with the sick, he became infected with leprosy, and died as a result of it. In 2009, Fr. Damian, who is called the "Apostle of the Lepers," or the "Leper Priest," was canonized by Pope John Paul II, becoming one of the few "American" saints. Although of Belgian origin, St. Damian is characterized as the 10th of the few American saints, having lived, worked and died within the U.S.A. I will remind the reader at this point that another – although not saintly – person, also accused of having leprosy, was Paul Gaugin, whose skin changes, at a certain stage of his disease, were suggestive of that disease. Or maybe, the idea that leprosy was the fourth stage of syphilis could have already reached Tahiti?

Fortunately, the hypothesis of leprosy being the fourth stage of syphilis did not find confirmation in the facts, and those ill with the latter avoided compulsory isolation in syphilisorias, although their status otherwise did not undergo any real change as a result. They continued to be treated as different from other ill people, as they were considered to have been responsible for own disease, and that what had befallen them was a deserved punishment. It wasn't enough that hospitals in which syphilitics were treated were situated at a distance from the town centers, but even the wards and their furnishings were far worse than those in which others were treated. This was not just in the early times of the pandemic, but also in modern times, as there has hardly been an instance of a venereology department that I have been able to visit, and that in various countries, where they were not customarily situated in distant, less representative parts of the hospital building. Outpatient venereal disease clinics have often been situated in buildings close to police stations, or, in the case of a clinic for prostitutes in one of the European capitals, in the building that also housed an "alcohol recovery room."

Another proof of the inferior treatment of those ill with venereal diseases was the avoidance by highly placed persons of visiting wards treating them. The custom of visiting the sick in hospitals has a long history, while those doing the visiting were commonly kings or their consorts wives, or representatives of the highest aristocracy. This type of activity augmented popularity among their subjects, or provided a sense of satisfaction in performing good deeds. Yet, one count on the fingers of one hand the visitation of wards of those sick with venereal diseases, even though this former type of activity did not stop during times of other epidemic infectious diseases. The Empress Elizabeth (Sissi), wife of the Emperor of Austro-Hungary, Franz Joseph, liked to visit the sick in hospitals to speak with them and to bring them presents. She was even so brave that at the time of the cholera epidemic of 1874, she visited the hospital in Munich, where she squeezed the hand of one of the patients, which was considered very risky because of the possibility of infection. (16)

I did not, however, find information anywhere saying that Sissi visited wards for syphilitics, although one could have expected that from her greater sympathy for people touched by this particular disease. Sissi wrote poems, while her poetry guru was Heinrich Heine, whom she tried to emulate. In her villa on the Greek island of Corfu, she placed a statue of Heine, who was described by those who saw him as having visible signs of the disease. Heine became infected with syphilis even in his youth, while the last years of his life he spent confined to his bed as a result of a serious form of *tabes dorsalis*. (15)

Speaking of the overt discrimination against the venereally diseased, it has to be added that even the specialization of dermatovenereology has often been considered as something inferior. Frequently, Jewish doctors, for whom it was difficult to specialize in other areas of medicine undertook the specialty. In fact, because among venereologists there were many Jews, the popularity of this disease among adherents to Judaism, resulted on their being blamed for the spread of the disease in Europe, even at the beginning of the pandemic and German Nazis claimed syphilis and typhus to be diseases spread by the Jews. An important role in this propaganda must be attributed to Hitler, himself, who, in *Mein Kampf*, the bible of the Nazis, blamed the Jews for the dissemination of disease and repeated mistaken views of the inescapable hereditary nature of syphilis, the inevitable consequences of which would reach to the 10th generation. Hitler's hatred of the Jews was said to have originated from the fact that in his youth, some Jewish prostitute was supposed to have infected him with a venereal disease, most probably gonorrhea.

I cannot say that discrimination against those venereally ill was the typical characteristic of totalitarian regimes, although there seems to be something to that. Visiting institutions treating those with venereal diseases in Moscow in the 1980s, I learned that, in the USSR (Union of Soviet Socialist Republics), those ill with syphilis were treated differently than other patients. First of all, in the (former) USSR, statistics pertaining to venereal diseases were not released to the public. These data were secret, and known only to select officials on the level of the Ministry of Health and, doubtless, the KGB. The physicians with whom I came in contact had some knowledge on the subject, but were not able to share their private observations with me, as only rarely did I have the opportunity to be with them privately. The method of treatment of syphilis in the USSR was different than in Europe and America at that time, as these diseases were treated with multi-week injections of crystalline penicillin several times daily. When I asked, somewhat in jest, whether the patients, mostly young people, weren't bored with being in the hospital for the long time required, the response was, no, as the patients had the obligation of working in the hospital, which filled their free time. I must have had a very surprised look on my face, as my respondents began nervously to explain that these were light tasks, which did not interfere with the treatment process. To my question why crystalline penicillin, which must be given intramuscularly several times daily, was used, and not procaine penicillin, which is given once daily, or long-acting Benzathine Penicillin G , which is given once weekly, I was told that it was done for the good of the patient, something that could not be said about capitalist public health, where the period of treatment was the shortest possible, in order to "get rid of the patient cheaply!" The fact is that crystalline penicillin enters the cerebrospinal fluid better than procaine penicillin or long-acting penicillin, but it is also true that this does not translate in any way into an increased number of late syphilis cases in countries where lues is treated with one or three injections (depending on the stage of the disease) of long-acting penicillin. The backwardness and archaic methods of treatment I found in the former USSR were caused by a certain isolation of the medical community there, as Soviet physicians rarely took part in international educational conferences – to which party activists or staff bureaucrats were the ones most often sent, and not professional physicians. During private contacts, my Soviet colleagues showed themselves to be wise and intelligent people, who were aware of the backwardness in which they remained in respect to the West, and questioned me about modern diagnostic and therapeutic methods that existed then in Western Europe and the U.S.A.

Writing about the relations between those ill with syphilis and the rest of society, one cannot ignore the role of prostitution in the spread venereal diseases. Boswell and his contemporaries wrote about this, as did authors both earlier and later. (17,18,19) Many defenders of this oldest profession in the world explained that prostitutes are necessary, based on their services, as were then considered to prevent the dangers of onanism! (20) Concerning the relationship of society to prostitution in the nineteenth century, the chapters of this book devoted to known artists from this period who were ill with syphilis, are quite informative. Most of them sporadically, and some, regularly, availed themselves of the services of prostitutes, and unfortunately, many of them paid for that with a loss of health and, often, of life. Naturally, the great artists were not the only clients of women employed in prostitution, and practically every male could buy sexual services that they could afford. I wish to stress that male prostitutes bestowing services to homosexuals were a rarity then, as were male prostitutes bestowing services upon women, about which practically nothing is written. Neglected wives made do in more traditional ways, romancing valets, neighbors or friends of their husbands, who at the same time frequented bordellos.

Over the course of history, a variety of attempts to liquidate or limit prostitution have been undertaken, but all actions in this direction have ended, sooner or later, in failure. One of the most important reasons for these types of undertakings was the fact that prostitutes were and still are a source of infection with venereal diseases. Over the course of centuries, the relationship of the law to this oldest profession in the world ranged, often radically, from very restrictive, brutal rules, to complete absence of control. Current jurisdiction relating to prostitution is also extremely varied, even in countries that are similar from the point of view of tradition or culture. In the U.S.A., for example, with the exception of one state, prostitution is punishable—the prostitutes being punished in all states, while both prostitutes and their clients in some. It must be admitted that the guardians of the law apply these rules with great reluctance, recognizing the low effectiveness of their actions. In European countries, prostitution is generally legal, and in some of them, for instance, most recently, Germany and Switzerland, there are attempts to make life easier, not only for the prostitutes and their clients, but also for the inhabitants of neighborhoods in which such services have been bestowed. A good example of such an approach are actions by the authorities in Zurich (Switzerland), in which, in order to move prostitutes from the center of town, they constructed "accommodations " something of the type of open garages, where one can park a car, have a place to lie down, a small table, a toilet and a bathroom with a shower. The room is equipped with an alarm system that the woman can use, in case the client were to threaten her in any way. On the walls of these rooms hang posters reminding of the advantages of using condoms, while in the neighborhood nearby, volunteers work in shifts, ready to provide assistance in case the prostitute or her clients were to need help. In some European countries, prostitution is taxed, which assures these women health insurance, as well as a right to a pension. In the majority of European countries, deriving advantage from prostitution by a third person (pimping) is punishable, as are utilizing underage prostitution, forcing into prostitution and human trafficking.

Hundreds of volumes have been written about prostitution, but this subject interests me solely in its epidemiologic aspects. It is obvious that for this group of women, venereal diseases are occupational diseases, and all actions must be undertaken that will allow the limitation of infections in this environment. One should put stress on the use of condoms and create organizational forms facilitating access of prostitutes to public health units that undertake the treatment of diseases transmitted by the sexual route. Very important is the conduct of informational campaigns to educate prostitutes about the signs and symptoms of venereal diseases, and enable them to identify signs of disease in their clients and themselves, and encourage early consultation of a physician. I believe that all attempts at penalizing women working in prostitution are unnecessary, and as history has already shown, are ineffective, while attempts at including criminal law only make control of prostitution more difficult, and are taken by these women as unnecessary harassment.

Looking at matters related to sex, it is not difficult to note that attempts at placing them into the arms of the law do not always end happily; even in countries considered modern and observant of human rights, one can find anachronistic or bizarre legal rules, and laws, which, fortunately, are not always observed. No one will be surprised if they read that in some countries of the Near East women, and more rarely men, are punished for such transgressions as fornication, cohabitation, adultery, and oral or anal sex. I think, however, that many readers will be surprised when they learn that even in highly developed country, one can go to prison for the same things. Depending on the state, severe punishments are threatened even for oral or anal sex with one's own wife, and for sex between cohabiting homosexuals. (21) The following is an example how this laws are observed: Among my patients at the V.D. clinic I had two homosexual policemen, who would come from time to time for a checkup. They were dressed in civilian clothes, but in conversations with me, they did not hide their profession. During one of their visits I decided to test their knowledge on this subject. While taking their medical histories, I asked the standard questions about the dates and types of their last sexual contacts, to which I received replies that had to be noted in their medical records. They stated that they had both oral and anal contacts, exclusively with men. When I showed them a publication containing information that, in the state where they were living, they were subject to up to five years in jail and/or a fine of $200 for their type of sexual activities, they did not want to believe their own eyes. I calmed them, by saying that the information they were giving me was covered by privacy within the physician-patient relationship, and that I had not the slightest intention of taking it to the police! I did add, however, that, regardless of the physician's confidentiality obligating us both, upon receiving a court order, our clinic would have to provide access to the information given by them. They did not seem especially worried by this, but probably came to the conclusion that it was not worth the risk, as I did not see them again. I also checked the status of legal requirements with the administration of our clinic, asking the director whether I would be required to inform the police myself, or whether I should delegate to one of the staff the fact that I had patients who had volunteered that they practiced oral and anal sex. The director looked at me very strikingly, as though to check whether the one asking the question needed psychiatric help, as every other patient of our clinic provided this type of information. When I showed her the publication saying that in our state such a law was in force, she was as surprised as the policemen just mentioned. She affirmed that at some time, in some place, she had heard something about this, but that it appeared to her that it did not actively pertain to our state. I asked some attorney friends, among whom some were equally surprised, while others knew something about it, and explained to me that this law had been passed over a hundred years ago, was currently not enforced, and was thus known as a so-called "dead law." I wish to calm the readers that such draconian laws are not in place in every state, and where they are, they are generally "dead." This does not change the fact, however, that should a sexual partner, or even a husband or a wife want to put his or her "other half" in jail, all that would be necessary would be to document the performance by one of them of the relations mentioned earlier (oral or anal), or as is described in legal language, of an "abominable and detestable crime against nature" (21) in order to be rid of a partner for some time. As a conclusion to this description of an attempt at control by law within the sphere of sexual life, I will remind the reader that in over a dozen states, the law obliges punishment for sex "between a man and a woman who are not married to one another." (21) I understand that this information may produce anxiety in some of my readers, but will try to calm them by suggesting that these are usually "dead laws." Yet, how else can one understand the old Latin proverb, *"Dura lex sed lex?"*

As a conclusion to considerations on the subject of the fear and shame of syphilis, I wanted to share my own observations on this phenomenon, i. e., the observations of a physician dealing with venereal diseases at the end of the twentieth and the beginning of the twenty-first centuries. As I already wrote, the introduction of penicillin to the treatment of syphilis made it one of many diseases that can be relatively easily and quickly cured, under the condition that therapy is begun in the early period of the disease. Unfortunately, that is not always what happens, as patients who learn about their disease many years after infection by accident, or sometimes by appropriately applied serologic testing. There are not too many of these patients, and they most often are without signs of late syphilis, inasmuch as modern use and abuse of antibiotics results in its inadvertent treatment, although not always cure, by chance. The old belief in the incurability of this disease has gone into oblivion, although, in rare cases, may remind us of itself.

The diagnosis of syphilis (lues) is established on the basis of signs of the disease, and confirmed by the results of laboratory testing, that is, tests discovering, among other things, antibodies that are found in blood serum. These tests are more or less specific only for syphilis, and those, which are positive not only in syphilis, but, also in other diseases, such as, occasionally, malaria, leprosy (Hansen's disease), or certain diseases with an immunologic basis. Positive results not specifically due to syphilis (i.e. those due to non-luetic diseases) are generally weakly positive – which permits distinguishing them from cases of syphilis in which, depending on the duration of the disease, they are usually strongly positive. Additionally, there are other tests less commonly done that are very specific, and thus permit either the exclusion or confirmation of infection with lues. It also happens that after correctly conducted anti-syphilitic treatment, the results of some tests remain positive in some patients, but at a very low level, which does not indicate that the disease has not been entirely cured. This sometimes creates a problematic situation, as some patients become convinced that their disease has not been finally eradicated. There remains in my memory the history of one patient, who was referred to our institution for consultation for this actual reason. This patient had weakly positive results in standard testing, and despite having undergone treatment in a private doctor's office, and maybe even several penicillin treatments, did not attain complete negativity. Very exact testing done by us excluded infection with syphilis, and, despite his demanding further treatment, and even treatment of his wife, in whom all test results were negative, he was released home. We explained to him at some length that additional treatment in his case was groundless, and it appeared that he finally understood, as he was a well-educated teaching employee at the engineering college. Over a year later, I met his wife at a mall, and asked about her husband. She was dressed in black, but did not look like a person in mourning. I was mistaken, however, as she told me that several months earlier her husband had died, by suicide. I felt bad and a bit embarrassed, as I thought to myself that my former patient had taken his life in the belief that he had "an incurable form of syphilis." His widow dispersed my doubts, however, clarifying for me that her husband had been ill with depression, and that had been the cause of his suicide. She said also that her husband had had psychiatric problems for a long time, but had not informed us.

Belief in having incurable syphilis and fear of this disease are currently rare, what cannot be said about feelings of shame or a certain abashedness as a result of having become infected with a sexually transmitted disease. This is linked to the fact that infection is often the result of marital infidelity or of being untrue to a sexual partner, of sexual contact with a prostitute, alcohol intoxication, or also use of narcotics. Taking advantage of the literature, or, lately, more frequently of the Internet, patients learn that syphilis, and also other venereal diseases can be contracted by other than sexual routes, for instance use of common objects, by touch, or by use of public toilets. The last suggestion gave rise to an anecdote known to every physician involved with venereal diseases. "After being examined by a physician, a wife tells her husband that she has been diagnosed with syphilis, but assures him that she was never unfaithful to him, and that she most probably became infected in a public toilet which she had used recently. The unbelieving husband asks the doctor if one can be infected with syphilis in a toilet, to which the latter replies, that one can, but it's not very comfortable." One can laugh at this, but to venereologists it isn't always funny, as quite often they have to answer this type of question, knowing that the questioner really isn't joking. Asked the same or similar question many times, I would always answer in the affirmative, out of the conviction that, although rare, non-sexual infections are possible, and that it is not I who should decide the fate of someone's relationship. I also often saw that patients regret having committed mistakes, which made it easier to take this type of approach.

In mentioning the Internet, it should be stressed that it is currently the main source of information about venereal diseases for many people. This has a huge meaning in the battle against these diseases, as, thanks to it, a patient suspecting infection may go to a physician in a much earlier stage of the disease. This is invaluable, both from the epidemiologic perspective, as he or she does not infect new partners, and the therapeutic point of view, as, in the early period, it is easier to cure lues, often avoiding serious later complications. Obtaining knowledge on the subject of venereal diseases exclusively from the Internet also has its negative side, as the brevity of information included there, and the impossibility of discussing it with a specialist (discussions on so-called fora/forums does not fulfill this role) causes us to have many patients at VD clinics, who go there due to a blemish on the skin of the genitalia, or burning upon urination, convinced that they have become infected with syphilis or gonorrhea, while not having these diseases. Despite everything, though, every physician prefers that a patient presents him- or herself even unnecessarily, rather than foregoing a visit in a case of genuine infection.

A different phenomenon associated with the Internet, is the somewhat changing clinical picture of venereal diseases, including syphilis, caused by the popularity of pornographic webpages, which propagate a variety of forms of performing sex, that are, let's say, distant from the traditional ones. Currently, every other patient, male or female, admits in his or her interviews, of participating in oral or anal sex, in addition to traditional (vaginal) relations. Formerly rare "rimming" or "fisting" are no longer as sporadic, while among women, use of a variety of mechanical toys (dildoes) while masturbating, is becoming increasingly prevalent. The appearance of various creams, ointments, and gels available on the market without prescription, which are supposed to potentiate sexual experiences, causes us to have to deal with formerly rarely observed signs or symptoms. Oral or anal sex, more and more frequently causes us to have to anticipate the appearance of primary luetic chancres on the lips or tongue, or likewise in the anal area, and that, not only among male homosexuals, but equally in women. More often than earlier, we observe patients presenting themselves as a result of injury in the genital and anal areas caused by teeth, mechanical toys or various attempts at genital adornment, associated with genital piercing, also equally in both women and men. (22)

The use of intimate gels causes allergic reactions in some patients, sometimes resulting in confusion with signs of venereal disease. (23) New anatomical discoveries and their popularization by the Internet, for example "point G," results in women presenting themselves to venerelogists or gynecologists with injuries to the anterior wall of the vagina caused by overly aggressive activity at this location by the partner, or during masturbation. I was told of a female patient who presented herself to a physician, convinced that she had syphilis, as she felt something like an ulcer in this area. Fortunately, this was not syphilis, while the ulceration on the anterior wall of the vagina was the result of scratching with long, artificial fingernails, such as women wear for decorative purposes. The inventiveness of patients searching for variety in their sexual life knows no bounds, whereas my citing examples concerning selective situations, in which patients infected themselves with syphilis in a non-traditional way or suspected syphilis in themselves, which was, in fact, a sequel to uncommon sexual practices, does.

In conclusion, I would like to relate an incident of which I was a witness, if not to say a participant, which took place in the late 1990s. One day, a patient presented himself to me with the complaint that, some time earlier, red spots had appeared on the skin of his penis and abdomen, and also enlarged nodes in his groin. He was very anxious and asked me what I thought about all this. I told him that I would reply to his question immediately after receiving the results of the blood test that we had drawn earlier. Consistent with my supposition, the RPR (Rapid Plasma Reagin) test was strongly positive, indicating that I was dealing with a patient with secondary syphilis. After his return to the office, I notified him that I had bad news for him, as he had syphilis, and that we would have to treat him with penicillin. In response to my words, the patient jumped from his chair, and threw himself at me, hugging and patting, then kissing me; he performed several circuits of the office with me in a dance that was reminiscent of something between a waltz and a polka. When, after a few minutes, he calmed down and was again seated on his chair, he informed me that he was delighted, and that he had never felt as happy as at the moment that I had told him that he had syphilis. For several days, he had walked around terribly depressed, as his friend (who was a hospital employee) had told him that the signs he had, indicated an infection with the HIV virus!

This occurrence apprised me of the change and evolution that have occurred in the attitude toward lues – a disease, which has taken millions of human beings from this world; a disease, the diagnosis of which had been a sentence of death or crippling for so long. Syphilis has been dethroned and replaced by other venereal disease such as AIDS. And in that very moment I thought to myself that 500 years had to pass for a diagnosis of syphilis not to frighten a patient but evoke joy and relief!

REFERENCES

Chapter 1

1. Simon Wiesenthal. "Sails of Hope," McMillan Publishing Co., Inc., New York. 1973. p. 139

2. Jakow Swiet. "Columbus" (translated from the Russian). National Publishing Institute, Warsaw 1982. p. 45.

3. Ibid. p. 63

4. Laurence Bergreen. "Columbus, the Four Voyages." Published by Viking Penguin. 2011. p. 70.

5. Manuel Fernandez Alvarez. "Izabela Katolicka" (Original title "Isabel la Catolica"). National Publishing Institute, Warsaw. 2003. p. 306.

6. Felipe Fernandez-Armesto." Columbus." Oxford University Press. 1991. p. 74.

7. Charles Duff." The Truth about Columbus and the discovery of America." Jarrolds, London. 1957. p. 149.

8. Claude Quetel. "*Niemoc z Neapolu czyli historia syfilisu.*" (The Sickness from Naples, or the History of Syphilis) (Original title, "*Le mal de Naples. Histoire de la syphilis.*" Translated from the French by Zofia Podgorska-Klawe), published by the Ossolineum National Foundation. Wroclaw, 1991, p. 36.

9. *Ibid.* pp. 59-60.

10. *Ibid.* p. 60.

11. Fernandez Oviedo, *in* Laurence Bergreen," Columbus". Viking Penguin 2011 p. 158.

12. Ambroise Pare, *in* Claude Quetel, *op. cit.*p. 46.

13. Claude Quetel, *op. cit.*, p.47.

14. Jean Fernel, *in* Claude Quetel, *op. cit.*, p. 72.

15. Claude Quetel, *op cit.*, pp. 51-53.

16. Tomasz F. Mroczkowski, Larry M. Millikan, Lawrence Parish. "Genital and Perianal Disease: A Color Handbook." CRS Press. 2013, sections 1 and 2.

17. Harper K.N., Ocampo P.S., Steiner B.M., *et al.*"On the origin of the Treponematoses. A Phylogenetic Approach." PLoS Neglected Tropical Diseases. Vol 2(1), Jan. 2008.

Chapter 2

1. Manuel Fernandez Alvarez. *"Izabela Katolicka."* (Original title *Isabel la Catolica*) National Publishing Institute, Warsaw. 2003. p. 328.
2. *Ibid.* p. 330.
3. Rachel Erlanger. "Lucrezia Borgia, A Biography." Hawthorne Books, Inc. 1978. p. 50-51.
4. Mario Puzo. *"Rodzina Borgiow."* (*The Borgia Family*)Translation from the English. Albatross Publishers, Warsaw, 2003. p. 89.
5. *Ibid.* p. 108.
6. *Ibid.* p. 110.
7. *Ibid.* p. 113.
8. Ivan Cloulas. „*Cezar Borgia, Syn Papieza, Ksiaze i Awanturnik.*" (Original title: *Cesar Borgia. Fils de Pape, Prince et Aventurier*) (Cezar Borgia, the Pope's Son, Prince and Adventurer). National Publishing Institute, Warsaw, 2005. pp.36-38.
9. *Ibid.* p. 40.
10. *Ibid.* p. 42.
11. Claude Quetel, *op.cit.* p. 15.
12. *Ibid.* p. 19.
13. Ivan Cloulas, *op.cit.* pp. 60 and 140.
13A. Rachel Erlanger, *op.cit.* pp. 300, 307, 322.
14. Ivan Cloulas. *op.cit.* p. 66.
15. Mario Puzo. *op.cit.* pp. 220-225.
16. *Ibid.* p. 259.
17. Rafael Sabatini. "The Life of Cesare Borgia." Houghton Mifflin Co. 1924. p. 158.
18. Mario Puzo. *op.cit.* p. 198.
19. *Ibid.* p. 300.

20. Tomasz F. Mroczkowski. "Sexually Transmitted Diseases." Igaku-Shoin Medical Publishers, Inc. 1990. Chapter 8, Syphilis, p. 164.
21. Ivan Cloulas. *op.cit.* p. 106.
22. Mario Puzo. *op.cit.* p. 295.
23. Ivan Cloulas. *op.cit.* p. 108.
24. *Ibid.* pp. 143-148.
25. *Ibid.* p. 165.
26. Claude Quetel. *op.cit.* pp. 16-23.
27. Parvi Rosaefontani, *Chronicon Johannis Regis Daniae.* 1560, *in* Claude Quetel. *op.cit.* p. 23.

Chapter 3

1. Sir George Pickering. Citation in T. Dormandy. "The White Death: A History of Tuberculosis," The Hambleton Press, London, 1999, p. 15.
2. Coradinus Gilinus. *De morbo quem gallicum nuncupant.* Ferrara, 1497, *in* Claude Quetel, *op.cit.* p.32.
3. Jahannis Widman from Tubingen. *Tractatus clarissimi medicinarum ... in* Claude Quetel, *op.cit.* p. 32.
4. Gasparis Torellae. *Tractatus cum cosiliis (contra) pudendagram, seu morbum Gallicum.* Rome, 1497. *in* Claude Quetel, *op.cit.* p. 33.
5. Cataneus, *in* w Claude Quetel, *op.cit.* p. 43.
6. Claude Quetel, *op.cit.* p. 98.
7. Michael J. O'Dowd. "The History of Medications for Women." Materia Medica Woman. New York 2001 p. 116. Cited *in* Robert Weston, Epistolary Consultations on Venereal Disease in Eighteenth Century France. p. 76, bibl. 39.
8. Claude Quetel, *op.cit.* p. 41.
9. Coradinus Gilinus, *op.cit.* p. 45.
10. Ambroise Pare *in* Claude Quetel, *op.cit.* p. 80.
11. Claude Quetel, *op.cit.* p. 44.

12. Manuel Fernandez Alvarez,"Emperor Charles V. A Man for Europe) (Original title *Carlos V. Un hombre para Europa*). National Publishing Institute. Warsaw. 2003. pp. 41-42.

12a. John Parascandola,"Sex, Sin and Science: A History of Syphilis in America." Praeger Publishers, 2008. p. 18.

12b. Richard M. Swiderski,"Quicksilver: A History of the Use, Lore and Effect of Mercury." McFarland nd Co., Inc. Publ. 2008. p. 95.

13. Ulrich von Hutten, *De guaiaci medicina et morbo gallico.*1519 *in* Claude Quetel, *op.cit.* p.39.

14. Sarsaparilla, http://www.herbco.com/c-179-sarsaparilla.aspx

14a. Jon Arrizabalaga, John Henderson, Roger French (editors),"The Great Pox: The French Disease in Renaissance Europe." 1997. p. 188.

15. Fallopio. *in* Claude Quetel, *op.cit.* p. 76.

16. Claude Quetel, *op.cit.* pp. 111-113.

17. *Ibid.* pp. 107-108.

18. *Ibid.* p. 124.

19. Giovanni Giacomo Casanova," Pamietniki" (Memoirs). Translation and selections by T. Evert. Siedmiogrod Publishers. Wroclaw, 1997.

19a. Lydia Flem. "Casanova The Man who loved Women". Translated by Catherine Temerson. Published by Ferrar, Straus, Giroux. New York. pp. 1113-114 and 180-183.

20. Uta Ranke-Heinemann. "No, and Amen" (original title *Nein und Amen. Anleitung zum Glaubenszweifel*). Publishing Agency URAEUS. Gdynia, 1994. p. 54.

21. Robert S. Morton., Evolution on venereology as a speciality. *In* Sexually Transmitted Diseases. King K. Holmes, Per-Anders Mardh, P. Frederick Sparling, Paul Wiesner (editors). McGraw-Hill Book Company. 1984. p. 30.

22. Andrzej Stapinski. "Fighting Syphilis and Gonorrhea in Poland." State Medical Publishers. Warsaw. 1979. p. 20.

22a. George R. Marek. "*Beethoven. Biografia Geniusza*" (original title: Beethoven: Biography of a Genius). National Publishing Institute. Warsaw, 1976. p. 318.

23. Mirabeau. *Observations d'un voyageur anglais sur la maison de force appelee ...* 1788. Citation *in* Claude Quetel, *op.cit.* pp. 127-128.

24. Claude Quetel. *op. cit.* pp.128-31.

25. *Ibid.* pp.132-133.

26. Rudolph H. Kampmeier. Early development of knowledge of sexually transmitted diseases. *In* Sexually Transmitted Diseases. King K. Holmes *et al* (editors) op.cit. p. 28.

27. *Ibid.* p. 26.

28. Claude Quetel. *op. cit.* p. 141.

29. *Ibid* pp. 142-143.

30. Homeopathy., http://en.wikipedia.org/wiki/Homeopathy

31. Syphilis: Symptoms, cause, diagnosis, homeopathic remedies & treatment, http://health.hpathy.com/syphilis-symptoms-treatment-cure.asp

31a. A. Lennox Thornburn, *Fritz Richard Schaudinn, 1872-1906.* Protozoolgist of syphilis. Brit.J.Vener.Dis. (1971) *47*:459.

32. Claude Quetel. *op.cit.* p. 174.

33. Molly Selvin. Changing medical and societal attitudes toward sexually transmitted diseases: A historical overview. *In* Sexually Transmitted Diseases. King. K. Holmes *et al.* op.cit. p. 6.

34. *Ibid.* p. 9.

35. Julius Wagner–Jauregg., http://www.whonamedit.com/doctor.cfm/2753.htmlJULES

36. Cynthia J. Tsay. Julius Wagner-Jauregg and the Legacy of Malaria Therapy for the Treatment of General Paresis of the Insane. Yale J. Biol. Med. 2013. *88*(2):245-254.

Chapter 4

1. Jean Molinet, Paris 1828. (*Chroniques de Jean Molinet*) in Claude Quetel, *Niemoc z Neapolu* ... etc. p.17.
2. A. Dickson Wright," Venereal Diseases and the Great." Brit. J. Vener. Dis. 1971, (47). pp. 295-306.
3. Pierre de Brantome." *Zywoty pan swawolnych* "(translated by Tadeusz (Boy) Zelenski). Warszawa. 1957
4. Alison Weir, "Mary Boleyn. The Mistress of Kings" Ballantine Books. The Random House Publishing Group. New York, 2011. p. 82-83
5. Manuel Fernandez Alvarez., "*Cesarz Karol V*" ("Emperor Charles V") (original title *"Carlos V, Un hombre para Europa."* National Publishing Institute. (Warsaw), 2003. p.91
6. *Ibid* p. 142.
7. *Ibid.* p. 272.
8. Molly Selvin." Changing medical and societal attitudes toward sexually transmitted diseases: A historical overview." *in* "Sexually Transmitted Diseases," Holmes K.K., Mardh P-A., Sparling P.F. Wiesner P.J. McGraw-Hill Book Company. 1984. p. 4.
9. George Bidwell., "*Rubaszny krol Hal*" (original title "Bluff King Hal"). *"Ksiaznica"* Publishers, Katowice, Poland, 2004.
10. Robert Hutchinson. *"Ostatnie lata Henryka VIII. Spiski i zdrady na dworze tyrana."* (original title "The Last Days of Henry VIII. Conspiracies, Treason and Heresy at the Court of the Dying Tyrant"). Wydawnictwo Amber.Sp.z.oo, 2005. p. 100.
11. *Ibid.* p.101.
12. *Ibid.* p.162.
13. Jerzy Besala. *"Najslynniejsze milosci krolow polskich"* ("The Most Famous Loves of Polish Kings"). Bellona SA Publishers, Warsaw, 2009. p. 211. (according to the text of Morsztyn.

14. *Ibid.* p. 213.
15. *Ibid.* p. 234. (*List Stefana Niemirycza do Fryderyka Wilhelma z 6 czrewca 1665 roku*) (Letter of June 6, 1665 from Stefan Niemirycz to Frederick Wilhelm)
16. *Ibid.* p. 238.
17. *Ibid.* p. 243.
18. Elwira Watala. "*Wielcy zboczency*" *Skandale Historii* ("Great Deviates." Scandals of History). "RYTM" Publishing Office, Warsaw. 2007. p. 149.
19. Laurence Brockliss and Colin Jones." Medical World of Early Modern France," p. 319.
20. Robert L. Weston. 2009, "Epistolary Consultations on Venereal Disease in Eighteenth-Century France," 2009. p. 72. *George Rudé Seminar*, http://www.h-france.net/rude/rudeTOC20092.html, 3,
21. Sain-Simon. "*Memoires.*" *La Pleiade*.vol.1, ch. XLIV *in* Claude Quetel "*Niemoc z Neapolu czyli historia syfilisu*" Ossolineum Publishers, Wroclaw, 1991. p. 118.
22. John T. Salvendy."*Buntownik z Mayerlingu. Portret psychologiczny arcyksiecia Rudolfa.*" (original title "The Royal Rebel. A psychological Portrait of Crown Prince Rudolf of Austria-Hungary." CZYTELNIK publishers, Warsaw. 1995. p. 194.
23. Brigitte Hamann. "*Cesarzowa Elzbieta*" ("The Empress Elizabeth") (original title "*Elisabeth Kaiserin wider Willen*" National Publishing Institute, Warsaw. 1999. p. 464.
24. Stanislaw Grodzinski. "*Franciszek Jozef I*" (Franz Joseph I). Ossolineum Publishers. Wroclaw, 1978. p.138.
25. Timothy Snyder. "*Czerwony Ksiaze*" (original title "The Red Prince: The Fall of a Dynasty and the Rise of Modern Europe." "*Swiat Ksiazki*" Publishers, Warsaw, 2010. p. 46.
26. Wladyslaw A. Serczyk. "*Katarzyna II*" ("Catherine II"). PLUS Publications LTD, London, 1995. p. 39.
27. R.S. Morton. "Did Catherine the Great of Russia have syphilis?" Genitourinary Medicine. 1991; *67*:498-502.

28. Wladyslaw A. Serczyk, *op.cit.* p. 8.
29. Ibid. p. 238.
30. Elwira Watala, *"Milosne igraszki rosyjskich caryc"* ("Love adventures of the Russian empresses"). "RYTM" publishing office, Warsaw, 2006. p. 426.
31. A. Dickson Wright. "Venereal diseases and the great." Brit. J. Vener. Dis. 1970. 47:303.

Chapter 5

1. Claude Quetel. *"Niemoc z Neapolu czyli historia syfilisu"* ("The Disease from Naples, or the History of Syphilis"). "Ossolineum." 1991. p.213
2. *Ibid.* p. 214.
3. Leon Daudet, *"Devant la douleur,"* publication from 1915. *In* Claude Quetel, *op. cit.*, p. 215.
4. A. Dickson Wright. "Venereal diseases and the great." British Journal of Venereal Diseases. 1971; 47:299.
5. Ralph G. Martin, "Jennie: The Life of Lady Randolph Churchill – The Romantic Years 1854-95," Vol. 1, Prentice-Hall Publishers. 1969

Chapter 5A

1. Michael Steen. *"Wielcy kompozytorzy i ich czasy"* (original title "The Lives and Times of the Great Composers"), "Rebis" Publishing House, Poznan (Poland). 2009. p. 237.
2. *Ibid.* p. 239
3. O.E.Deutsch. "Schubert: Memoirs by his friends." A. and C. Black, London. 1958. p. 131.
4. Newman Flower. "Franz Schubert" The Man and His Circle." Tudor Publishing Co., New York. 1939. p. 53
5. O.E. Deutsch. *in* Michael Steen, *op.cit.* p. 248.

6. *Ibid.* pp. 121,126.
7. Newman Flower, *op.cit.* p. 133.
8. Georg R. Marek. "Schubert." Viking Penguin Inc. 1985. p. 135.
9. Newman Flower. *Op. cit.* pp. 130-145.
10. Tomasz F. Mroczkowski."Sexually Transmitted Diseases. Chapter 8, "Syphilis." Igaku-Shoin Medical Publishers.1990. p. 183.
11. Michael Steen. *op. cit.* p. 252.
12. *Ibid.* p. 253.
13. Newman Flower, *op. cit.* p.169.
14. Michael Stein, *op. cit.* p. 258.
15. Maurice J. E. Brown. "Schubert" W. W. Norton and Co., New York (The New Grove). 1983. p. 67.
16. Alfred Einstein. "Schubert. A Musical Portrait." Oxford University Press, New York, 1951. p. 315.
17. Newman Flower. *op. cit.* p. 269.
18. *Ibid.* p. 271.
19. Michael Steen, *op. cit.* p. 324.
20. H. Weistock. "Donizetti and the World of Opera." Methuen, London, 1964 p. 105.
21. Enid Peschel and Richard Peschel. "Donizetti and the music of mental derangement: Anna Bolena, Lucia di Lammermoor, and the composer's neurobiological illness." Yale Journal of Biology and Medicine, 1992; 65:189-200.
22. Michel Steen, *op. cit.,* p. 326.
23. H. Weinstock. "Rossini: A Biography." Oxford University Press, London. 1968. p. 184.
24. R. Osborn. "Rossini." (Master Musicians). J. M. Dent Publishers. London 1986. p. 94.
25. Michael Steen, *op. cit.,* p. 331.
26. *Ibid.* p. 332.
27. Ronald Taylor. "Robert Schumann. His Life and Work." Universe Books. New York.1982. p. 56.
28. Michael Steen, *op. cit.,* p. 441.

29. Peter Ostwald. "Music and Madness." Gollancz , London. 1985. p. 42.

30. *Ibid.* p. 191.

31. J. Chissell. "Schumann." (Master Musicians), J.M. Dent Publishers, London. 1948. p. 12.

32. Eric Jensen. "Schumann." (Master Musicians). Oxford University Press, Oxford. 2001. p. 66.

33. Anton Neumayr, Vol II, p. 256 (citation in Deborach Hayden. 2003. p. 101.

34. Deborah Hayden. "Pox. Genius, Madness and the Mystery of Syphilis." Basic Books . 2003. p. 102.

35. Peter Ostwald, cited in Deborah Hayden. *op. cit. p.* 102.

36. Robert Taylor, *op. cit.* p. 69.

37. Deborah Hayden, *op. cit.* p. 104.

38. Eric Jensen, *op. cit.* p. 74.

39. Styra Avins. "Johannes Brahms.Life and Letters." Oxford University Press, Oxford. 1977. p. 759.

40. J. Chissell, cited in Michael Steen, *op. cit.*, p. 455.

41. Michael Steen, *op. cit.*, p. 455.

42. *Ibid.* p. 459.

43. J.Chissell, *op. cit.*, p. 460.

44. Michael Steen, *op. cit.*, p. 462.

44a. H. Nogushi and J.W. Moore. "A demonstration of *Treponema pallidum* in the brain in cases of general paresis," Journal of Experimental Medicine. 1913

45. Claude Quetel, *op. cit.*, p. 201.

46. Michael Steen, *op. cit.*, p. 463.

47. Ronald Taylor, *op. cit.*, p. 327

48. Michael Steen, *op. cit.*, p. 465.

49. Allan Walker *et al.* "Robert Schumann. The Man and His Music." Harper and Row Publishers, Inc. 1974, pp. 412-414.

50. Franz Hermann Franken, cited in Deborah Hayden, *op. cit.*, p. 100.

51. J. Clapham. ""Smetana" (Master Musicians). J.M. Dent , London. 1972. p. 24.
52. *Ibid.* p. 43.
53. *Ibid.* p. 50.
53a. wikipedia.org/wiki/BedřichSmetana. Ref. p. 84.
54. H.F. Redlich. "Bruckner and Mahler" (Master Musicians). J.M. Dent , *op. cit.*, 1963, p.114.
55. Ernest Newman, cited in Deborah Hayden, *op. cit.*, p. 314.
56. A. Einstein. "Music in the Romantic Era." J.M. Dent Publishers, London 1947, p. 153.
57. Michael Steen, *op. cit.*, p. 632.

58. Percy Grainer. "The Personality of Frederick Delius." *in* "A Delius Companion." Christopher Redwood, ed. John Calder, London. 1976. p. 122.
59. Diana Mc Veagh. "Delius, Frederick Theodor Albert (1863-1934)." Oxford Dictionary of National Biography. Oxford University Press. 2004. 59a. n.wikipedia.org/wiki/Frederick_Delius/ Ref. p. 30.
60. Eric Fenby. "Delius As I Knew Him." Faber and Faber, London, 1981. pp. 31-33.
61. Eric Fenby. "The Great Composers: Delius." Faber and Faber, London. 1971. pp. 88-89.
62. Eric Fenby. "Delius As I Knew Him." *op. cit.* p. 208.
63. Edward A. Berlin. "King of Ragtime. Scott Joplin and His Era." Oxford University Press, New York, Oxford. 1994. p. 4.
64. James Haskins with Kathleen Benson. "Scott Joplin." Doubleday and Co., Inc., New York. 1978. p. 32.
65. Katherine Preston,"Scott Joplin." Chelsea House Publishers, New York. 1988. p. 107.
66 .*Ibid.* p. 23.
67. Edward A. Berlin, *op. cit.*, p. 7.
68. James Haskins with Kathleen Benson, *op. cit.*, p. 61.
69. Edward A. Berlin, *op. cit.*, p. 31.

70. *Ibid.* p. 126.
71. Mark Evans. "Scott Joplin and the Ragtime Years."
Dodd, Mead & Co., New York. 1976. p. 104.
72. Peter Gammond. "Scott Joplin and the Ragtime Era."
St. Marti's Press, New York. 1975. p. 80.
73. Edward A. Berlin, *op. cit.*, p. 84.
74. *Ibid.* p. 142.
75. *Ibid.* pp. 223-224.
76. *Ibid.* p. 104.
76a. wikipedia.org/wiki/Scott_Joplin, ref. 68.
77. Edward A. Berlin, *op. cit.* p. 238.
78. Dieter Kerner. "*Krankenheiten grosser Musiker*"
("Illnesses of the Great Musicians"), 3rd. ed., Stuttgart-New
York. 1973. *In* Anton Neumayr. "*Muzyka i cierpienie*" (Music
and Suffering), original title "*Musik und Medizin*". FELBERG
SJA Publishers, Warsaw. 2002. p. 475.
79. Anton Neumayr, *op. cit.*, p. 80.
79a. Dan Olmsted, Mark Blaxill. "The Age of Autism:
Mercury, Medicine, and Man Made Epidemic," chapter on
"Genius Interrupted." McMillan, 2010.
80. Anton Neumayr, *op. cit.*, p. 33.
81. *Ibid.* p. 95.
82. *Ibid.* p. 93.
83. Georg R. Marek, *op. cit.*, p. 318.
84. *Ibid.* p. 314.
85. Anton Neumayr, *op. cit.*, pp. 144,188.
86. *Ibid.* p. 77.
87. *Ibid.* p. 188.
88. George R. Marek, *op. cit.*, p. 315.
89. L. Lesinski, F. Miedzinski, J. Towpik. "Wspolczesna
Syfilidologia" ("Contemporary Syphilidology"). PZWL,
Warszawa. 1970. p. 268.
90. George R. Marek, *op. cit.*, p. 315.
91. Anton Neumayr, *op. cit.*, p. 190.
92. *Ibid.* p. 189.
93. *Ibid.* pp. 115-215.

94. George R. Marek, *op. cit.*, pp. 313-318.
95. *Ibid.* p. 317.
96. Anton Neumayr, *op. cit.*, p. 143.
97. Michael Stein, *op. cit.*, p. 205.
98. George R. Marek, *op. cit.*, pp. 225-318.
99. *Ibid.* p. 316.
100. Anton Neumayr, *op. cit.*, p. 197.
101. Deborah Hayden, *op. cit.*, p. 86.
102. Anton Neumayr, *op. cit.*, p. 204.
103. *Ibid.* p. 146.

Chapter 5b

1. Adam Zamoyski. "Chopin" (original title "Chopin. A biography"). Panstwowy Instytut Wydawniczy. Warsaw. 1990. p. 119.
2. Jules and Edmond de Goncourt. "Dziennik." (original title *"Journal. Memoires de la vie litteraire"* PZWL. Warsaw. 1988. p. 51.
3. http://www.chessville.com/misc/History/PastPawns/deMusset.htm
4. Mosby's Medical, Nursing and Allied Health Dictionary. 5th Ed., Kenneth N. Anderson, ed. Mosby-Year Book Inc. 1998. p. 1064.
5. A.Dickson Wright. "Venereal diseases and the great." Brit. J. Vener.Dis.1971;47:298
6. Alex de Jonge, "Baudelaire: Prince of Clouds." Paddington Press, New York, 1938. p. 55.
7. http://www.thedailybeast.com/articles/2013/05/07/baudelaire-s-femme-fatale-muse.html
8. Roger L. Williams. "The Horror of Life." University Chicago Press. 1980. Str.43
9. *Ibid.* p. 10.

10. *Encyklopedia Powszechna* (Encyclopedia). PWN (*Polskie Wydawnictwo Naukowe*), Warsaw. 1973. p. 223.
11. Jules and Edmond de Goncourt, *op. cit.*, p. 136.
12. Roger L. Williams, *op. cit.*, p. 30.
13. *Ibid.* p. 52.
14. Joanna Richardson. "Baudelaire: A Biography." St. Martin's Press, New York. 1994. p. 415.
15. *Ibid.* p. 434.
16. *Ibid.* p. 437.
17. *Ibid.* p. 452.
18. Alex de Jonge. "Baudelaire. Prince of Clouds." Paddington Press Ltd., New York. 1976. p. 225.
19. Geoffrey Wall. "Flaubert. A Life." Farrah, Straus and Giroux. New York. 2001. p. 80.
20. Enid Starkie. "Flaubert. The Making of the Master." Atheneum Press, New York. 1967. p. 98.
21. *Ibid.* p. 103.
22. Benjamin F. Bart. "Flaubert." Syracuse University Press, Syracuse, New York. 1967. p. 89-96.
23. Frederic Brown. "Flaubert. A Biography." Little, Brown Company, New York. 2006. pp.138-144.
24. Jules and Edmond de Goncourt, *op. cit.* p. 214.
25. Francis Steegmuller. "The Letters of Gustave Flaubert 1830-1857." The Belknap Press of Harvard University Press, Cambridge, Massachussets and London. 1980. p. 129.
26. Jean-Louis Douchin, *"La vie erotique de Flaubert."* Carrere-J.J. Pauvert. 984 *in* Claude Quetel, *op. cit.*, p. 160.
27. http://en.wikipedia.org/wiki/Gustave_Flaubert
28. J. Lesinski., F. Miedzinski, J. Towpik, *op. cit.*, p. 37.
29. Tomasz F. Mroczkowski,"Syphilis" *in* "Sexually Transmitted Diseases." Igaku-Shoin Medical Publishers, New York, Tokyo. 1990. pp.164-226.
30. Renata Lis. *"Reka Flauberta"* ("The Hand of Flaubert"). Sic! Publishers, Warsaw. 2011. p. 161.
31. *Ibid.* p. 174.

32. Francis Steegmuller, *op. cit.*, p. 46.
33. Renata Lis, *op. cit.*, p. 175.
34. *Ibid.* p. 177.
35. *Ibid.* p. 180.
36. *Ibid.* pp. 257-258.
37. *Ibid.* pp. 265-266.
38. Jules and Edmond de Goncourt, *op. cit.*, p. 59.
39. *Ibid.* p. 423.
40. *Ibid.* p. 287.
41. *Ibid.* p. 214.
42. Francis Steegmuller, *op. cit.*, pp. 239-240.
43. Henri Troyat. "Flaubert." Viking Penquin, New York. 1992. p. 282.
44. Jules and Edmond de Goncourt, *op. cit.*, p. 337.
45. Renata Lis, *op. cit.*, p. 222.
46. Jules and Edmond de Goncourt, *op. cit.*, pp. 436-437.
47. *Ibid.* p. 89.
48. *Ibid.* p. 388.
49. *Ibid.* p. 25.
50. I*bid.* p. 529.
51. *Ibid.* p. 67.
52. *Ibid.* p. 152.
53. *Ibid.* p. 294.
54. *Ibid.* pp. 295-303.
55. *Ibid.* p. 392.
56. A. Dickson Wright. "Venereal diseases and the great." Brit. J. Vener. Dis. 1971;47:295
57. Jules and Edmond de Goncourt, *op. cit.*, pp. 526, 532.
58. *Ibid.* p. 441.
59. Ewa K. Kossak. *"W strone Misi z Godebskich"* ("About Misia of the Godebskis). *Czytelnik*, Warsaw. 1978. p. 136.
60. Jules and Edmond de Goncourt, *op. cit.*, pp. 531-533.
61. *Ibid.* p. 538.
62. *Ibid.* pp. 533,539,557,559.

63. Claude Quetel, *op. cit.*, p. 161.

64. Frank Harris. *"Ma vie mes amours"* (My Life, My Loves). Gallimad Press. 1960 *in* Claude Quetel, *op. cit.*, p. 161.

65. Claude Quetel, *op. cit.*, p. 161. (Fragment of the *Goncourt Journal* from Sunday, February 1, 1891).

66. Francis Steegmuller. "Maupassant. A Lion in the Path." Random House, New York. 1949. p. 86.

67. Claude Quetel, *op. cit.*, pp. 161-162.

68. Francis Steegmuller, *op. cit.*, p. 224.

69. Claude Quetel, *op. cit.*, p. 156.

70. Robert H. Sherard, "The Life, Work and Evil Fate of Guy de Maupassant," Published by Brentano's, New York. 1926. pp. 203-208.

71. Jules and Edmond de Goncourt, *op. cit.*, p. 533.

72. Michael G. Lerner. "Maupassant." George Braziller, Inc., New York. 1975. p. 241.

73. Robert H. Sherard, *op. cit.*, p. 372.

74. Jules and Edmond de Goncourt, *op. cit.*, p. 548.

75. Robert H. Sherard, *op. cit.*, p. 378.

76. Richard Ellmann. "Oscar Wilde." Alfred A. Knopf . Publishers, New York. 1988. p. 92.

77. Neil Mc Kenna, "The secret life of Oscar Wilde." Basic Books, Publishers, New York. 2005. p. 86.

78. *Ibid.* p. 8.

79. *Ibid.* p. 86.

80. *Ibid.* p. 16.

81. *Ibid.* p. 17.

82. *Ibid.* p. 23.

83. Frank Harris. "Oscar Wilde." Michigan State University Press, 1959. p. 52.

84. Jules i Edmond de Goncourt, *op. cit.*, p. 455.

85. Neil McKenna, *op. cit.*, p. 38.

86. *Ibid.* p. 50.

87. *Ibid.* p. 70.

88. *Ibid.* p. 73.

89. *Ibid.* p. 80.
90. *Ibid.* p. 82.
91. *Ibid.* p. 86.
92. *Ibid.* p. 118.
93. *Ibid.* p. 122.
94. Ibid. p. 223.
95. Ibid. p. 283.
96. *Ibid.* p. 324.
97. *Ibid.* p. 331-332.
98. *Ibid.* p. 356.
99. *Ibid.* p. 372.
100. Ibid. p. 373.
101. Richard Ellmann, *op. cit.*, p. 580.
102. Frank Harris, *op. cit.*, p. 315.
103. Richard Ellmann *op. cit.*, p. 581.
104. *Ibid.* p. 579.
105. Tomasz F. Mroczkowski, *op. cit.*, p. 188
106. Stan Gebler Davis, "James Joyce A Portrait of the Artist." Stein and Day, Publishers. New York. 1975. pp. 314-315
107. *Ibid.* p. 12.
108. Chester G. Anderson, "James Joyce and His World." A Studio Book: The Viking Press, New York. 1967. p. 10.
109. Stan Gebler Davis, op. cit., p.27
110. *Ibid.* p. 29-30.
111. Richard Ellmann, "James Joyce" New and Revised Edition, Oxford University Press. 1982. p. 48.
112. Edna O'Brien, "James Joyce." A Lipper/Viking Book, New York, 1999. p. 18-19.
113. Chester G. Anderson, *op. cit.*, p. 40
114. *Ibid.* p. 46.
115. James Joyce. "Ulysses." Random House, New York. 1986. p.534.
116. Stan Gebler Davis, *op. cit.*, p. 92.
117. Richard Ellmann, *op. cit.*, p. 150.
118. Deborah Hayden, *op. cit.*, p. 241.

119. Stuart Gilbert, "Letters of James Joyce," vol. I. The Viking Press, 1966. p. 54.

120. Stan Gebler Davis, *op. cit.*, p. 111.

121. *Ibid.* p. 107.

122. John McCourt. "The Years of Bloom. James Joyce in Trieste 1904-1920." The University of Wisconsin Press, 2000. p. 122.

123. Tomasz F. Mroczkowski, *"Choroby Przenoszone Droga Plciowa"* ("Sexually Transmitted Diseases"). "Czelej", Lublin (Poland). 2013.

124. Chester G. Anderson, *op. cit.*, p. 68.

125. *Ibid.* p. 73.

126. Stan Gebler Davis, *op. cit.*, p. 170.

127. *Ibid.* p. 171.

128. *Ibid.* p. 206.

129. *Ibid.* p. 165.

130. J. Lesinski, F. Miedzinski, J. Towpik, *op. cit.*, pp302-306i

131. Richard Ellmann, *op. cit.*, p. 451.

132. Stan Gelber Davis, *op. cit.*, pp. 244, 246.

133. *Ibid.* p. 249.

134. *Ibid.* p. 244.

135. *Ibid.* p. 276.

136. http://www.karenblixen.com/

137. Aage Henriksen, "Isak Dinesen/Karen Blixen. The Work and the Life." St. Martin's Press, New York. 1988. p. 125.

138. Kaare Weismann. "Neurosyphilis, or Chronic Heavy Metal Poisoning: Karen Blixen's Lifelong Disease." Sexually Transmitted Diseases 1995;22:137-144.

139. Linda Donelson. Excerpted from "Out of Isak Dineson in Africa " http://archive.is/Ks3wa

140. J. Lesinski, F. Miedzinski, J. Towpik, *op. cit*, pp. 125-131.

Chapter 5c

1. Michael Stein. "*Wielcy Kompozytorzy i ich Czasy*" (original title "The Lives and Times of the Great Composers"). REBIS Publishing House, Poznan. 2009. p. 549.
2. Beth Archer Brombert. "Edouard Manet. Rebel in a Frock Coat." Little, Brown and Co. 1996. pp. 74-75.
3. *Ibid*. p. 27.
4. *Ibid*. p. 28.
5. Peter McPhee. "A Social History of France 1780-1880.", London. 1992. p. 203.
6. Adam Zamoyski. "Chopin" (original title: "Chopin. A Biography"). *Panstwowy Instytut Wydawniczy* (National Publishing Institute), Warsaw. 1990. p. 78.
7. Emil Zola. "Nana." *Panstwowy Instytut Wydawniczy* (National Publishing Institute), Warsaw 1976. Vol. 2, p. 44.
8. Michael Stein, *op. cit.*, p. 281.
9. Alain Corbin. "*Les Filles de Nice, misere sexuelle et prostitution 19e et 20e siecles*" ("The Women of Nice, Poverty and Prostitution in the 19th and 20th Centuries"). Paris, 1978, p. 138. *In* Beth Archer Brombert, Edouard Manet, *op. cit.*, p. 91.
10. Otto Friedrich. "Olympia: Paris in the Age of Manet." Aurum Press, London. 1922. p. 281.
11. *Ibid*. p. 282.
12. Samuel Richardson. "Pamela: Or, Virtue Rewarded." Oxford University Press. 2001. (First edition, 1740). p. 1.
13. Beth Archer Brombert, *op. cit.*, p. 140.
14. *Ibid*. p. 141.
15. Michael Stein, *op. cit.*, p. 290.
16. Beth Archer Brombert, *op. cit.*, p. 262.
17. Anne Higonnet. "Berthe Morisot." New York 1990. p. 56. *In* Beth Archer Brombert, *op. cit.*, p. 262.

18. Beatrice Farwell. "Manet, Morisot, and Propriety. Perspectives on Morisot." T.J. Edelstein, ed. New York. 1990. p. 46. *In* Beth Archer Brombert, *op. cit.*, p. 236.

19. Beth Archer Brombert, *op. cit.*, p. 288.

20. Adolphe Tabarant. *"Manet et ses oeuvres"* ("Manet and His Works"). Paris. 1947. p. 191.

21. Beth Archer Brombert, *op. cit.*, p. 374.

22. Denis Rouart, ed. "Correspondance de Berthe Morisot avec sa famille et ses amis") ("Correspondence of Berthe Morisot with Her Family and Friends"). Paris. 1950. p. 102. *In* Beth Archer Brombert, *op. cit.*, p. 176.

23. Beth Archer Brombert, *op. cit.*, p. 401.

24. *Ibid.* p. 412.

25. Denis Rouart, ed., *op. cit.*, pp. 21-117. *In* Beth Archer Brombert, *op. cit.*, p. 444.

26. Beth Archer Brombert, *op. cit.*, p. 444.

27. *Ibid.* p. 448.

28. *Ibid.* p. 452.

29. Otto Friedrich, *op. cit.*, p. 281.

30. Henri Loyrette. "Degas." Paris. 1991. p. 489.

31. Jean-Luc Coatalem. "In Search of Gauguin." Weidenfeld and Nicolson, London. 2004. p. 14.

32. *Ibid.* p. 15

33. Henri Perruchot. "Gauguin" (original title "La vie de Gauguin" ("The Life of Gaugin"). World Publishing Co., Cleveland. 1963. pp. 51-52.

34. Howard Greenfeld. "Paul Gauguin." Harry N. Abrams Inc., Publishers. 1993. P. 21.

35. Henri Perruchot, *op. cit.*, p. 84.

36. Howard Greenfeld, *op. cit.*, p. 24.

37. *Ibid.* p. 30.

38. Henri Perruchot, *op. cit.*, p. 129.

39. *Ibid.* p. 142.

40. *Ibid.* p. 143.

41. I*bid.* p. 148.

42. Howard Greenfeld, *op. cit.*, p. 36.

43. Henri Perruchot, *op. cit.*, p. 163.
44. David Sweetman. "Paul Gauguin. A Life." Simon and Schuster, New York. 1995. p. 195.
45. *Ibid.* p. 197.
46. Henri Perruchot, *op. cit.*, p. 164.
47. Howard Greenfeld, *op. cit.*, p. 42.
48. *Ibid.* p. 45.
49. Henri Perruchot, *op. cit.*, p. 204.
50. Bengt Danielsson. "Gauguin in the South Seas." Doubleday and Co., Inc., New York. 1966. p. 45.
51. Marta Tomczyk-Maryon. "Wyspianski." National Publishing Institute, Warsaw. 2009. p. 118.
52. *Ibid.* p. 207.
53. Bengt Danielsson, *op. cit.*, p. 204.
54. Howard Greenfeld, *op. cit.*, p. 60.
55. Bengt Danielsson, *op. cit.*, p. 75 (citation from Claverie: 130-3, p. 46).
56. *Ibid.* p. 75 (citation from Desfontaines: 118 p. 47).
57. *Ibid.* p. 75.
58. *Ibid.* p. 89.
59. Henri Perruchot, *op. cit.*, p. 229.
60. David Sweetman, *op. cit.*, p. 307.
61. Bengt Danielsson, *op. cit.*, p. 43.
62. Lawrence and Elisabeth Hanson. "Noble Savage. The Life of Paul Gauguin." Random House, New York. 1955. p. 205.
63. *Ibid.* pp. 206-207.
64. Bengt Danielsson, *op. cit.*, p. 129.
65. Henri Perruchot, *op. cit.*, p. 249.
66. Howard Greenfield, *op. cit.*, p. 71.
67. *Ibid.* p. 72.
68. David Sweetman, *op. cit.*, p. 403.
69. *Ibid.* p. 391.
70. Henri Perruchot, *op. cit.*, p. 258.
71. Marta Tomczyk-Maryon, *op. cit.*, p. 120.
72. David Sweetman, *op. cit.*, p. 407.

73. Henri Perrucho, *p. cit.*, p. 266.

74. Bengt Danielsson, *op. cit.*, p. 195 (oral information from M. Ma'ari a Teheiura).

75. Jean-Luc Coatalem, *op. cit.*, p. 199.

76. Bengt Danielsson, *op. cit.*, p. 203.

77. Howard Gfreenfiels, *op. cit.*, p. 80.

78. Bengt Danielsson, *op. cit*, p. 243.

79. Lawrence and Elisabeth Hanson, *op. cit.*, pp. 268-9.

80. Bengt Danielsson, *op. cit.*, p. 256.

81. *Ibid.* p. 257.

82. Lawrence and Elisabeth Hanson, *op. cit.*, p. 270.

83. Bengt Danielsson, *op. cit.*, p. 274.

84. *Ibid.* p. 275.

85. *Ibid.* p. 284.

86. Henri Perruchot, *op. cit.*, p. 343.

87. Derek Fell. "Van Gogh's Women. His Love Affairs and Journey into Madness." Carroll & Graf Publishers, New York. 2004. p. xvii.

88. *Ibid.* p. xviii.

89. *Ibid.* p. 4.

90. *Ibid.* p. 7.

91. *Ibid.* pp. 8-10. (letters of November 3, 7, 9. 1881)

92. Steven Naifeh and Gregory White Smith. " Van Gogh. The Life." Random House Trade Paperback Edition, New York. 2011. 239.

93. *Ibid.* p. 249.

94. Derek Fell, *op. cit.*, p. 37.

95. *Ibid.* p. 39 (letter of December. 21. 1881)

96. Steven Naifeh and Gregory White Smith, *op. cit.*, p. 294.

97. *Ibid.* p. 404.

97a. Albert J. Lubin. "Stranger on the Earth. A Psychological Biography of Vincent van Gogh." Da Capo Press, New York. 1996. p. 116.

98. Deborah Hayden, *op. cit.*, p. 158.

99. Steven Naifeh, *op. cit.*, p. 478.

100. Julia Frey. "Toulouse-Lautrec. A Life." Viking
Penguin Group Publishers, USA. 1994. p. 205.
101. Derek Fell, *op. cit.*, p. 80.
102. *Ibid.* p. 81.
103. *Ibid.* p. 93.
104. *Ibid.* p. 131.
105. *Ibid.* p. 150 (letter of April 30, 1889).
106. *Ibid.* p. 166.
107. *Ibid.* p. 167.
108. *Ibid.* p. 182.
109. *Ibid.* pp. 177-178.
110. Bogumila Welsh-Ovcharow. "Van Gogh in Provence
and Auvers." University Publishing, 2008. p. 182.
111. Lawrence and Elisabeth Hanson. "Passionate
Pilgrim. The Life of Vincent van Gogh." Random House, New
York. 1955. p. 265.
112. Philip Callow. "Vincent van Gogh. A Life." Ivan R.
Dee, Inc., Chicago. 1990. P. p. 274.
113. Derek Fell, *op. cit.*, p. 231.
114. Steven Naife, *op. cit.*, p. 866.
115. Julia Frey, *op. cit.*, pp. 10-11.
116. Jackie Rosenhek., Oct.2009. http://www.toulouse-
lautrec-foundation.org/biography.html
117. Henri Perruchot. "Toulouse-Lautrec. A Definitive
Biography." World Publishing Co., Cleveland. 1960. p. 52.
118. Wikipedia., http://www.toulouse-lautrec-
foundation.org/biography.html
119. Henri Perruchot., *op. cit.*, p. 78.
120. *Ibid.* p. 121.
121. *Ibid.* p. 129.
122. *Ibid.* p. 130.
123. Jacques Lassaigne. "Lautrec, Biographical and
Critical Studies." SKIRA Art Books, 1953. pp. 42-52.
124. *Ibid.* p. 61.
125. Henri Perruchot, *op. cit.*, p. 103.
126. *Ibid.* p. 143.

127. *Ibid.* p. 149.
128. *Ibid.* p. 173.
129. *Ibid.* p. 156.
130. *Ibid.* p. 157.
131. *Ibid.* p.169.
132. *Ibid.* p.167.
133. Julia Frey, *op. cit.*, p. 203.
134. Jaroslaw Iwaszkiewicz. "*Dzienniki* (Diaries) *1964-1980.*" *Czytelnik.* Warszawa. 2011. p. 107.
135. Ewa K. Kossak, *op. cit.*, p. 140.
135a. *Ibid.* p. 183.
136. *Ibid.* p. 381.
137. Arthur Rubinstein. "My Many Years." A Hamish Hammilton Paperback, London. 1987.
138. *Ibid.* p. 107.
139. *Ibid.* p. 108.
140. Henri Peruchot, *op. cit.*, p. 240.
141. *Ibid.* p. 199.
142. Yvette Guilbert. "*Le Chanson de Vie* ("The Song of Life"). *In* Henri Perruchot, *op. cit.*, p. 190.
143. Henri Perruchot, *op. cit.*, p. 200.
144. *Ibid.* p. 205.
145. Gerstle Mack. "Toulouse-Lautrec" Alfred A. Knopf Publishers, New York. 1952. p. 322.
146. *Ibid.* p. 133.
147. Henri Perruchot, *op. cit.*, p. 221.
148. *Ibid.* p. 232.
149. *Ibid,* p. 236.
150. *Ibid.* p. 251.
151. *Ibid.* p. 261.
152. *Ibid.* p. 265.
153. *Ibid.* p. 268.
154. *Ibid.* p. 275.

Chapter 6

1. Steven Otfinowski. "Alexander Fleming: Conquering Disease with Penicillin. Facts on File". New York. 1992. p. 5.
2. John Rowland. "The Penicillin Man. The Story of Alexander Fleming." Roy Press, New York. 1957. p. 27.
3. Ronald W. Clark. "The Life of Ernst Chain. Penicillin and Beyond." St. Martin's Press, New York. 1985. p. 43.
4. Steven Otfinowski *op. cit.*, p. 77.
5. *Ibid.* p. 64.
6. J.F. Mahoney, R.C. Arnold and A. D. Harris. Penicillin Treatment of Early Syphilis: A Preliminary Report. *American Journal of Public Health* 1943;33: 1387-1391.
7. J.F. Mahoney., R.C. Arnold., B.L. Sterner, *et al.* Penicillin treatment of early syphilis. *JAMA* 1944; 126 (2):63-67.
8. J.H. Stokes, T. Sternberg, W. Schwartz, *et al.* The Action of penicillin in late syphilis. *JAMA* 1944; 126 (2):73-80.
9. Richard A. Koch and Ray Lyman Wilbur. Promiscuity as a factor in the spread of venereal disease. *Journal of Social Hygiene* 1944;30: 517-529.
10. Allan M. Brandt and David Shumway Jones. Historical Perspectives on Sexually Transmitted Diseases: Challenges for Prevention and Control. *in* King K. Holmes, Per-Anders Mardh, P. Frederick Sparling, *et al.* "Sexually Transmitted Diseases." McGraw-Hill, New York. 1999. pp. 15-21.
11. Tomasz F. Mroczkowski. "Choroby przenoszone droga plciowa" ("Sexually Transmited Diseses"). Czelej Publishers . S.z.o.o. Lublin. 2012. p. 3
12. *Ibid.* p. 49.
13. Erin Santa and Joya Sahu. "Syphilis" *in*"Genital and Perianal Diseases. A Color Handbook," Tomasz F. Mroczkowski, Larry E. Millikan and Larry Ch. Parish (editors). CRC Press, Taylor and Francis Group. 2013. p. 23.

Chapter 7

1. Claude Quetel, *op. cit.*, p. 67.
2. Wikipedia. Girolamo Fracastoro.
3. Norbert Finzch, Robert Jutte. "Institutions of Confinement: Hospitals, Asylums and Prisons in Western, Cambridge University Press. pp. 102-115.
4. Stephanie Koscak. Michigan Feminist Study. "Morbid Fantasies of the Sexual Marketplace: 'Lascivious Appetites,' 'Luxury' and *Lues Venerea* in England1750-1800." Vol.21, No.1. Fall 2007-Spring 2008. Bibliogr. p.30.
5. *Ibid.* p. 33.
6. *Ibid.* p. 68.
7. Frederick A. Pottle. Boswell's London Journal, 1762-1763. McGraw-Hill Book Company, Inc. 1950. p. 164.
8. Kiran Rana. James Boswell and a History of Gonorrhea. The guardian.com, Wednesday, June 13, 2012.
9. Frderick A. Pottle, *op. cit.*, p. 178.
10. *Ibid.* p. 155.
11. Frederick A. Pottle. James Boswell. The Earlier Years, 1740-1769. McGraw-Hill Book Company, 1966. p. 345.
12. Stephanie Koscak, *op. cit.,* p. 99.
13. *Ibid.* p. 107.
14. Frederick A. Pottle, *op. cit.,* p. 157.
15. Dickson Wright, A. Venereal diseases and the great, *Brit. J. Vener.Dis.*1971;*47*: 295.
16. Brigitte Hamann. *Cesarzowa Elzbieta* (original title: *Elisabeth: Keiserin wider Willen*), Panstwowy Instytut Wydawniczy (National Publishing Institute), Warsaw. 1981. p. 247.
17. Marek Karpinski. *Najstarszy zawod swiata. Historia prostytucji* (The world's oldest profession. A History of prostitution). Wydawnictwo Iskry (Iskra Publishers), Warsaw, 2010.
18. Stephanie Koscak, *op cit.* pp.36, 37.

19. *Ibid.*, p. 39.
20. *Ibid.*, p. 49.
21. Laws regulating sexual behavior between consenting adults. *In* Bruce M. King, Human Sexuality Today. Prentice-Hall, Inc., 1996. Table 16-1, p. 393.
22. Michael Waugh. Genital adornment. *In* Genital and Perianal Diseases, A Color Handbook. Tomasz F. Mroczkowski, Larry E. Millikan, Larry Ch. Parish, eds. CRS Press, 2013. p. 241.
23. Roman J. Nowicki. Allergic Dermatitis, Irritant Dermatitis and Drug reactions. *In* Genital and Perianal Diseases, A Color Handbook, Tomasz F. Mroczkowski, Larry E. Millikan, Larry Ch. Parish, eds. CRS Press, 2013. p. 163.